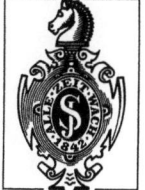

Raffaele De Simone

Atlas of Transesophageal Color Doppler Echocardiography and Intraoperative Imaging

With Contributions by
Rüdiger Lange and Siegfried Hagl

With 185 Figures in 608 Separate Illustrations, Mostly in Color

Springer-Verlag

Berlin Heidelberg New York
London Paris Tokyo
Hong Kong Barcelona
Budapest

Dr. Raffaele De Simone
University of Heidelberg
Department of Cardiac Surgery
Im Neuenheimer Feld 110

D-69120 Heidelberg

ISBN-13:978-3-642-78958-8   e-ISBN-13:978-3-642-78956-4
DOI: 10.1007/978-3-642-78956-4

CIP data applied for

© Springer-Verlag Berlin Heidelberg 1994
Softcover reprint of the hardcover 1st edition 1994

Reproduction of the figures: Universitätsdruckerei H. Stürtz AG, Würzburg

SPIN: 10465406   23/3130-5 4 3 2 1 0 – Printed on acid-free paper

Dedicated to my father, Luigi De Simone

Foreword

This Atlas of transesophageal echocardiography represents four years' clinical experience with perioperative color Doppler echocardiography performed at the Department of Heart Surgery of the University of Heidelberg. Four years ago we started a training program in echocardiography with the purpose of utilizing the information derived from transesophageal and epicardial echocardiography for intraoperative diagnosis and surgical decisions. The great impact of echocardiographic information on the surgical procedures disclosed to us an increasing number of applications of TEE and its enormous diagnostic potential. At the moment, intraoperative transesophageal echocardiography represents, in our Institution, an indispensable diagnostic technique for assessing the adequacy of heart surgery. The aim of this Atlas, which was conceived primarily to deal with intraoperative imaging, goes beyond the purpose of making the cardiac surgeon familiar with this technique. The clinical cardiologist will find immense advantages from the description of many rare diseases and from the direct verification of the echocardiographic diagnoses by the operative findings. We hope that our experience will contribute to supporting all colleagues who are engaged in the treatment of heart disease.

Prof. Dr. Siegfried Hagl
Department of Heart Surgery
University of Heidelberg
Germany

Preface

Why an atlas?

This book was conceived primarily as a short manual to introduce cardiac surgeons to the basics of color Doppler echocardiography. With the increasing range of applications of intraoperative transesophageal echocardiography (TEE) the collection of figures expanded until it covered a wide variety of heart diseases. In its final form, this Atlas represents a comprehensive handbook of transesophageal echocardiography which is directed not only to the cardiac surgeon but also to the clinical cardiologist and to everyone involved in the diagnosis and treatment of heart disease. The echocardiographic figures were chosen with the purpose of showing the anatomy and function of the heart in a single picture, thus enabling a diagnosis "at first glance". The concise self-explanatory form of this Atlas aims to reproduce the situations in which the surgeon must quickly evaluate the echocardiographic information necessary for operative decisions.

The authors have attempted to treat the spectrum of intraoperative applications of TEE comprehensively, but as in any ambitious undertaking the final outcome never appears complete. Since the introduction of echocardiography into the surgical theater is still fairly recent, many of its potential applications have not yet been investigated.

Special attention is given to the evaluation of cardiac valve repairs, the most frequent use of echocardiography in adult cardiac surgery, since TEE provides a reliable method for intraoperative diagnoses of residual valve regurgitation and stenosis. The adjustment of suture annuloplasty under echocardiographic control is an example of active interaction between intraoperative TEE and surgical procedures. The use of TEE in patients undergoing heart transplantation and in experimental surgery, as well as in patients with dynamic cardiomyoplasty, reveals new aspects of these diseases and contributes to their surgical treatment.

Congenital heart disease represents a quite new application for TEE. Hitherto, only few experiences with pediatric TEE are reported in the literature. Conventional echocardiography can still be considered the method of choice since high-quality images can easily be obtained in most children by the transthoracic approach. Despite the new application of TEE in pediatric patients, the series of images shown in the respective section covers a broad spectrum of congenital heart diseases.

The content of this Atlas summarizes our experience with perioperative echocardiography at the Department of Cardiac Surgery, University of Heidelberg, Germany. We address this manual to all those engaged in the diagnosis and management of heart disease, and hope that it will contribute to further exploit of the great diagnostic potential of this technique.

Dr. Raffaele De Simone

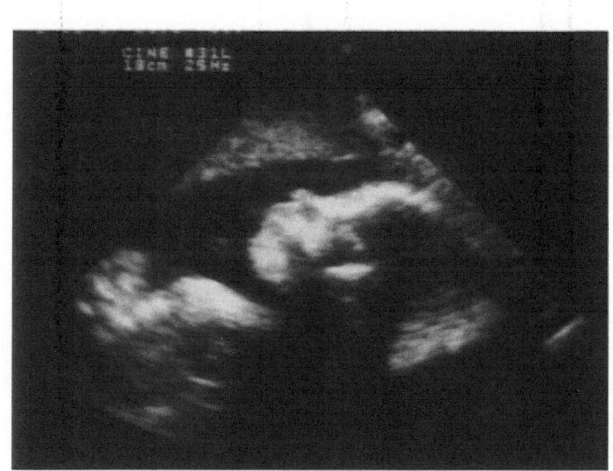

Prenatal echography, Lara's
profile at the age of –3 months.

Acknowledgements

The accomplishment of this Atlas reflects the clinical and research activity of the Department of Cardiac Surgery of the University of Heidelberg and involves the support of several colleagues who directly or indirectly contributed to the completion of this work. The precious contributions of Prof. Siegfried Hagl and Dr. Rüdiger Lange have been decisive for the elaboration and development of the Atlas. In addition, they also perceived the important role of echocardiography in cardiac surgery, promoted the use of TEE in the operating room and encouraged the investigation of new clinical applications. I would like to express my gratitude to many other colleagues who were engaged in the surgical treatment of the patients. In particular I would like to thank Prof. Emmeram Gams, Dr. Bodo Hasper, Dr. Heinz Jakob, Prof. Werner Saggau, Dr. Ahmed Tanzeem, and Dr. Christian Vahl who also actively contributed with criticism and constructive discussions. I am thankful to Mr. Manfred Heinen for the technical assistance, to Ms. Edith Schierz-Crusius, and Mr. Jörg Rodrian for the photographic artwork, to Ms. Jutta von Bergmann for the drawings, to Mr. Rüdi Götz and Mr. Bernd Köstering (Aloka Inc.) for the technical assistance of the echocardiographs. We would like to thank St. Jude Medical Inc. for having provided our institution with the echocardiographic equipment.

Dr. Giovanni Paolella, staff scientist of the European Molecular Biology Laboratories, deserves particular mention for having shared the onerous enterprise to produce a computer-based CD-ROM version of the Atlas. This difficult task could never be accomplished without his devotion to the experimental method and his great competence in computing science. His wife, Dr. Vittoria Barone, kindly hosted and tolerated our sleepless nocturnal programming sessions.

Prof. Aldo Iacono guided my training in cardiology at the University of Naples with great clinical experience and dedication. He bears the responsibility for having introduced me to the management of the patients with heart disease. The European Society of Cardiology promoted the realization of this book by awarding the project "Intraoperative Transesophageal Echocardiography, New Clinical Applications" with the "ESC Research Fellowship" 1991.

Finally, I wish to thank my wife, Dr. Eliana De Simone, for the constant incentive and the precious methodological suggestions. This book would have never been written without her help and the tolerance of my daughter Lara (see figure at next page), who accepted with patience my absence during the preparation of the manuscript.

Dr. Raffaele De Simone

Contents

Abbreviations

Most of the abbreviations used in the figures are commonly used in the cardiological practice. Nonstandard abbreviations are explained in the legends to the figures. The standard abbreviations are listed below:

A, AO,	Aorta
ASD,	Atrial septal defect
LA,	Left atrium
LV,	Left ventricle
LVOT,	Left ventricular outflow tract
M, MV,	Mitral valve
P, PV,	Pulmonary valve
PA,	Pulmonary artery
RA,	Right atrium
RV,	Right ventricle
RVOT,	Right ventricular outflow tract
T, TV,	Tricuspid valve
VSD,	Ventricular septal defect

1 Techniques

This section describes the techniques used for intraoperative imaging and the basics of two-dimensional transesophageal echocardiography (TEE) and color Doppler flow imaging. In addition the following chapters present schematic diagrams of the standard views and the pattern of normal intracardiac flow.

Intraoperative Echocardiography

Recent technological advances such as the advent of color Doppler flow mapping and the development of safe transesophageal transducers make possible clinical applications of cardiac sonography.

Clinical Applications

The use of transesophageal and epicardial color Doppler echocardiography in the operating room provides information for assessing the outcome of heart surgery immediately after the surgical procedure. Up to now, many decisions made in evaluating cardiac repairs have been based on subjective judgments. Conventional methods such as the measurement of pressures and oxygen saturation provide an indirect and relatively insensitive appraisal of the adequacy of cardiac repairs. In contrast, two-dimensional echocardiography, used in combination with Doppler and two-dimensional Doppler (color flow imaging), provides real-time data on morphology, hemodynamics, and blood flow in the beating heart immediately after the surgical procedure and before closure of the chest.

However, optimal use of this technique requires a long training. The high-quality images obtained by intraoperative epicardial and transesophageal echocardiography can be easily interpreted by echocardiographers, but they are not immediately understandable by non-experienced users. Our institution initiated a clinical program to optimize the application of this method in heart surgery and to enable the surgical team to use and interpret operative echocardiography.

Transesophageal Approach

TEE has only recently been introduced into clinical practice. The first application of M-mode TEE dates from 1972. With the introduction of flexible endoscopes and the advent of phased-array technology and transducer miniaturization, around 1980, the interest in the new clinical applications of the technique began to increase considerably. Most of the commercially available machines use 5.0-MHz transducers fixed to the tip of a modified flexible gastroscope. The proximity of the esophagus to the heart and aorta allows high-quality imaging without interference from ribs and lungs.

The transesophageal probe in intubated patients undergoing cardiac surgery can be introduced under direct laryngoscopy or even "blindly" by directing the tip of the esophagoscope into the posterior part of the pharynx and allowing the probe to flex passively. Catheters within the esophagus, such as a nasogastric tube, should be removed to ensure satisfactory images and to avoid potential kinking or knotting of the device. Intraoperative TEE can be performed continuously during surgery without interfering with the surgical procedures (Fig. 1.1).

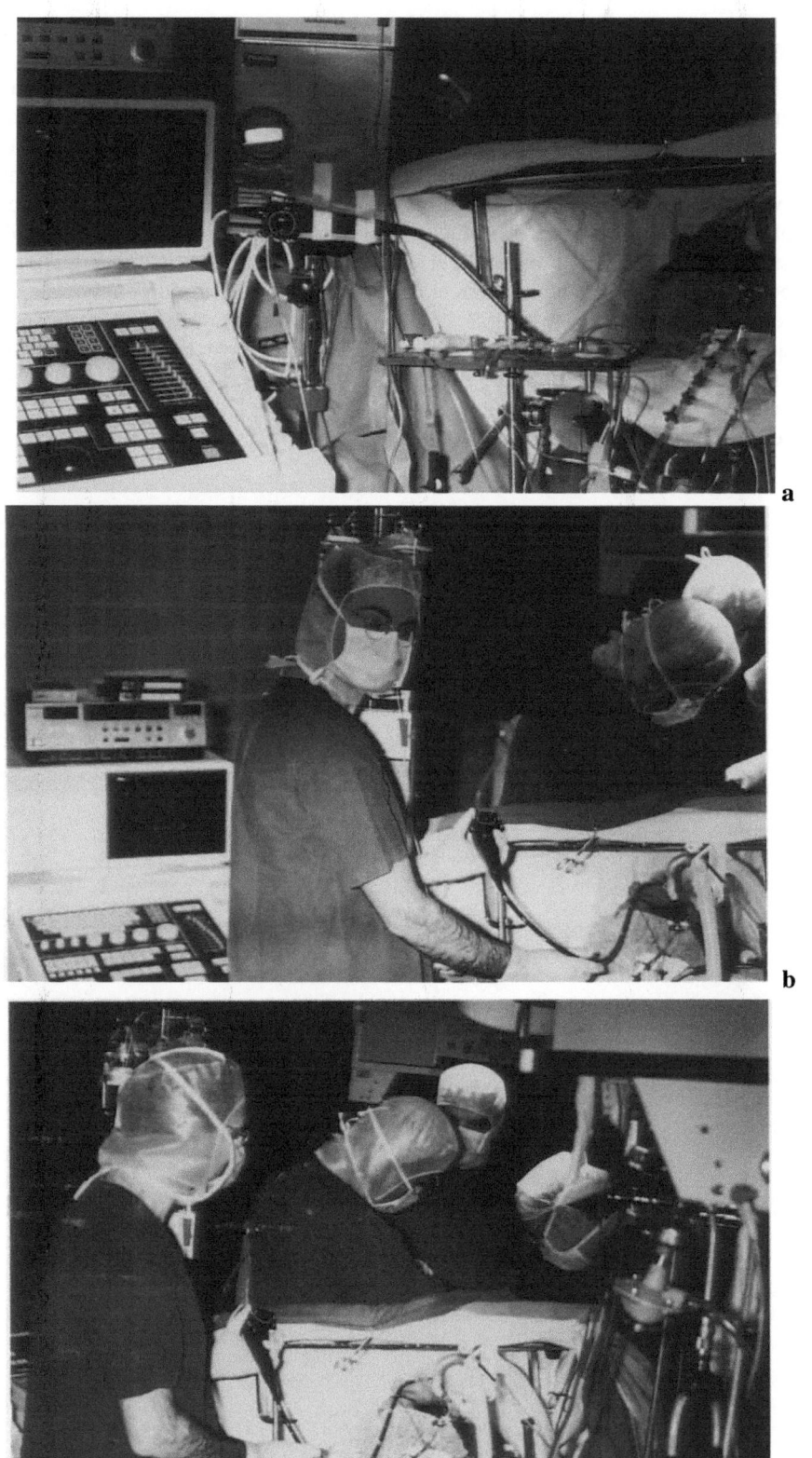

Fig. 1.1 a–c. Intraoperative TEE. View of the surgical theater. The examination can be performed contin-uously during surgery without interfering with the surgical procedure.

Epicardial Approach

Epicardial echocardiography is another valuable technique for performing intraoperative echocardiographic examinations. Epicardial echocardiography can be performed with normal transducers sterilized by a cold gas technique or with a nonsterile transducer placed inside a sterile plastic cover. Ultrasound gel should be placed between the head of the transducer and the sleeve to eliminate the air space (Fig. 1.2). This procedure requires a team of two persons. The acquisition of data is made by the surgeon in the sterile field, while another person operates the instrument controls of the echocardiographic machine.

The major advantages of intraoperative epicardial echocardiography are its ability to provide multiple tomographic planes and its easy availability. The principal limitations of the epicardial technique are poor visualization of the apex of the left ventricle and interruption of the operation during the examinations. The patient can be studied after thoracotomy. Four standard imaging planes are suggested for visualizing the various cardiac structures: the parasternal equivalent view, the aortopulmonary sulcus view, the subcostal equivalent view, and aorta-superior vena cava view. These have been derived from the standard views of conventional transthoracic echocardiography.

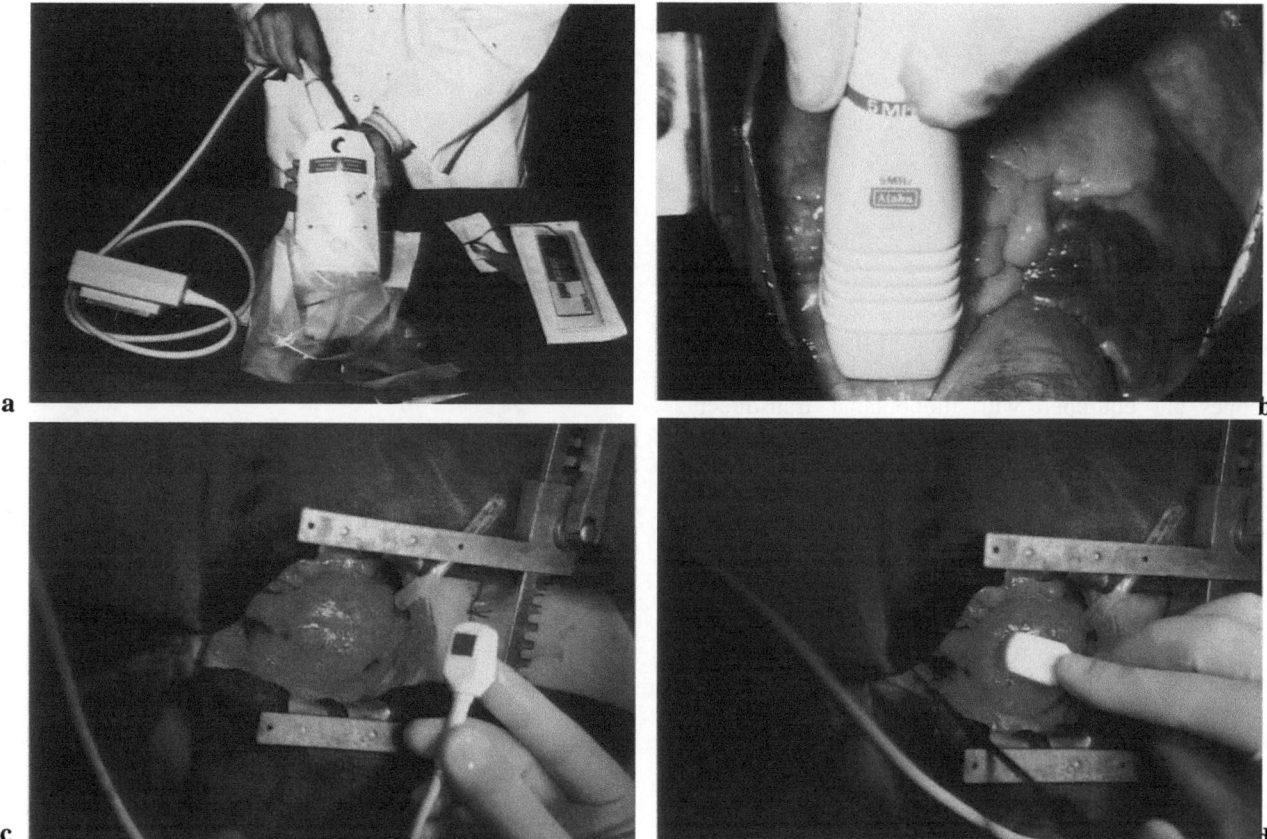

Fig. 1.2a–d. Epicardial echocardiography. **a** A non-sterile transducer is introduced into the sterile sheath. **b** The transducer has been sterilized and can be placed directly onto the epicardial surface of the heart. **c, d** Special miniaturized transducer for epicardial echocardiography.

Two-Dimensional TEE

TEE examinations include transversal and longitudinal views of the heart. The most common TEE endoscopes are equipped with monoplanar transducers which provide only transverse views. With the recent advent of new biplanar probes, an additional longitudinal plane can be visualized along with the transverse one. The second longitudinal plane adds further useful information for spatial localization of intracardiac blood flows and for three-dimensional imaging of the cardiac chambers.

Monoplanar Imaging

TEE examination includes three primary standard views: the basal short-axis, the four-chamber, and the transgastric view. The thoracic portion of the descending aorta and the first 2–3 cm of the supravalvular ascending aorta can be imaged systematically. The upper portion of the ascending aorta cannot be visualized due to the interposition of the left bronchus between the esophagus and the aorta. Monoplanar TEE provides a single transverse imaging plane. However, intermediate views, or "off-axis" views, may be obtained by manipulating the tip of the endoscope (advancement, withdrawal, retroflexion, anteflexion, and rotation). These views are very useful for visualizing the structures of interest.

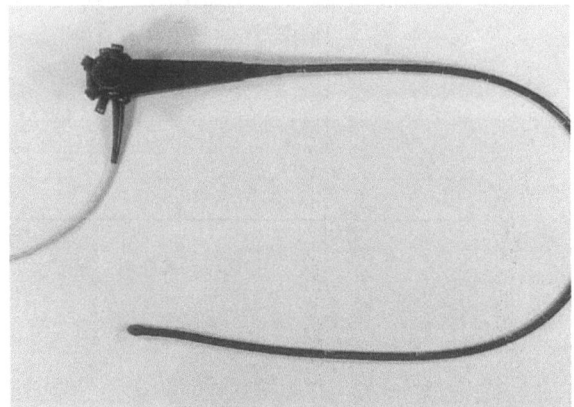

a

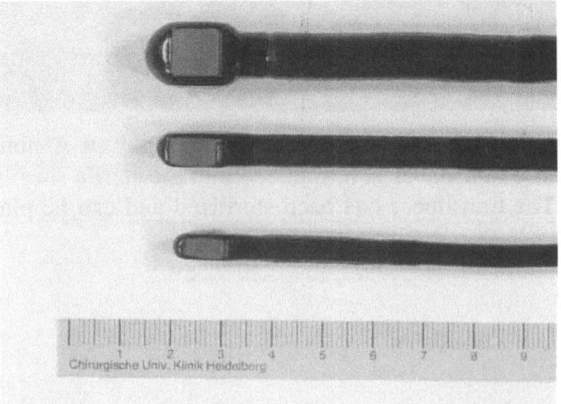

b

Fig. 1.3a, b. Monoplanar endoscopes for TEE. Different sizes for adults, children, and newborns.

Transversal Views

Three primary standard transversal views can be obtained by monoplanar TEE. The basal short-axis, the four-chamber, and the transgastric view. Standard TEE examinations should begin with the four-chamber view since this represents a useful landmark for orientation.

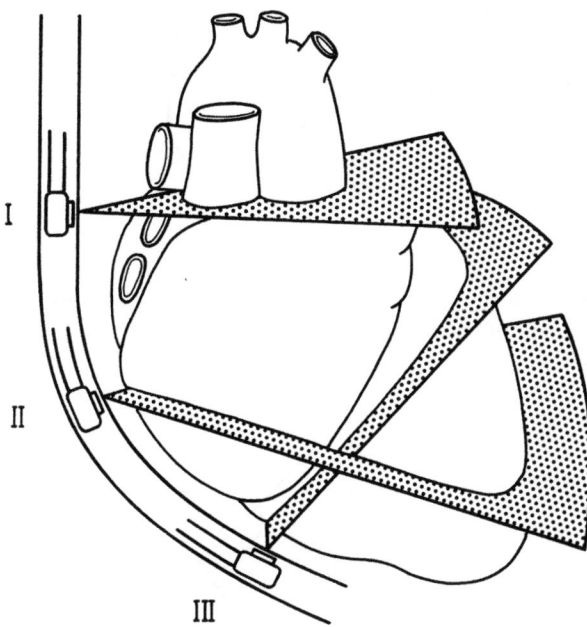

Fig. 1.4. Standard transversal views. Schematic diagram of the three primary transversal views: basal short-axis view (*I*), four-chamber view (*II*), and transgastric view (*III*).

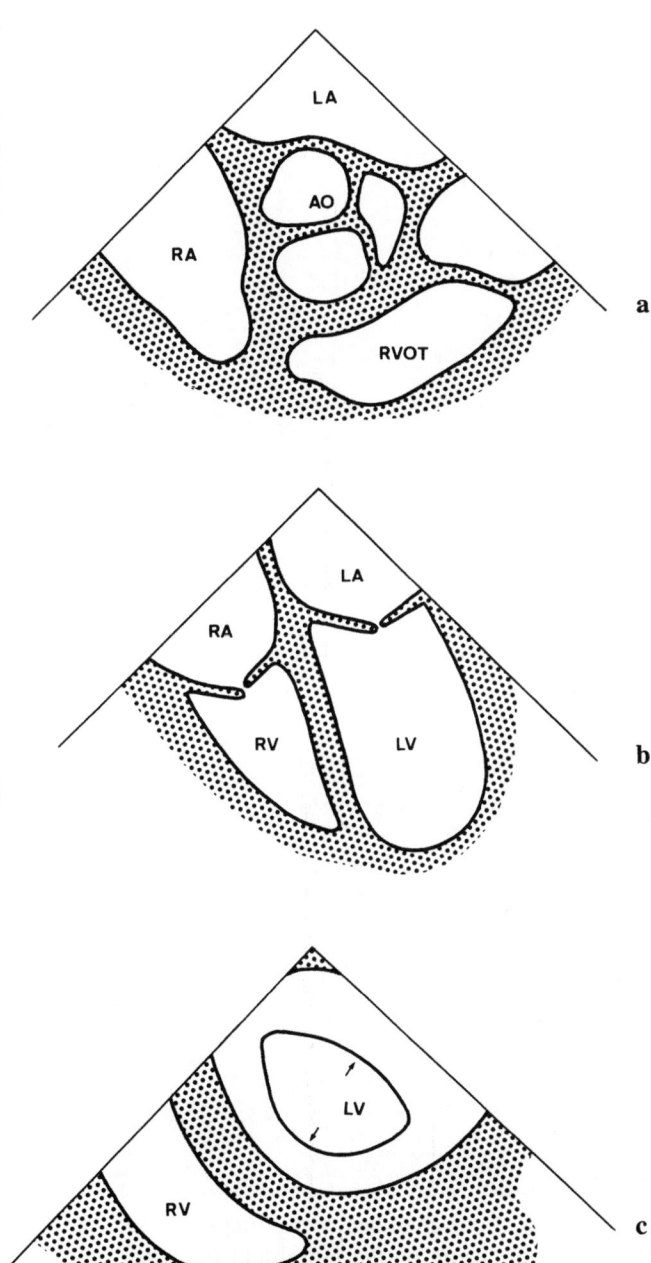

Fig. 1.5a–c. Standard transversal views. **a** Basal short-axis view. **b** Four-chamber view. **c** Transgastric view.

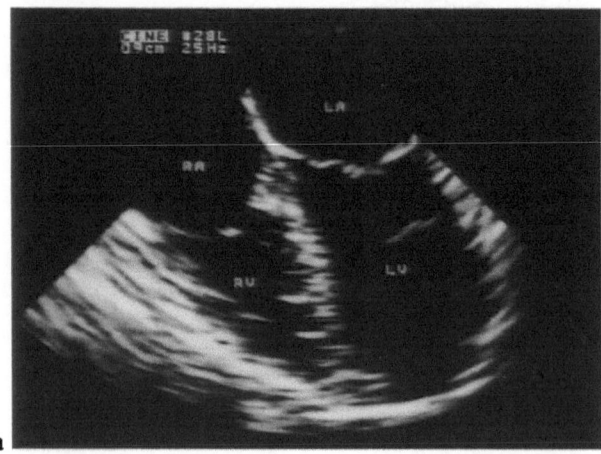 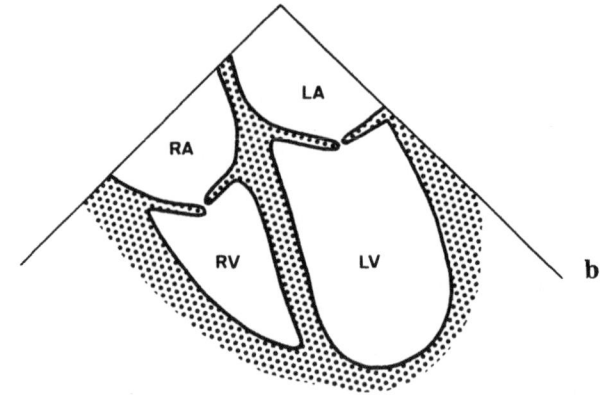

Fig. 1.6a, b. Four-chamber view, obtained by placing the transducer posterior to the left atrium, at the level of the atrioventricular valves. Mitral valve, tricuspid valve, and both atria can be visualized.

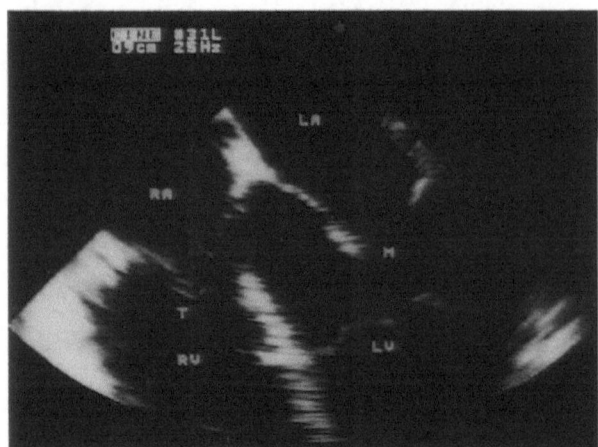 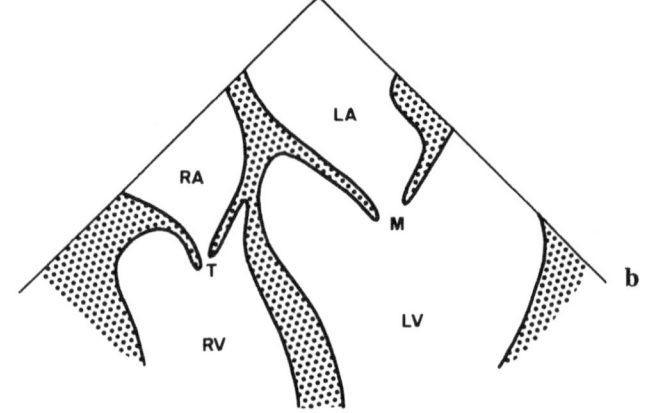

Fig. 1.7a, b. Four-chamber view, magnification of the Fig. 1.6 focusing on the mitral and tricuspid valves.

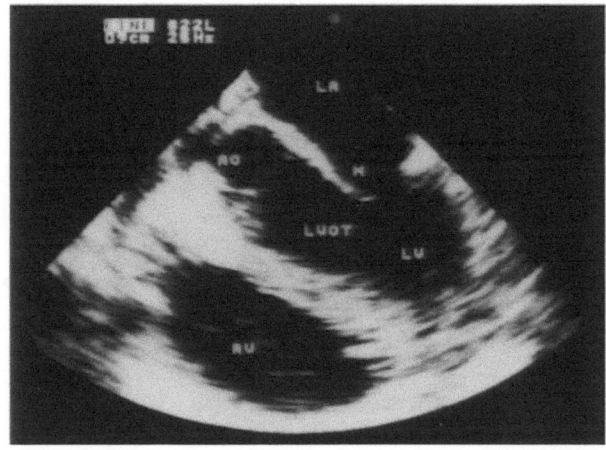
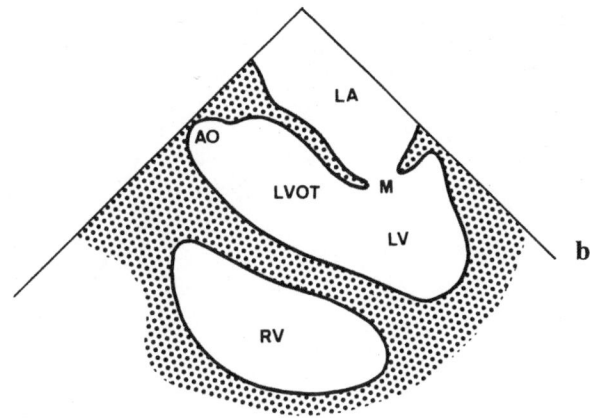

a

b

Fig. 1.8a, b. LVOT view, obtained from the four-chamber view position by slightly anteflexing the tip of the endoscope. This view is useful for evaluating aortic valve regurgitation and LVOT obstruction.

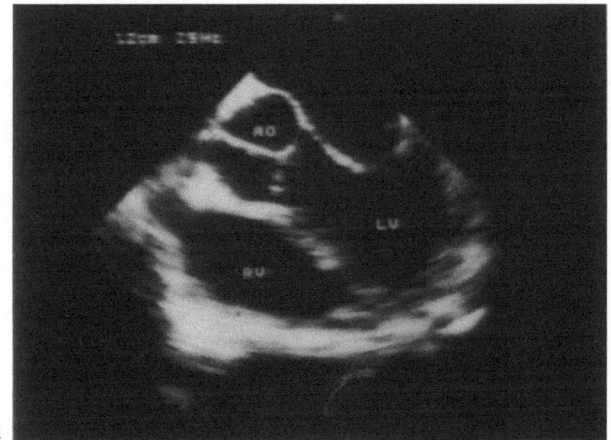
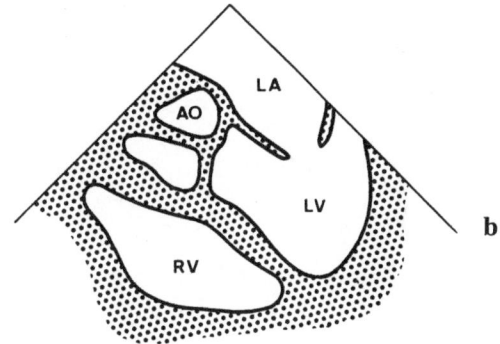

a

b

Fig. 1.9a, b. LVOT view at a level higher than in Fig. 1.8, obtained from the previous position by slightly withdrawing the probe toward the basis of the heart.

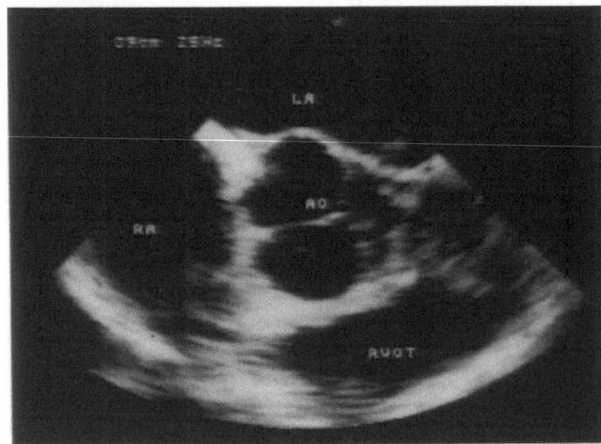
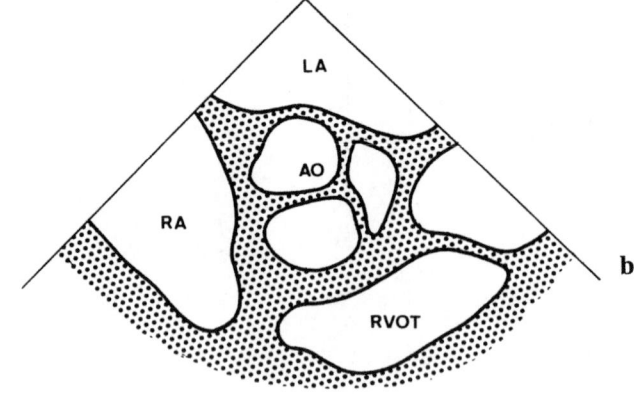

Fig. 1.10a, b. Basal short-axis view, obtained by placing the tip of the endoscope at the level of the basis of the heart. It can be derived from a four-chamber view by withdrawing the endoscope. The aortic valve leaflets, both atria, and the RVOT can be visualized.

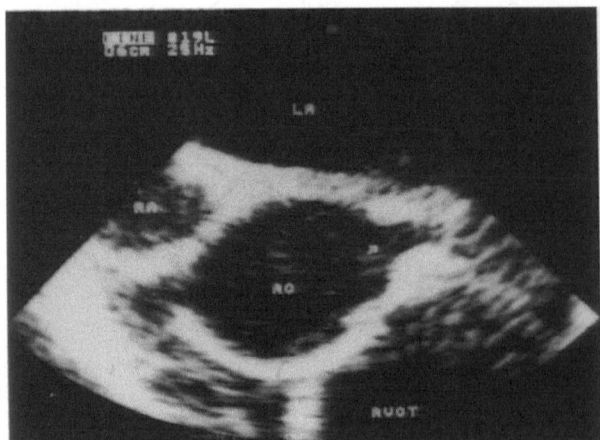
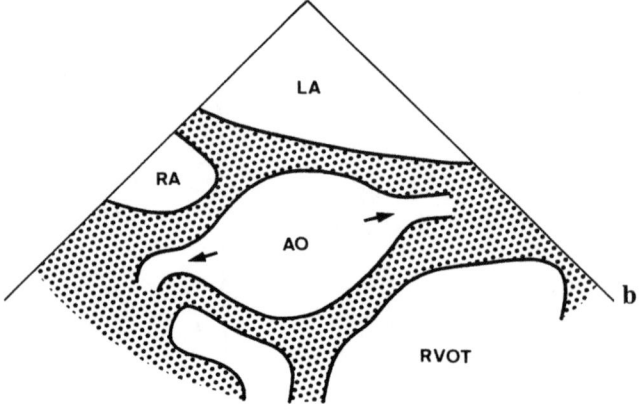

Fig. 1.11a, b. Basal short-axis view, obtained from the projection in Fig. 1.10 by further withdrawing the endoscope. The ascending aorta and the orifices of the coronary arteries can be visualized (*arrows*).

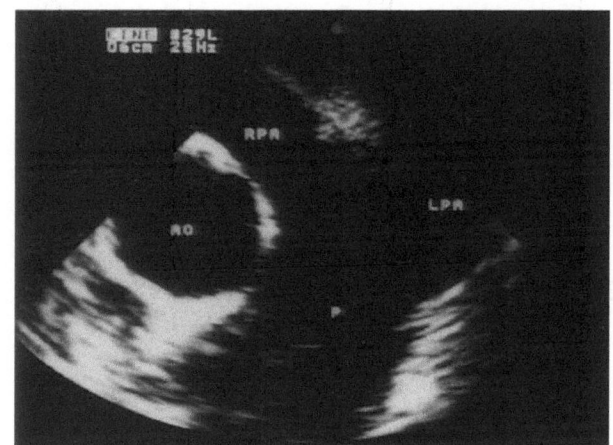 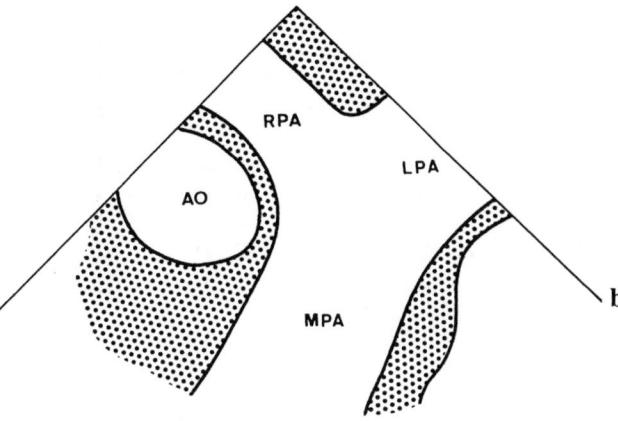

a   b

Fig. 1.12a, b. Basal short-axis view, allowing the visualization of the main pulmonary artery (*P*), right
(*RPA*) and left (*LPA*) pulmonary arteries, and ascending aorta. This imaging plane cannot always be obtained because of the interposition of the left bronchus between the esophagus and the great arteries of
the heart.

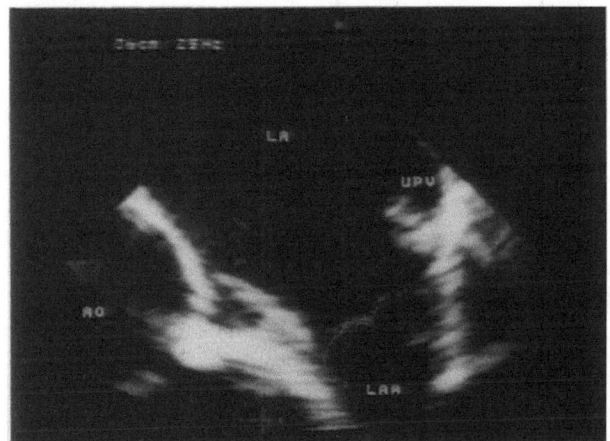 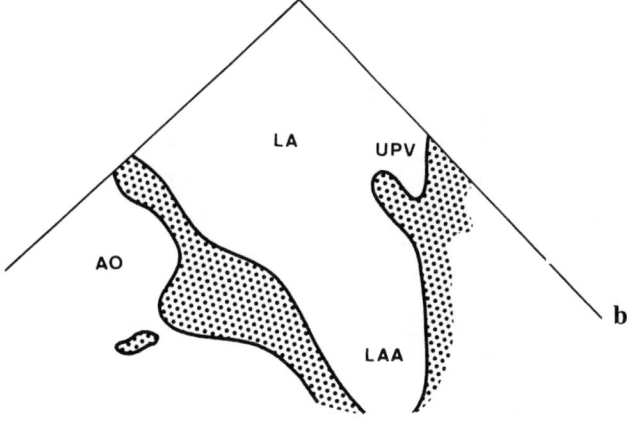

a   b

Fig. 1.13a, b. Basal short-axis view, left atrial appendage, obtained from the projection in Fig. 1.12 by
flexing the tip of endoscope anteriorly. Thrombotic
formations within the left atrium can be easily detected. *LAA*, Left atrial appendage; *UPV*, upper pulmonary vein.

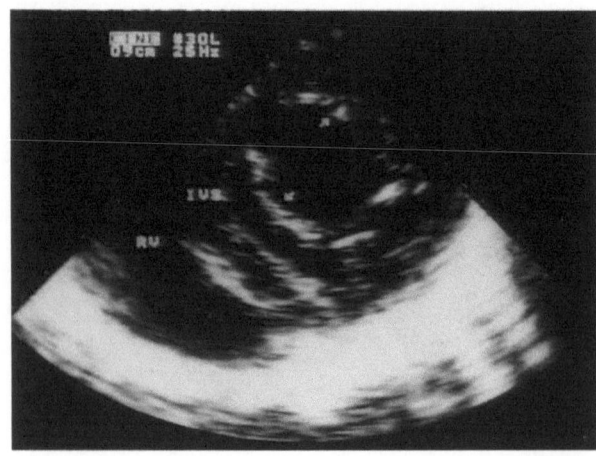

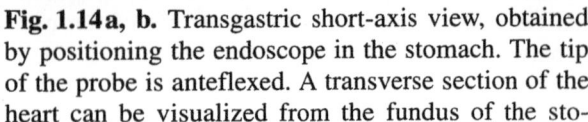

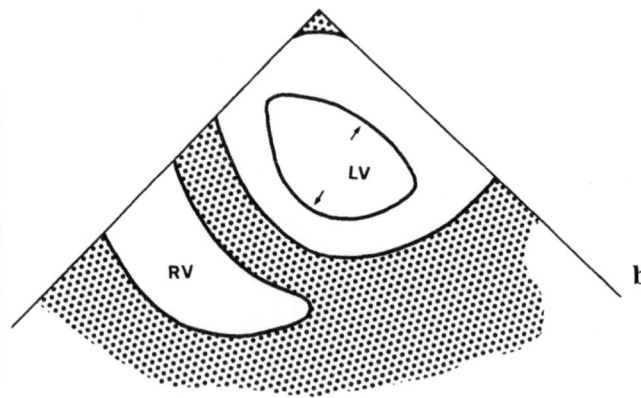

Fig. 1.14a, b. Transgastric short-axis view, obtained by positioning the endoscope in the stomach. The tip of the probe is anteflexed. A transverse section of the heart can be visualized from the fundus of the stomach. This view is taken at the level of the mitral valve and shows the diastolic opening of the anterior and posterior leaflet (*arrows*).

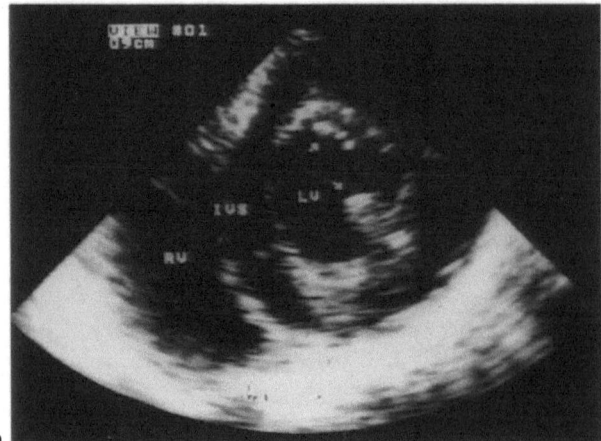

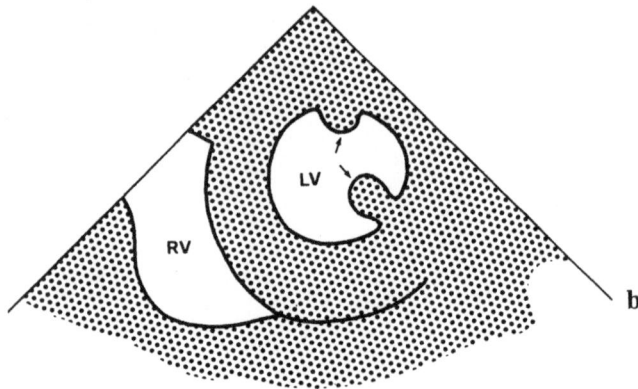

Fig. 1.15a, b. Transgastric short-axis view at the level of the papillary muscles (*arrows*), obtained from the view in Fig. 1.14 by slightly retroflexing the tip of the endoscope.

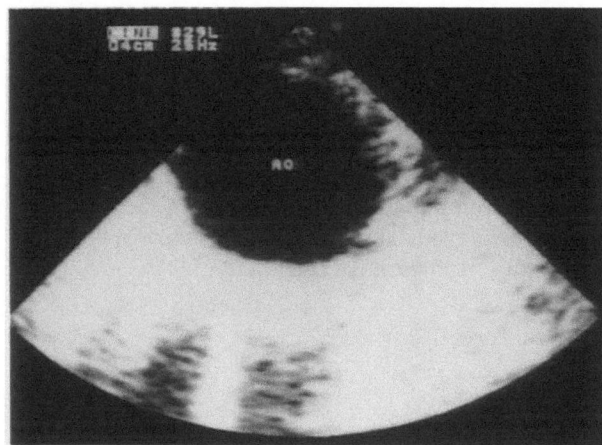
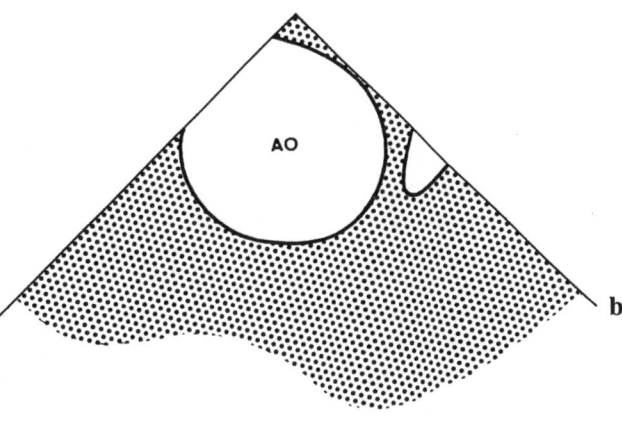

Fig. 1.16a, b. Transverse view of the descending aorta, obtained by rotating the endoscope posteriorly. Complete visualization of the descending aorta at different levels can be performed. The depth of the tip of the endoscope from incisor teeth should be recorded for orientation.

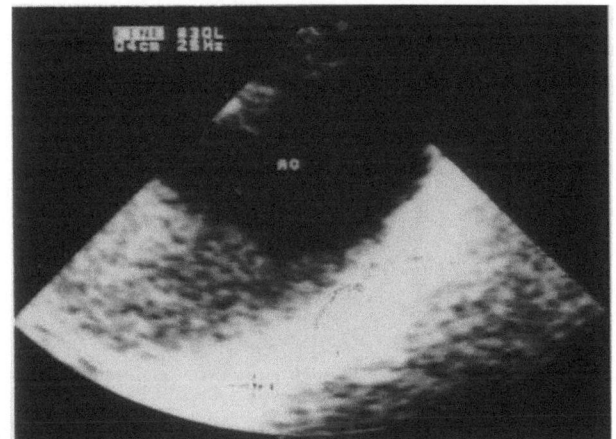
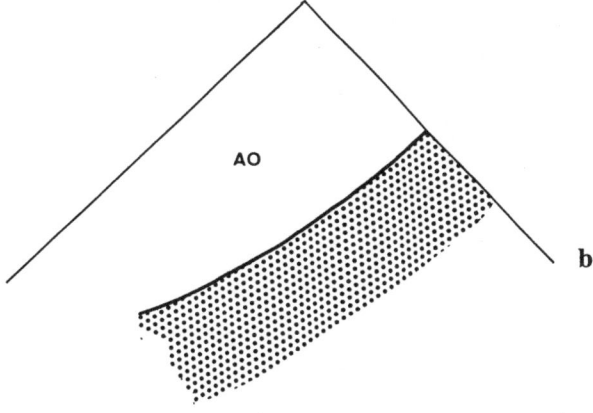

Fig. 1.17a, b. Transverse view of the aortic arch, obtained by rotating the endoscope posteriorly and by withdrawing the endoscope along the descending aorta to its proximal extremity.

Biplanar Imaging

Biplanar and multiplanar transducers have been recently built into the new TEE endoscopes. Biplanar imaging is now the current standard for TEE examinations. Two imaging planes (transversal and longitudinal) can be visualized from the same location without moving the probe.

A series of longitudinal views can be obtained from each standard transversal view. Four standard longitudinal views can be obtained by placing the transducer posterior to the left atrium, at the level of the corresponding transversal four-chamber view, by rotating the endoscope from left to right. The longitudinal views taken at the level of the corresponding four-chamber view are: the left ventricular-left atrial (LV-LA) long-axis view, the right ventricular outflow tract (RVOT) long-axis view, the ascending aorta-atrial septal long-axis view, and the caval-atrial septal long-axis view. Longitudinal views can even be obtained with the transducer at the level of the corresponding basal and transgastric short-axis views.

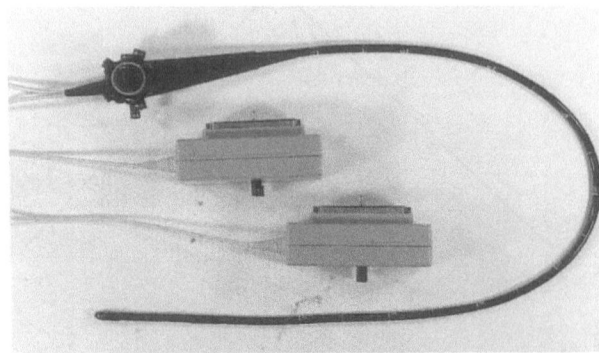

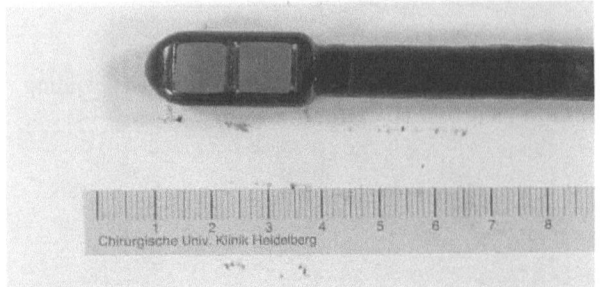

Fig. 1.18a, b. Biplanar TEE endoscopes. Two transducers are mounted at the tip of the endoscope; the distal transducer provides a transversal imaging view and the proximal a longitudinal imaging plane.

Longitudinal Views

Four primary standard longitudinal views can be obtained by biplanar TEE. The LV-LA long-axis view, the RVOT long-axis view, the ascending aorta-atrial septal long-axis view, and the caval-atrial septal long-axis view. These can be obtained at the level of the corresponding four-chamber view. A line on the two-dimensional transversal echocardiogram indicates the plane on which the corresponding longitudinal view will be displayed. The four-chamber view represents a necessary landmark for orientation.

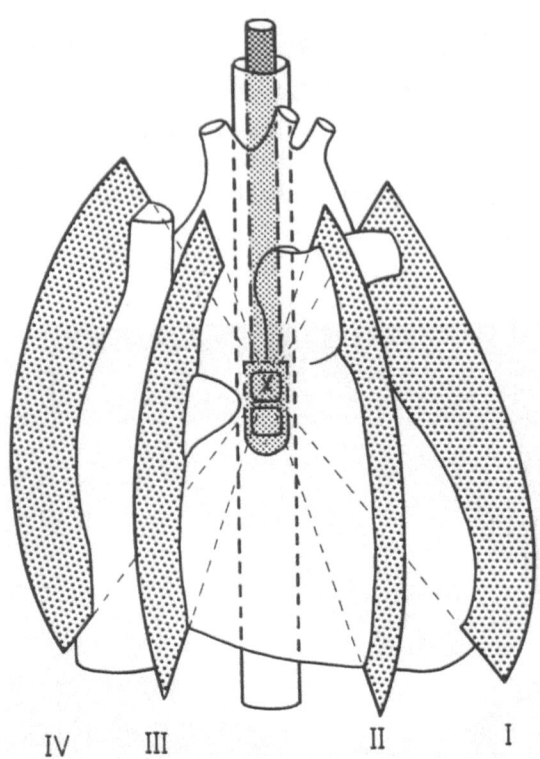

Fig. 1.19. Standard longitudinal views. Schematic diagram of the standard longitudinal views derived from the four-chamber view: LV-LA long-axis view (*I*), RVOT long-axis view (*II*), ascending aorta-atrial septal long-axis view (*III*), caval-atrial septal long-axis view (*IV*).

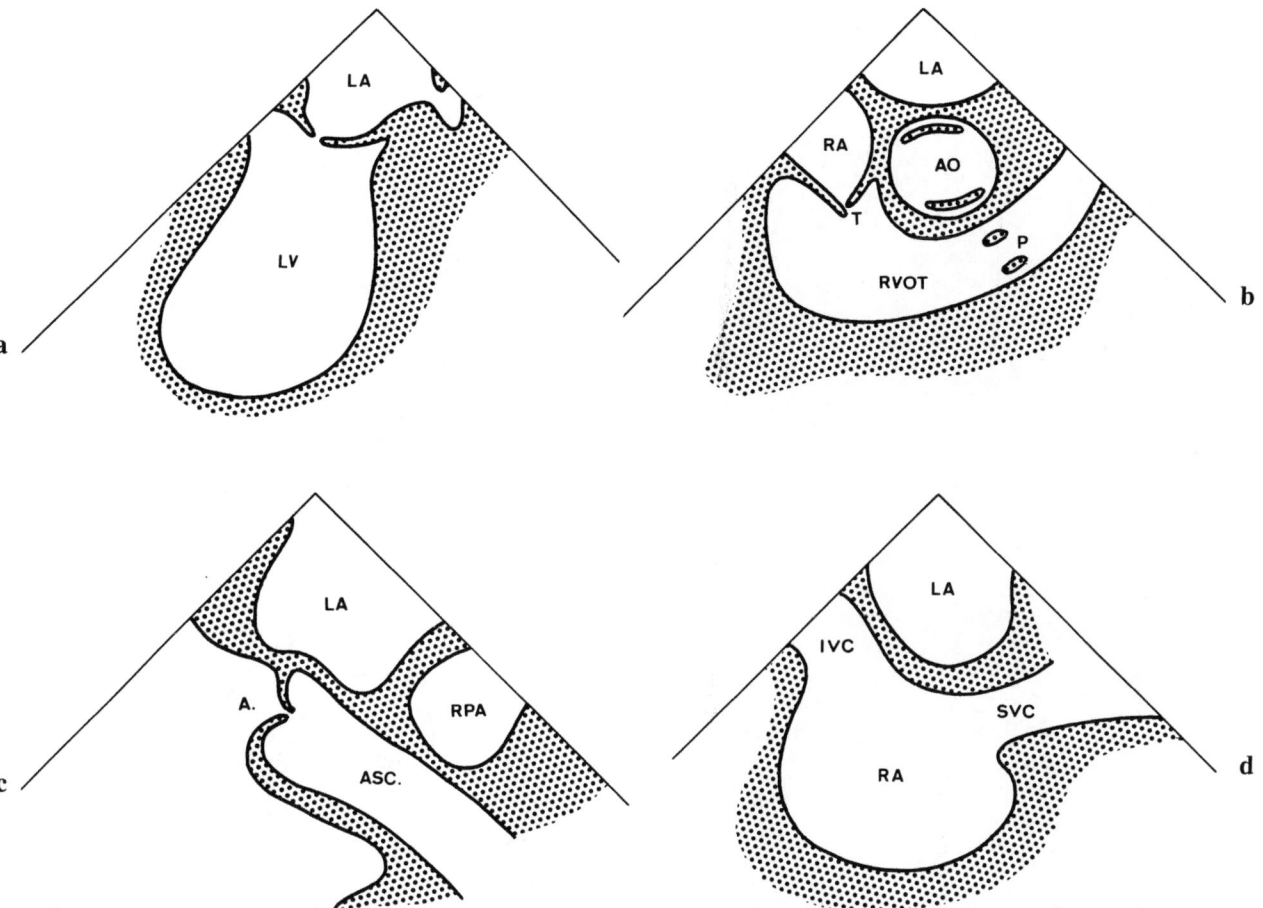

Fig. 1.20a–d. Standard longitudinal views, obtained at the level of the transversal four-chamber view by rotating the endoscope from the left side toward the right side of the heart. **a** LV-LA long-axis view. **b** RVOT long-axis view. **c** Ascending aorta-atrial septal long-axis view. **d** Caval-atrial septal long-axis view.

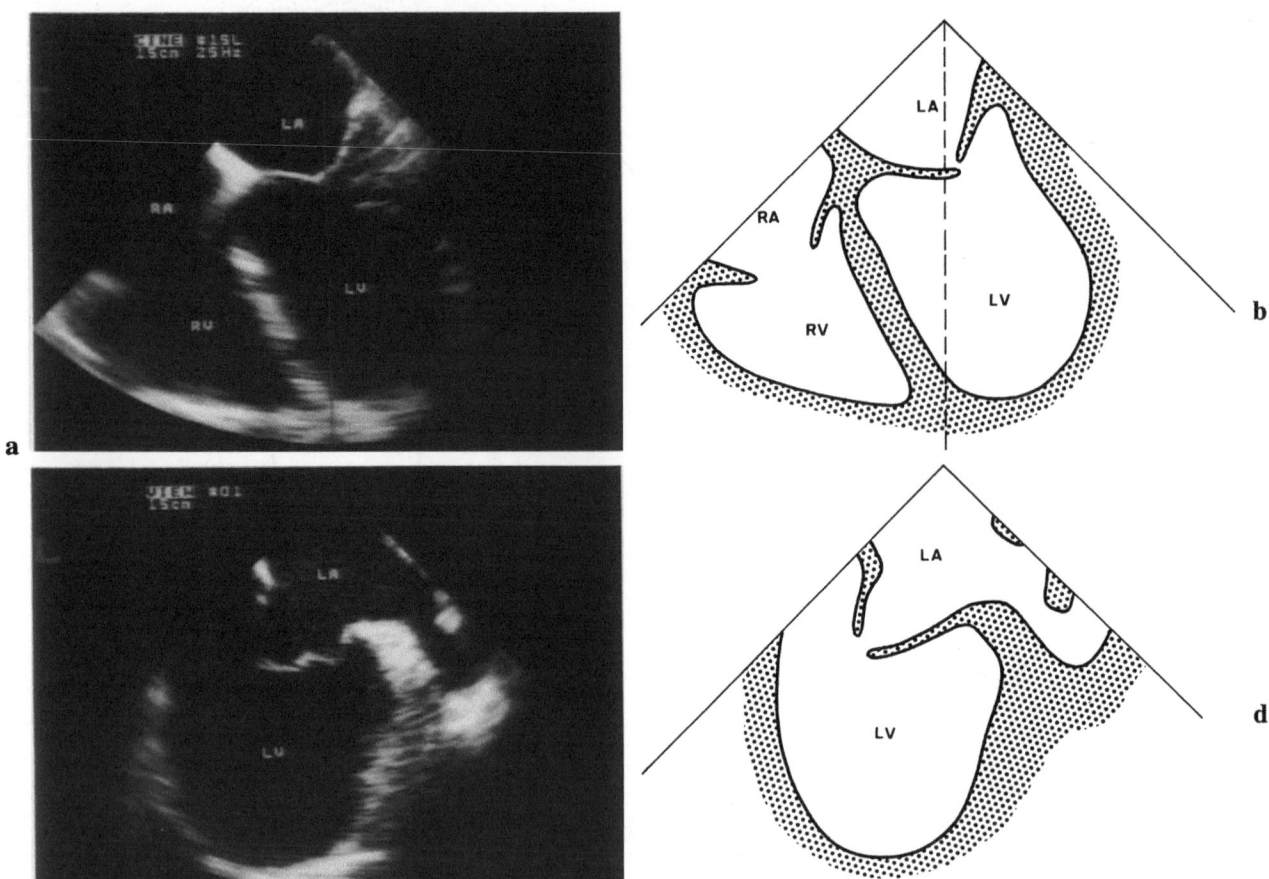

Fig. 1.21a–d. LV-LA long-axis view, transversal view (*above*) and corresponding longitudinal view (*below*). *Line* (transversal view) indicates the imaging plane where the corresponding longitudinal view is visualized. **a, b** Transversal four-chamber view. **c, d** Corresponding LV-LA long-axis view. *T*, Transversal view; *L*, longitudinal view.

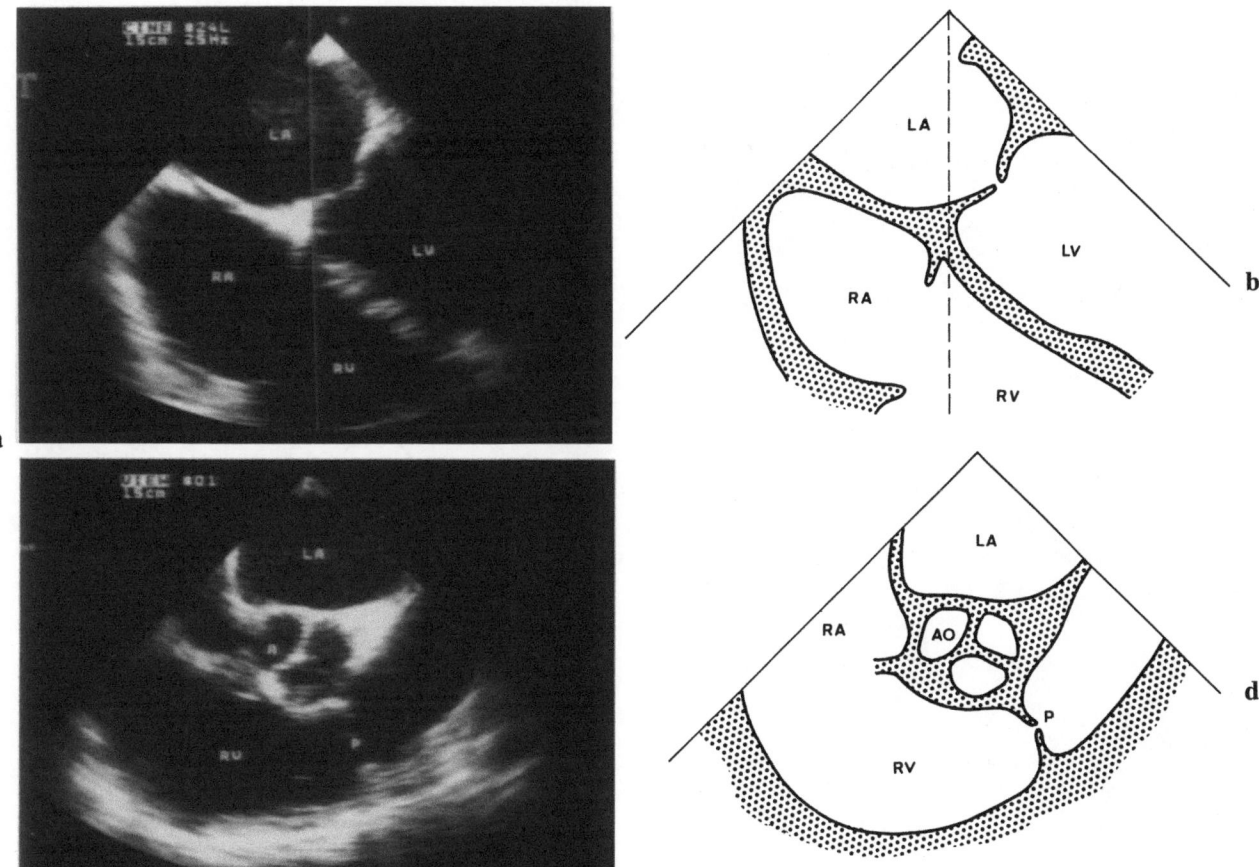

Fig. 1.22a–d. RVOT long-axis view, transversal view (*above*) and corresponding longitudinal view (*below*). *Line* (transversal view) indicates the imaging plane where the corresponding longitudinal view is visualized. **a, b** Transversal four-chamber view. **c, d** Corresponding RVOT long-axis view. *T*, Transversal view; *L*, longitudinal view.

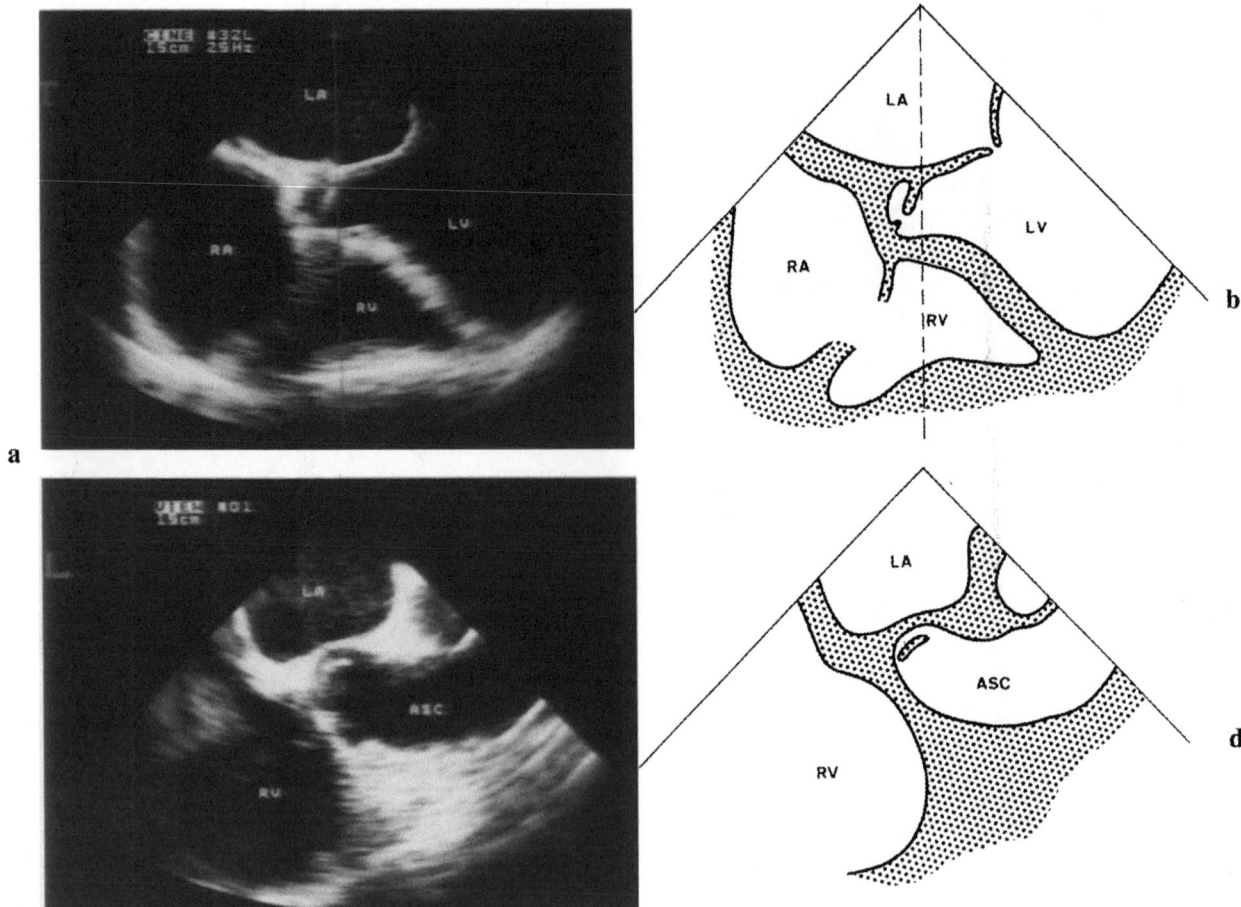

Fig. 1.23a–d. Ascending aorta-atrial septal long-axis view, transversal view (*above*) and corresponding longitudinal view (*below*). *Line* (transversal view) indicates the imaging plane where the corresponding longitudinal view is visualized. **a, b** Transversal four-chamber view. **c, d,** Corresponding ascending aorta-atrial septal long-axis view. *T*, Transversal view; *L*, longitudinal view.

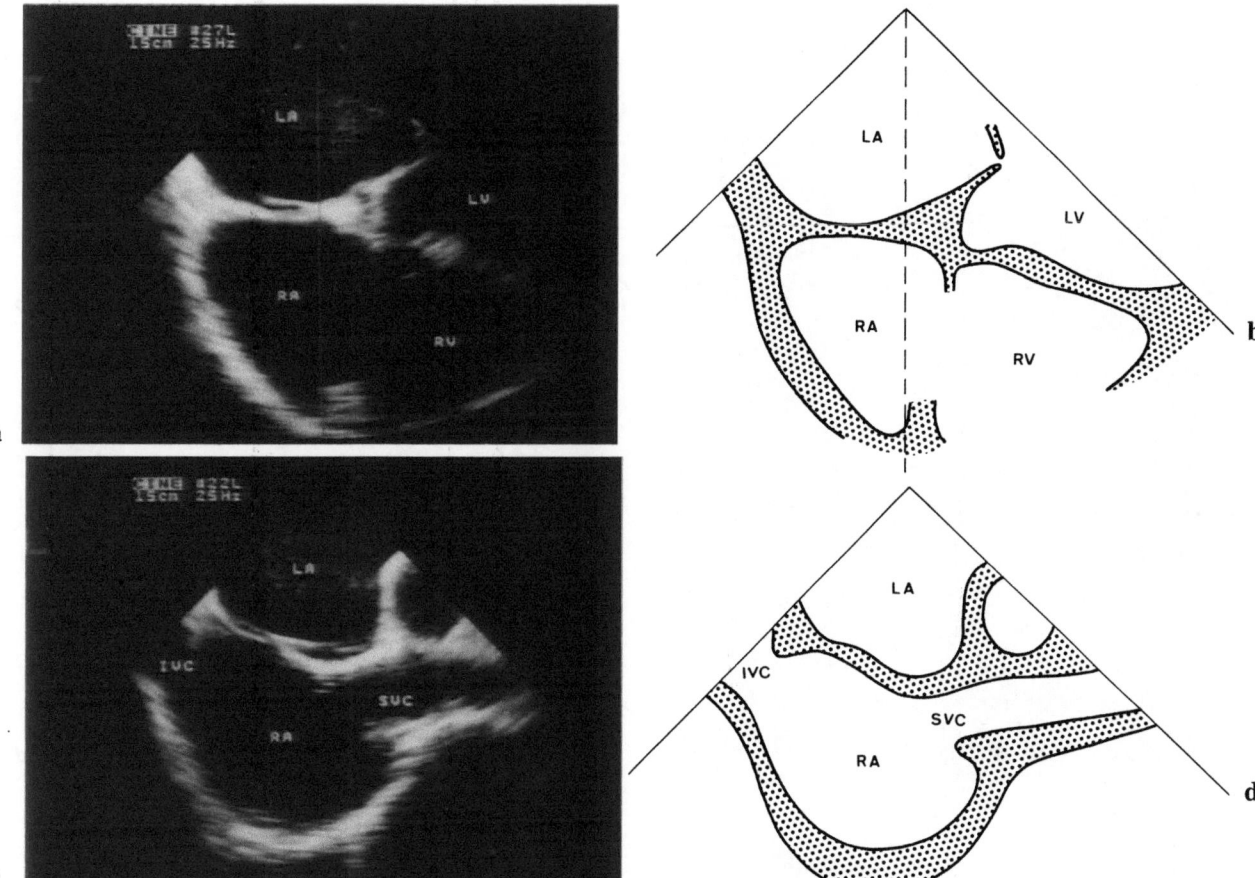

Fig. 1.24a–d. Caval-atrial septal long-axis view, transversal view (*above*) and corresponding longitudinal view (*below*). *Line* (transversal view) indicates the imaging plane where the corresponding longitudinal view is visualized. **a, b** Transversal four-chamber view. **c, d** Corresponding caval-atrial septal long-axis view. *T*, Transversal view; *L*, longitudinal view.

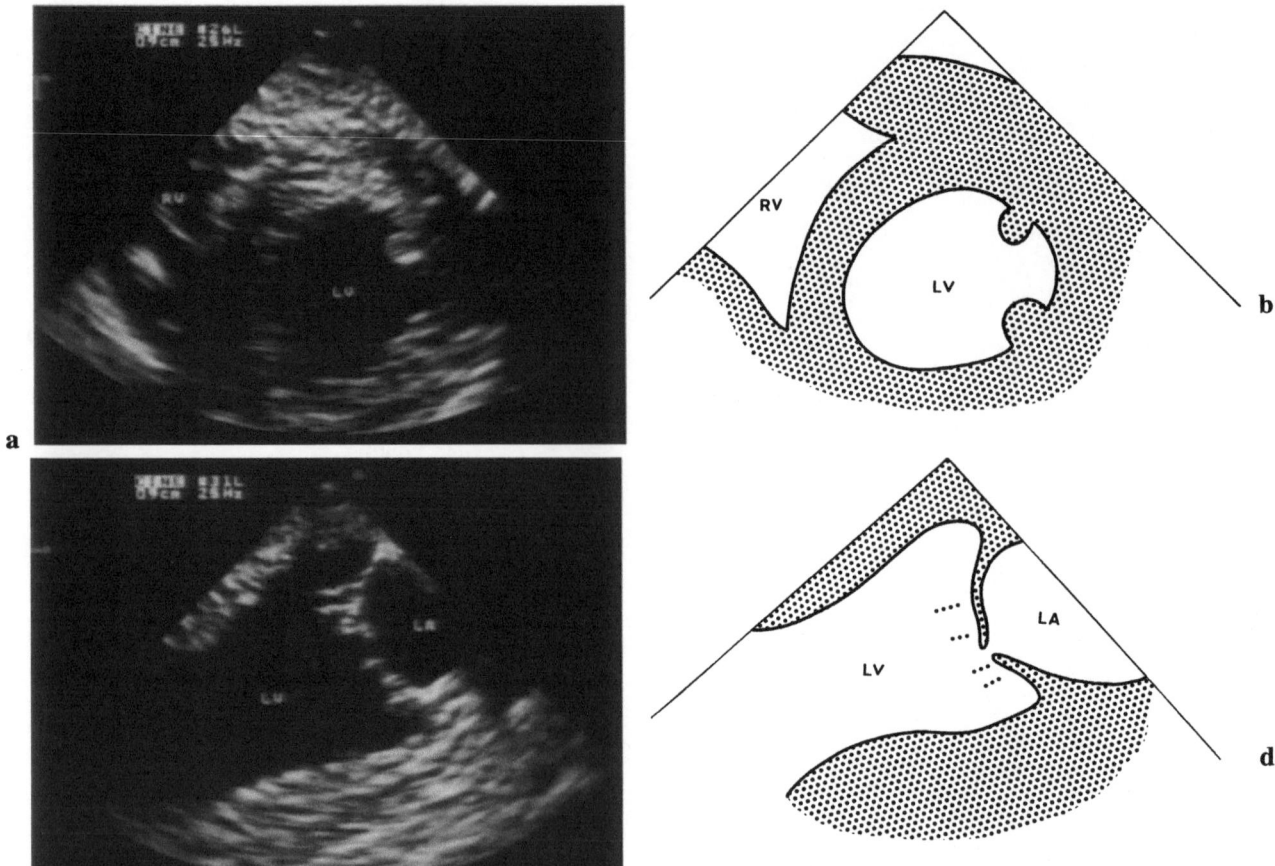

Fig. 1.25 a–d. Transgastric long-axis views, transversal view (*above*) and corresponding longitudinal view (*below*). The longitudinal view of the left ventricle can be obtained from the transgastric position. The subvalvular apparatus and the chordae of the mitral valve can be visualized more in detail by this view. **a, b** Transgastric short-axis view. **c, d** Corresponding transgastric long-axis view. The subvalvular apparatus and chordae tendineae can be clearly visualized. *T*, Transversal view; *L*, longitudinal view.

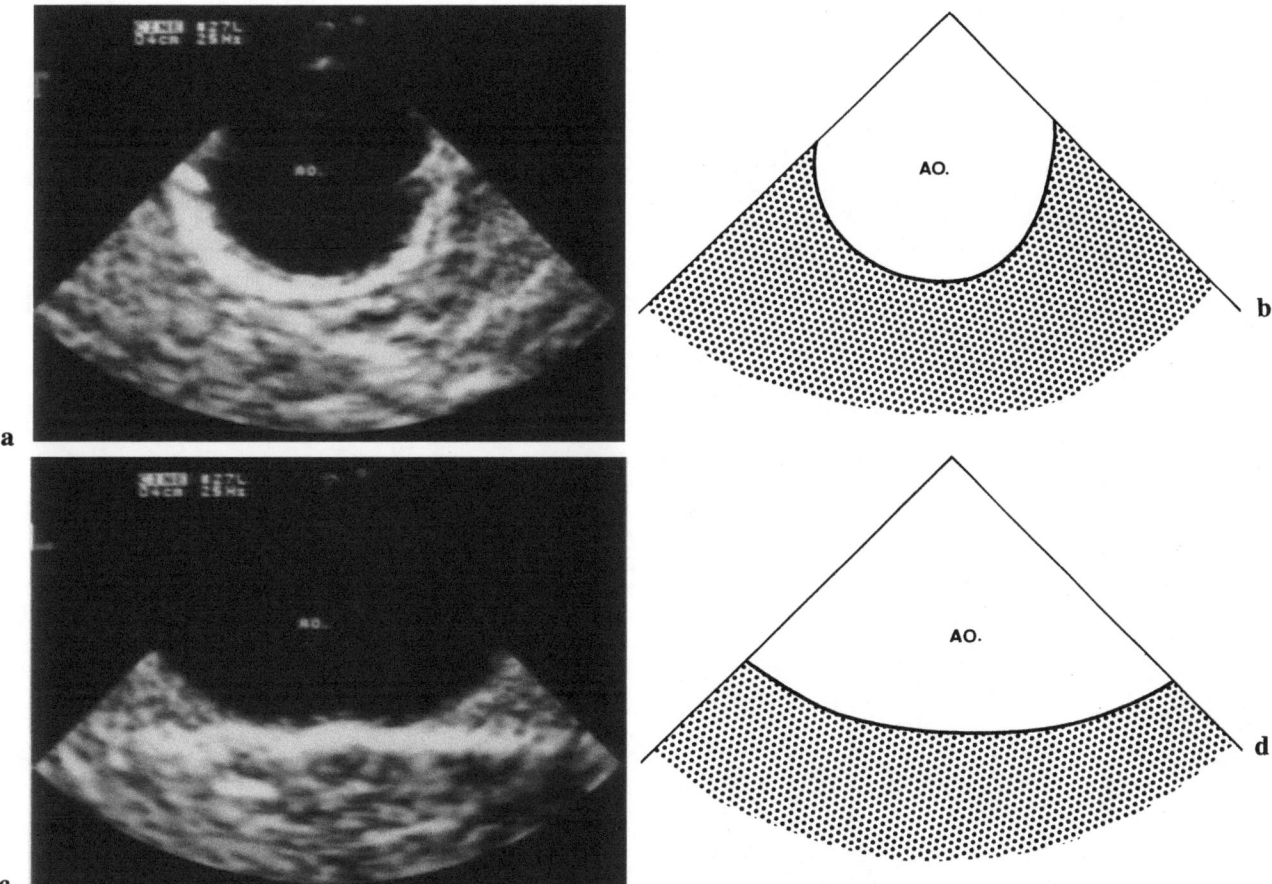

Fig. 1.26a–d. Longitudinal view of the descending aorta, transversal view (*above*) and corresponding longitudinal view (*below*). Longitudinal views of the descending aorta can be obtained from the corresponding transversal views. The descending aorta can be visualized at different depths of the transducer from the incisors. **a, b** Short-axis view of the aorta. **c, d** Corresponding longitudinal view of the aorta. *T*, Transversal view; *L*, longitudinal view.

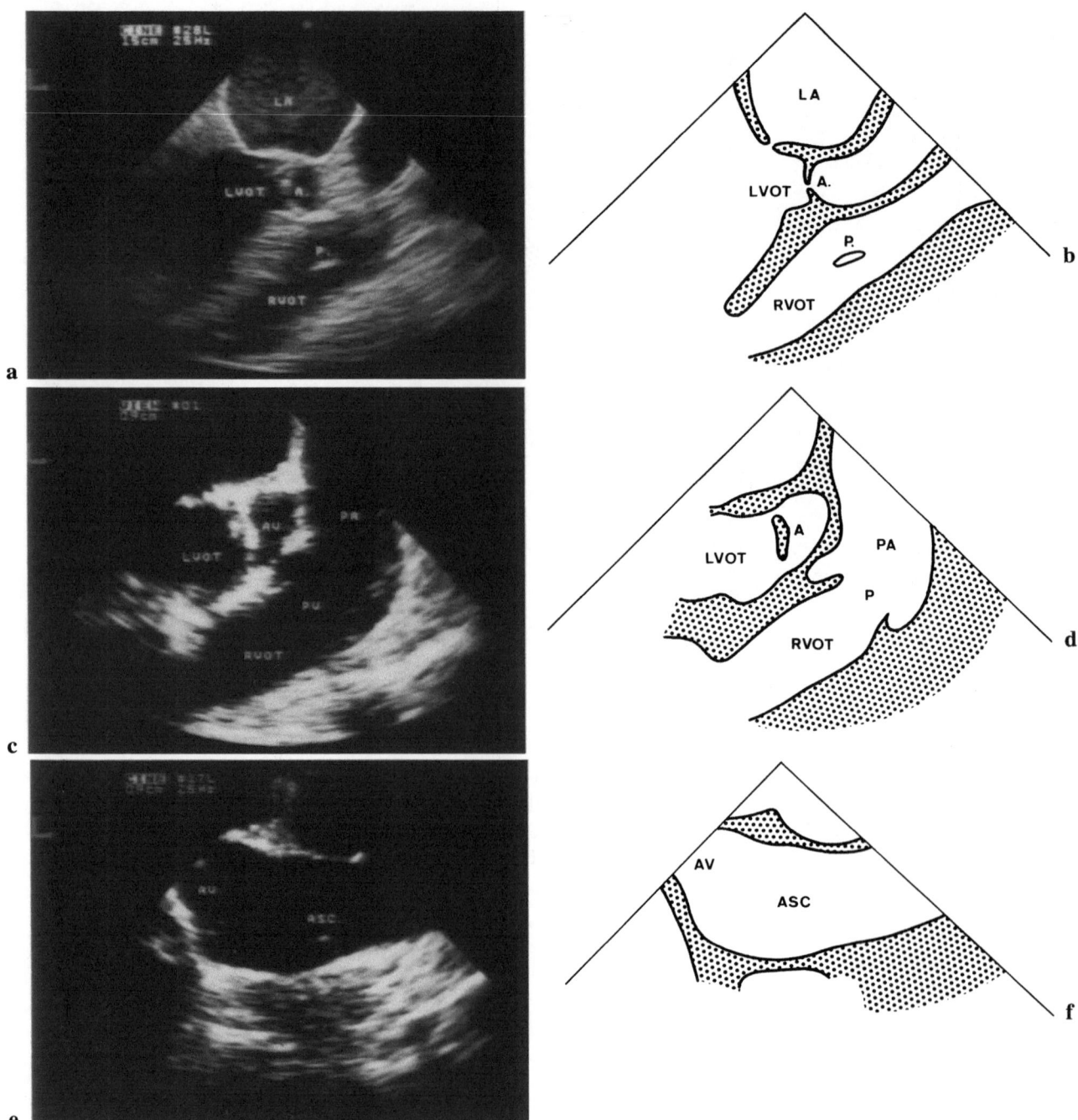

Fig. 1.27a–f. Off-axis longitudinal views. Nonstandard views are useful for visualizing particular structures. They can be obtained by slight movements of the transducer into the esophagus. **a, b** LVOT and RVOT are imaged in the same frame. **c, d** The pulmonary valve and main pulmonary artery are well visualized in this view. **e, f** A long portion of the ascending aorta can be visualized up to the arch. *L,* Longitudinal view.

Color Doppler Flow Imaging

Color Doppler flow imaging is based on pulsed wave Doppler technology. Blood flow velocity can be measured by analyzing the velocity of the red blood cells in a small area, called a *sample volume*, along a scan line superimposed on the two-dimensional echocardiogram.

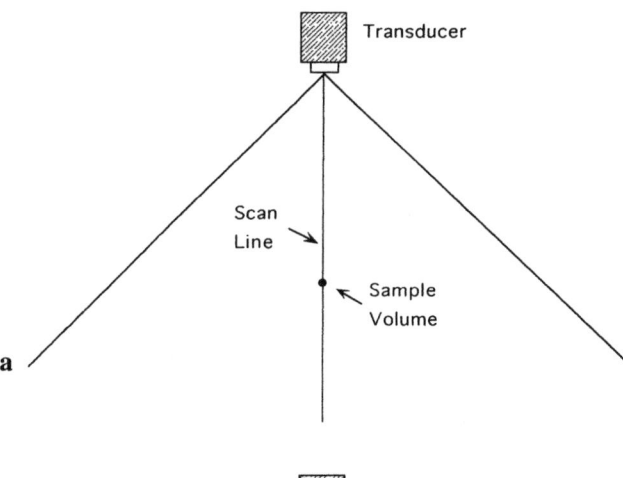

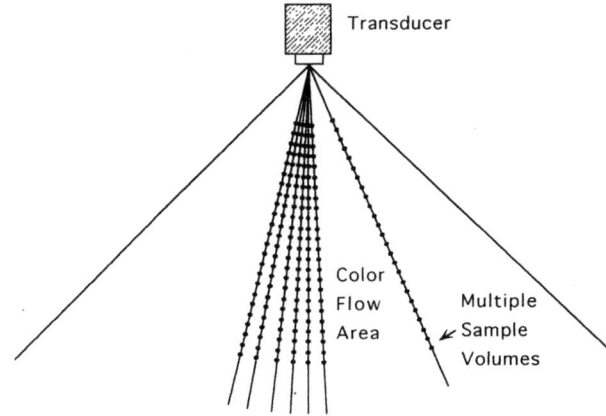

Fig. 1.28a, b. Pulsed-wave Doppler and color flow imaging. **a** Pulsed Doppler. Intracardiac blood flow is measured in a small area (sample volume) along a scan line. **b** Color Doppler. A sector with multiple sample volumes (color flow area) is superimposed on the two-dimensional echocardiogram.

Basics

Color Doppler consists of multiple sample volumes along multiple sample lines. These lines form a sector containing a large number of sample volumes (Fig. 1.28). The Doppler shift signal measured at each sampling point is transformed into color-coded information. A sector with multiple pulsed-wave sample sites (color flow area) is superimposed on the two-dimensional echocardiogram, providing real-time imaging of intracardiac blood flow (Fig. 1.29). The characteristics of blood flow that can be evaluated by color Doppler imaging are *direction*, *velocity*, and *variance*. Blood flow *direction* is usually displayed with the colors red and blue. Red represents the flow toward the transducer, and blue the flow away from the transducer. The *velocity* of blood flow is represented by the brightness: the higher the velocity, the brighter is the color displayed. The *variance*, or degree of dispersion in the velocity of the single blood cells, indicates the amount of turbulent or disturbed flow; this is displayed by adding another col-

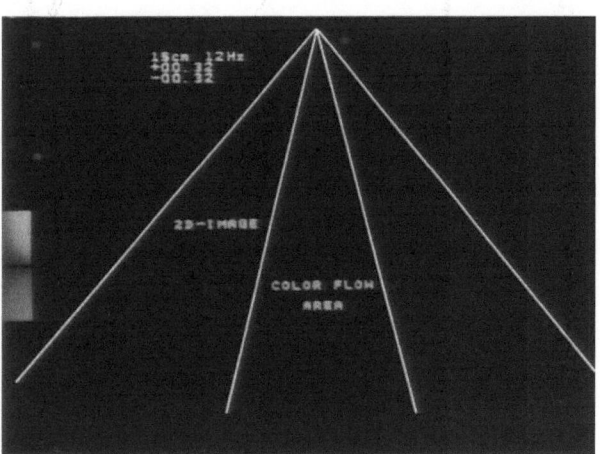

Fig. 1.29. Color flow area superimposed on the two-dimensional echocardiogram (*2-D image*) as it appears on the screen of the echo machine.

or, usually green, to the principals. Each commercial color Doppler imaging system visualizes flow information using different colors (Fig. 1.30).

The *frequency* of color image display (frame rate) depends on the cross-sectional area of the color flow sector. The generation of real-time color flow images requires the calculation of all data points (sample volumes) which constitute the sector of color flow area within a very short time (a few milliseconds). The larger the angle of color flow area, the greater the number of data points to be calculated and displayed, and hence the slower is the frequency of color picture generation. The *depth* of color Doppler examination does not affect the frame rate of color flow pictures since the number of data points to be displayed remains the same at different depths. However, the higher the depth of Doppler examination, the lower is the resolution and the maximal blood flow

Table 1.1. Relationship between frequency of color image display and angle of color Doppler sector.

Angle of color Doppler	Frequency of display
30	25 Hz
50	12 Hz
80	6 Hz
30/80*	17 Hz
45/80*	12 Hz

* The first angle refers to color flow area, the second to the sector of two-dimensional echocardiogram.

velocity which is measurable. The relationship between the frequency of color image display and the angle of color Doppler sector in a commercially available system is shown in Table 1.1.

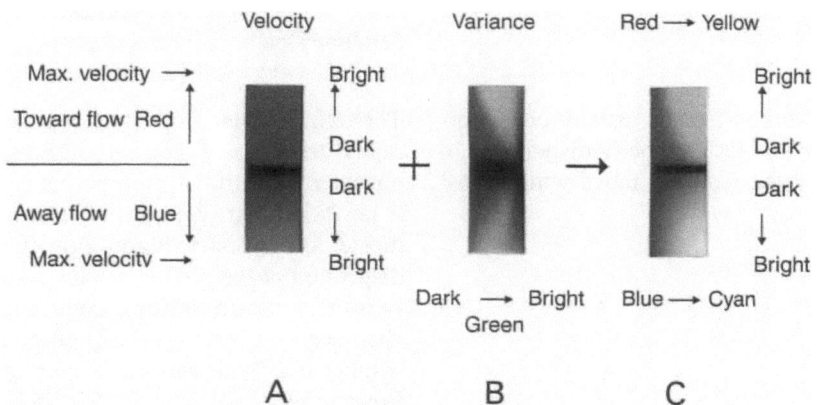

Fig. 1.30. Information derived from color-coded signals. The color flow Doppler signal is formed by the three fundamental colors: red, blue, and green. *A,* Flow direction is represented by *red* (toward flow) and *blue* (away flow). Flow velocity is displayed by varying the *brightness* of red or blue. *B,* Variance, or the degree of flow velocity dispersion, is obtained by adding *green.* (Blue + green = *yellow*; red + green = *cyan*). *C,* Color bar shows complete flow information.

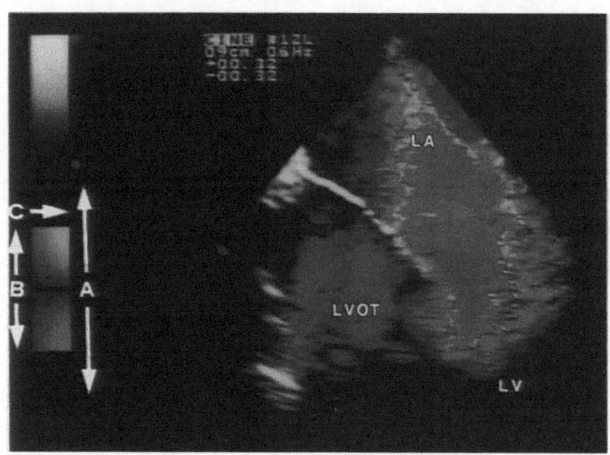

Fig. 1.31. Color Doppler echocardiography, examples of different color flow patterns. Color bar (*left*) shows the flow information. *A,* Flow direction; *red,* toward the transducer; *blue,* away from the transducer. *B,* Flow velocity; high flow velocity is displayed with *bright colors. C,* Variance; disturbed flow is displayed by adding *green* to the principal color (blue + green = *yellow*; red + green = *cyan.*

Normal Flow

Normal intracardiac blood flow is usually characterized by low velocity and little velocity dispersion. In laminar flow most of the red cells move with almost equal velocity.

Laminar Flow

The term *laminar* flow has been used in echocardiography to indicate normal intracardiac blood flow; however the term is improper since intracardiac flow is never laminar. We use the term laminar flow to indicate low-velocity blood flow with little velocity dispersion of the red cells. This flow pattern is usually displayed as a uniform color signal. From a four-chamber view, tricuspid and mitral diastolic flows are displayed in blue and pulmonary and aortic ejection flows in red.

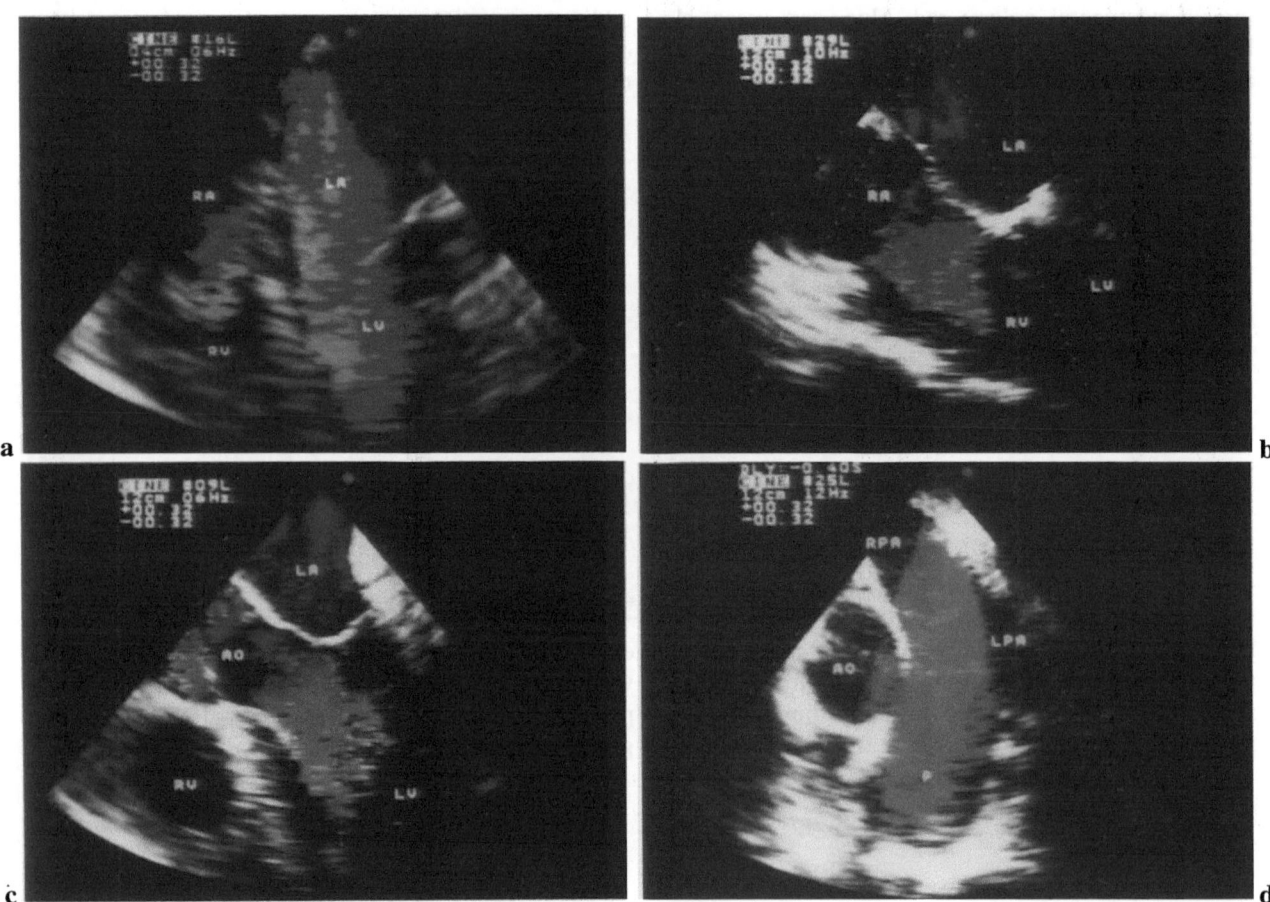

Fig. 1.32a–d. Laminar flow, color Doppler, normal diastolic and systolic flows. **a** Left ventricular inflow. The flow (*blue*) is directed away from the transducer (ideally placed at the top of the figure), from the left atrium into the left ventricle. **b** Right ventricular inflow. The flow (*blue*) is directed away from the transducer, from the right atrium into the right ventricle. **c** Left ventricular ejection flow. The flow (*red*) is directed toward the transducer. The systolic flow in the LVOT is displayed in *red*. **d** Pulmonary ejection flow. The systolic flow in the main pulmonary artery is displayed in *red*. *AO*, Aorta; *P*, main pulmonary artery; *RPA*, right pulmonary artery; *LPA*, left pulmonary artery.

Pulsed Doppler

Intracardiac blood flow can be analyzed with pulsed-wave Doppler by placing the sample volume in the color flow area. The pulsed-wave Doppler curves of laminar flow show little velocity dispersion. The single blood cell velocities are displayed along the contour of the curve. An empty zone with no Doppler signals can be observed in the inner part of the curve.

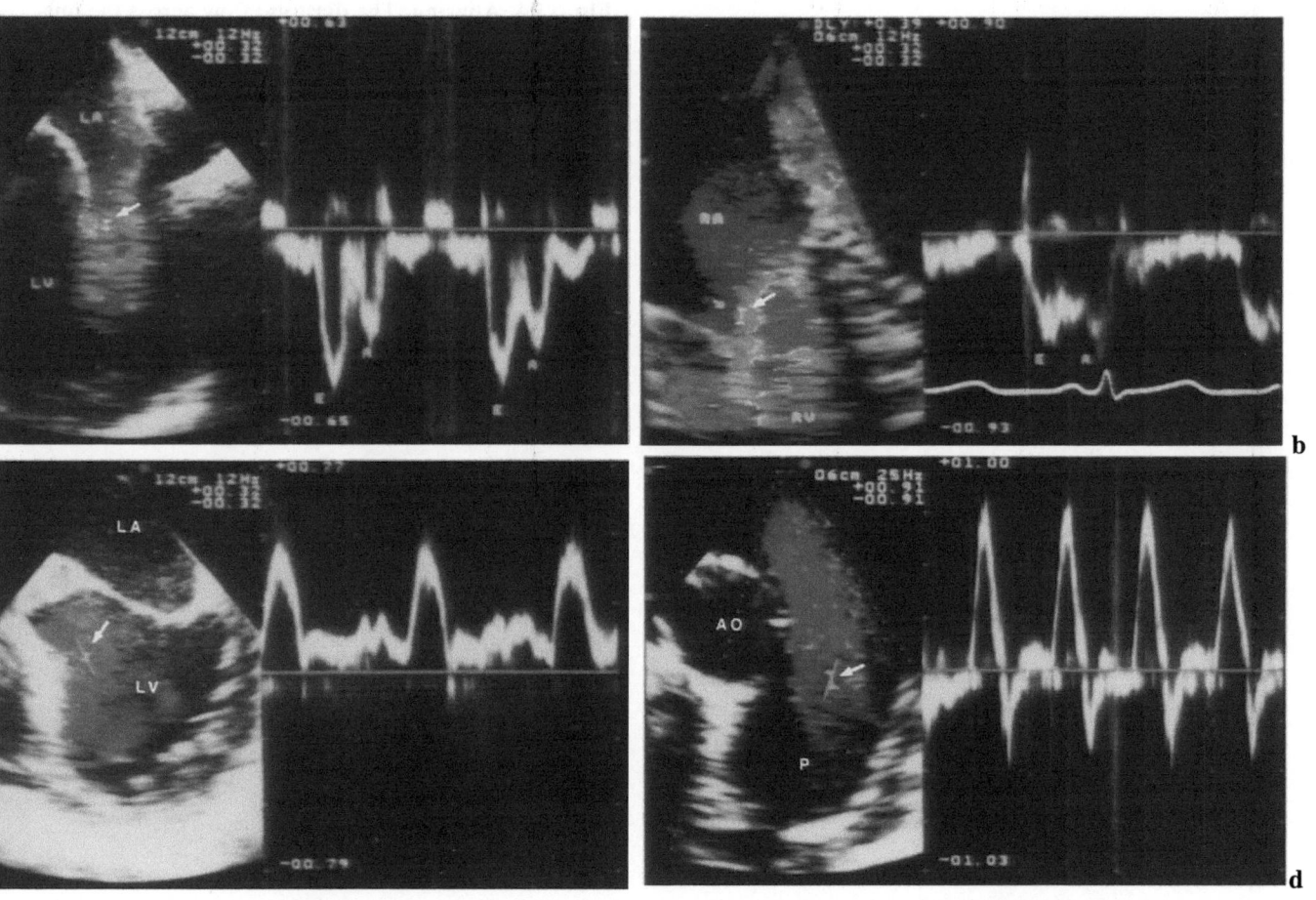

Fig. 1.33a–d. Pulsed Doppler, normal diastolic and systolic flow. **a** Left ventricular diastolic inflow. The sample volume is placed at the level of the mitral valve. *E*, Early diastolic filling velocity; *A*, Late diastolic filling, due to atrial contraction. **b** Right ventricular diastolic inflow. The sample volume is placed at the level of tricuspid valve. **c** Left ventricular ejection flow. The sample volume is placed in the LVOT. **d** Pulmonary ejection flow. The sample volume is placed in the main pulmonary artery.

Aliased Flow

Both pulsed-wave Doppler and color Doppler are unable to measure high flow velocities. The higher measurable velocity, called *Nyquist limit*, depends on the pulse repetition frequency of the transducer and on the depth of the flow to be measured. If the flow velocity exceeds the Nyquist limit, a reversed flow with opposite direction, is displayed. This phenomenon is called *aliasing*. In aliased flows both positive and negative color Doppler signals are observed. *Aliasing does not mean turbulent or abnormal flow.* Aliased flow indicates normal flow with velocity exceeding the maximal measurable flow velocity.

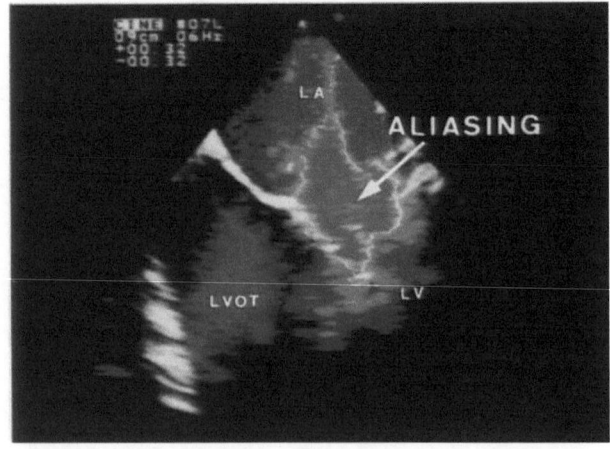

Fig. 1.34. Aliasing. The diastolic flow across the mitral valve, directed from the left atrium into the left ventricle, is displayed in *blue* (flow away from the transducer). *Arrow*, aliasing within the left ventricular diastolic flow. This phenomenon is due to acceleration of the blood flow at the level of the mitral valve leaflets.

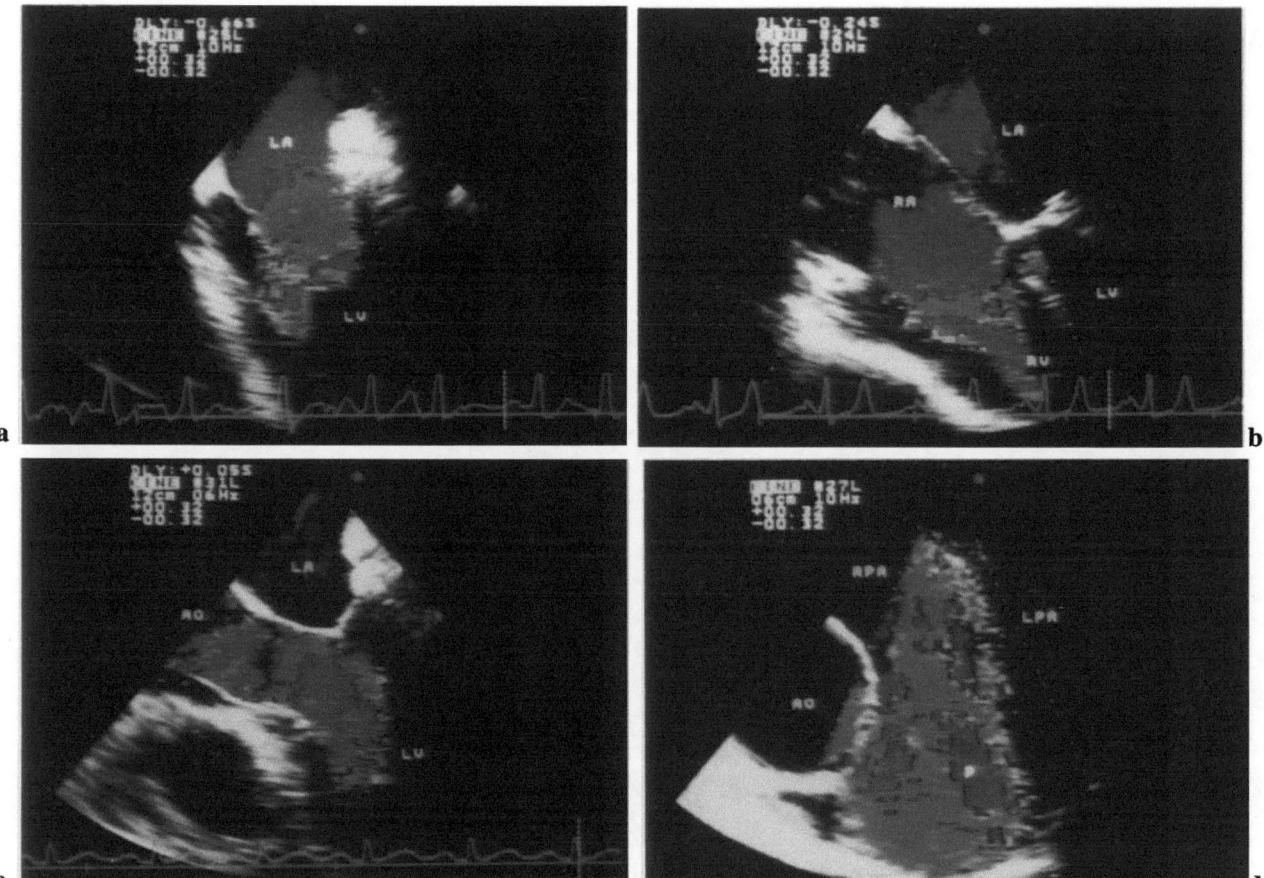

Fig. 1.35a–d. Aliased flow, color Doppler, diastolic and systolic flow. **a** Left ventricular inflow, directed from the left atrium into the left ventricle, is displayed in *blue; red,* aliasing. **b** Right ventricular inflow. The flow (*blue*) is directed from the right atrium into the right ventricle; *red,* aliased flow. **c** Left ventricular ejection flow. *Red,* systolic flow in the LVOT; *blue,* aliasing. **d** Pulmonary ejection flow. *Red,* systolic flow in the main pulmonary artery; *blue,* zones of aliased flow. *AO,* Aorta; *P,* main pulmonary artery; *RPA,* right pulmonary artery; *LPA,* left pulmonary artery.

Abnormal Flow

Disturbed intracardiac blood flow is frequently characterized by high velocity and/or turbulence. Abnormal flow is generally displayed as a *mosaic* effect.

This effect derives from the combination of the aliasing phenomenon (due to the high velocity) and the high dispersion of the blood cell direction (high variance). High-velocity turbulent flows, such as regurgitant or post-stenotic flow, are displayed as a mosaic effect and are called *jets*.

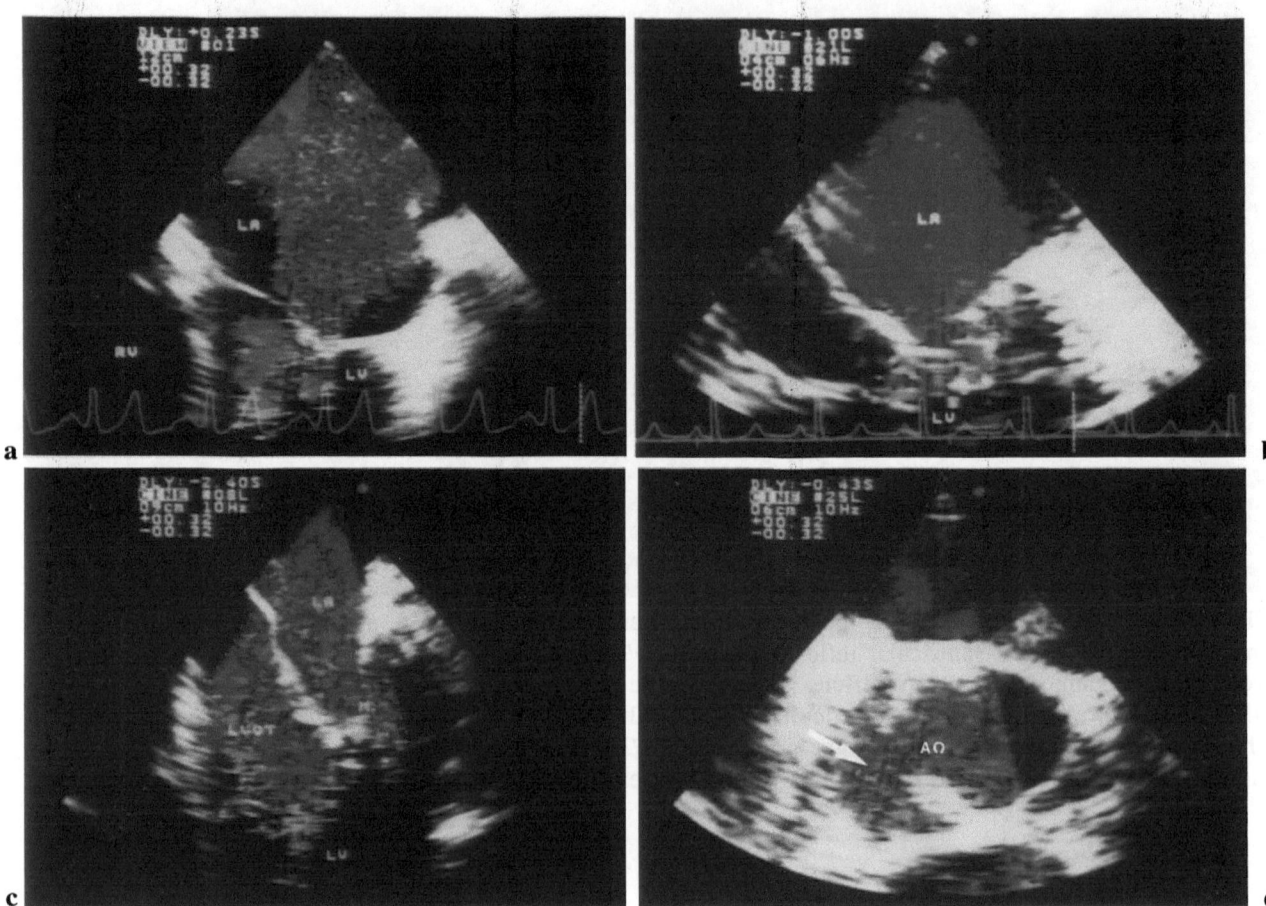

Fig. 1.36a–d. Abnormal flow. **a** Mitral valve regurgitation. A wide multicolored regurgitant jet (*mosaic*) spreads into the left atrium. **b** Mitral valve stenosis. Turbulent diastolic flow (*multicolored jet*) across the stenotic mitral valve. **c** Aortic regurgitation. The regurgitant jet (*mosaic*) in the LVOT obstructs the diastolic flow across the mitral valve causing "functional" stenosis. Disturbed diastolic flow (*mosaic*) at the level of the mitral valve. **d** Aortic stenosis. Turbulent systolic ejection flow (*mosaic*) beyond the stenotic aortic cusps (*arrow*).

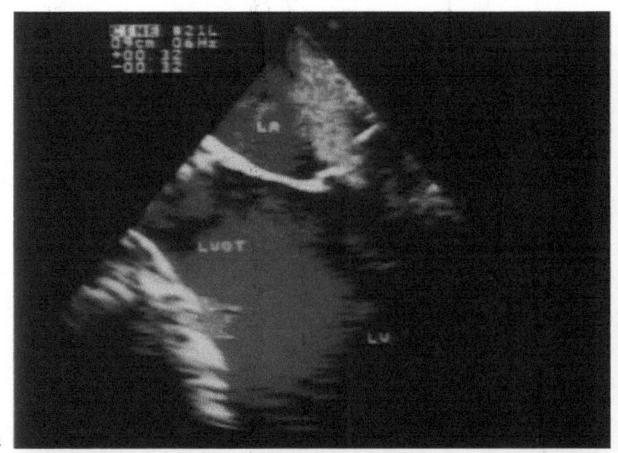

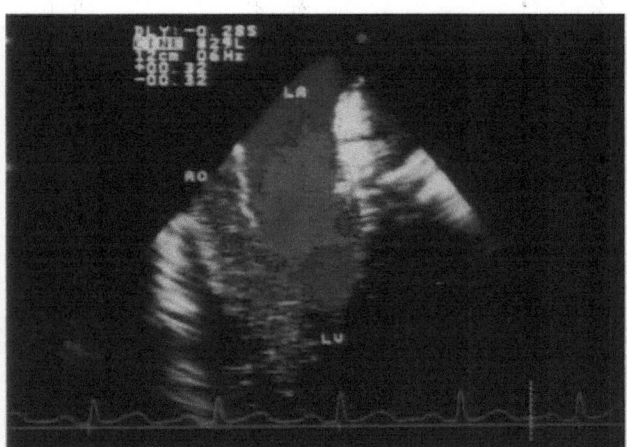

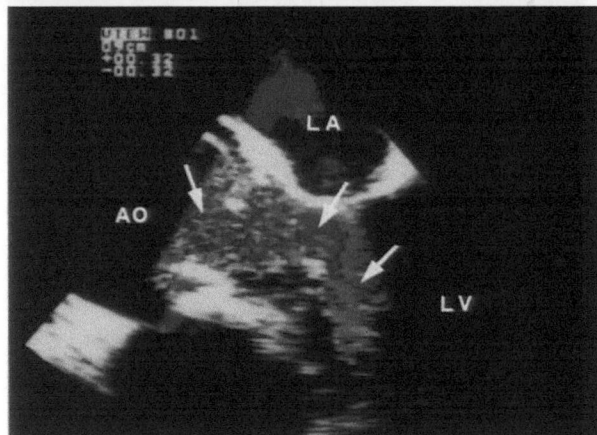

Fig. 1.37 a–c. Abnormal flow, presence of normal and abnormal flow in the same frame. **a** Mitral insufficiency. Normal systolic ejection flow (*red*) in the LVOT and mitral regurgitant jet (*mosaic*) in the left atrium. **b** Aortic insufficiency. Normal diastolic flow across the mitral valve (*aliased flow*) and aortic regurgitant jet (*mosaic*) in the LVOT. **c** Subaortic stenosis. Left ventricular ejection flow (*red*) turns first into aliased flow (*blue*) and then into turbulent-high velocity flow (*mosaic*) beyond the subvalvular obstruction.

2 Acquired Heart Disease

This section considers the most frequent and useful applications of echocardiography in acquired diseases of the heart. Many examples are drawn from intra- or perioperative examinations performed to assess the adequacy of surgical repair.

Valvular Heart Disease

The study of valvular function represents one the most diffuse and valuable applications of cardiac sonography. The advent of TEE has markedly improved the diagnostic potential of this technique, allowing clear visualization of the valvular apparatus and assessment of its function. TEE is the most useful diagnostic tool for intraoperative assessment of the heart valve function.

Mitral Valve

Visualization of the mitral valve and evaluation of its function are among the most profitable applications of TEE. Residual valve regurgitation and the pressure gradient across the mitral valve can be accurately evaluated by intraoperative TEE.

Valvuloplasty

Up to now assessment of the adequacy of valve regurgitation has been based on the detection of fluid leaks into the open atrium while the heart is arrested and the patient is on cardiopulmonary bypass. However, the dynamics of the valve apparatus is quite different in the actively beating heart, and residual regurgitation may therefore occur after cardiopulmonary bypass, even though no leaks are detected by intraoperative testing. Valve regurgitation may also be detected by palpation of a systolic thrill on the atrial free wall or by measurement of the atrial pressure and the size of the "V" wave on the pressure curve. However, these methods are subjective and may not reflect the severity of residual regurgitation. Color Doppler flow imaging provides more reliable information on valve motion and blood flow dynamics in the beating and ejecting heart.

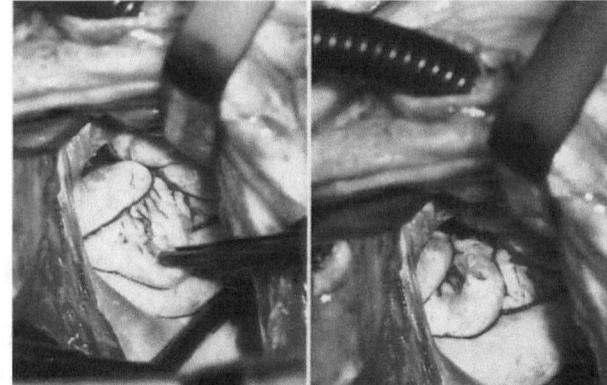
a

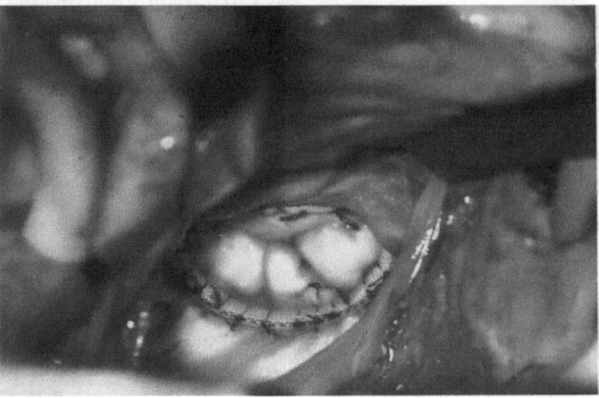
b

Fig. 2.1a, b. Mitral valve prolapse, operative view. **a** Prolapse of the posterior mitral leaflet before valvuloplasty. **b** Mitral valvuloplasty. The patient underwent quadrangular resection of the posterior leaflet and implantation of a Carpentier-Edwards ring.

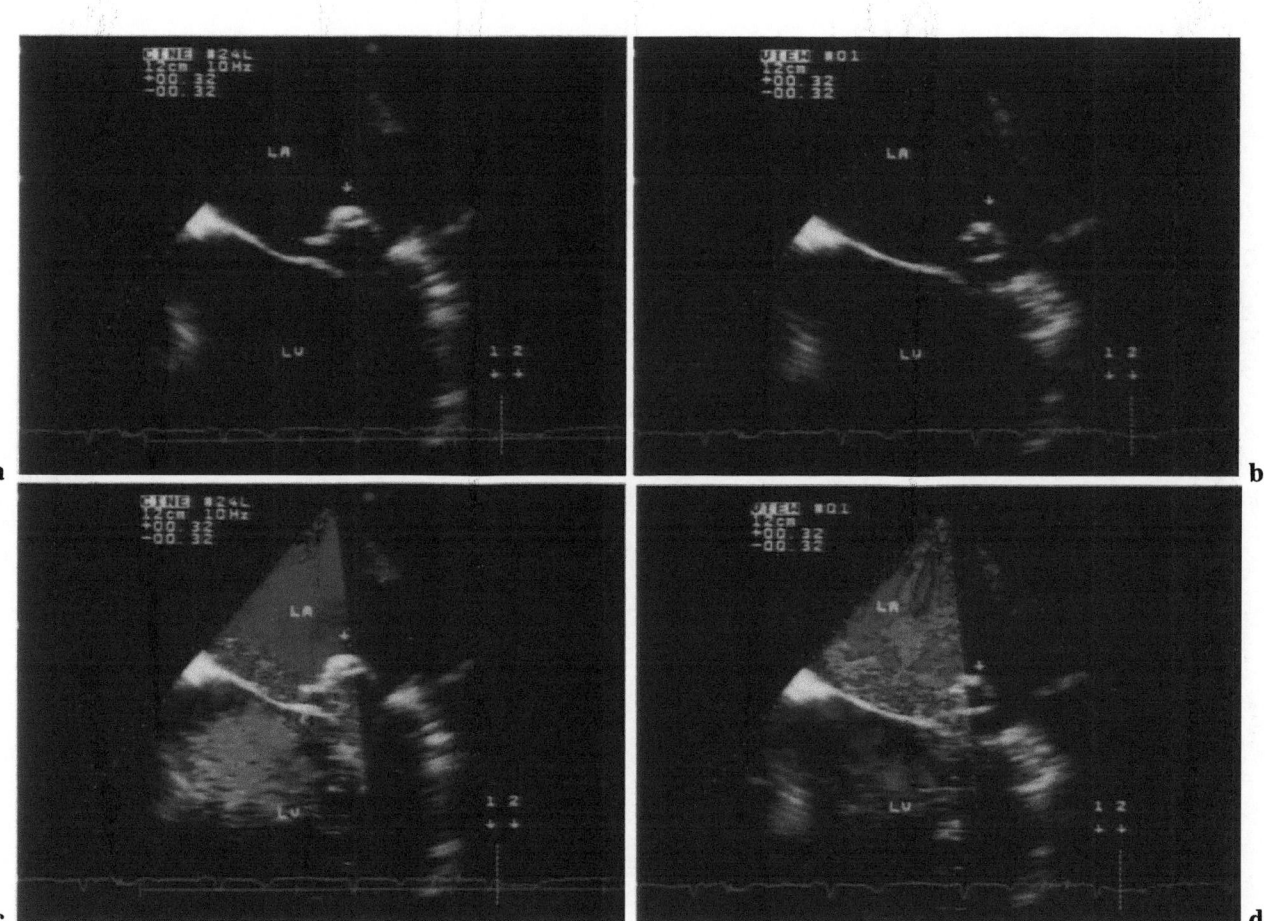

Fig. 2.2a–d. Mitral valvuloplasty. Intraoperative TEE prior to surgery; Same patient as in the Fig. 2.1. **a, b** Two-dimensional TEE shows the prolapse of the posterior mitral leaflet at two different points in time during systole (*1, 2* on the ECG). **c, d** Color Doppler shows the mitral regurgitant jet directed away from the prolapsed leaflet.

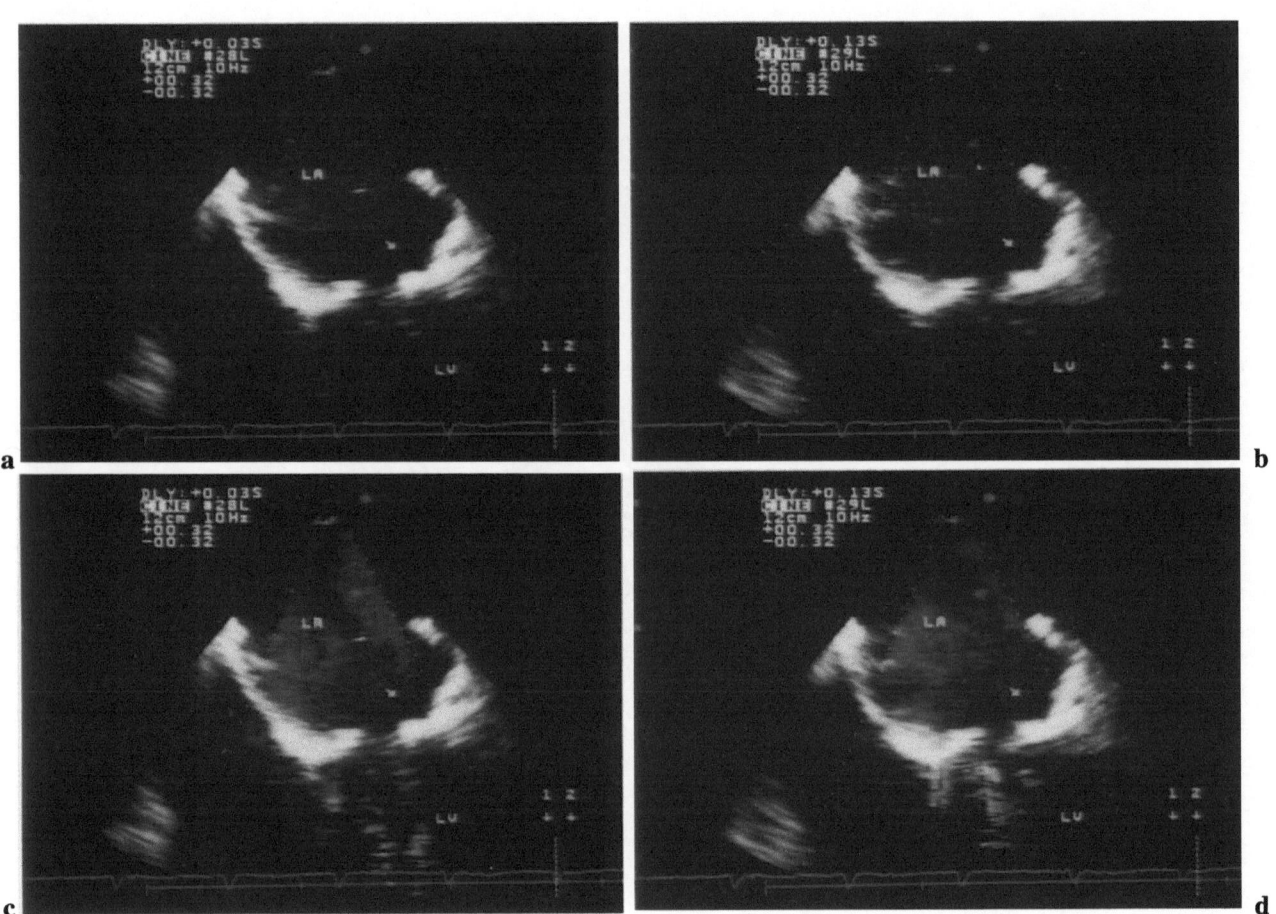

Fig. 2.3a–d. Mitral valvuloplasty, TEE after surgery; same patient as in the Figs. 2.1, 2.2. **a, b** Disappearance of the prolapse of the posterior mitral leaflet (*arrow*). **c, d** Color Doppler shows the disappearance of mitral valve regurgitation after valvuloplasty (*1, 2* on the ECG).

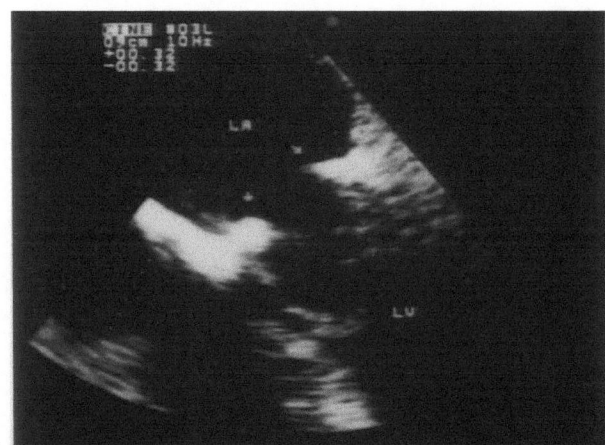

Fig. 2.4a–c. Mitral valvuloplasty and ring implantation. Same patient as in the Figs. 2.1–2.3. **a** Two-dimensional TEE, four-chamber view. *Arrows*, position of the annulus. **b** Pulsed-wave Doppler. The sample volume (*arrow*) is placed immediately behind the repaired mitral valve. No regurgitation can be detected after valvuloplasty. **c** M-mode color Doppler. The M-mode line (*white arrow*) is placed across the mitral valve orifice. After valvuloplasty no residual mitral regurgitation can be observed during the entire systole (*between the two arrows*).

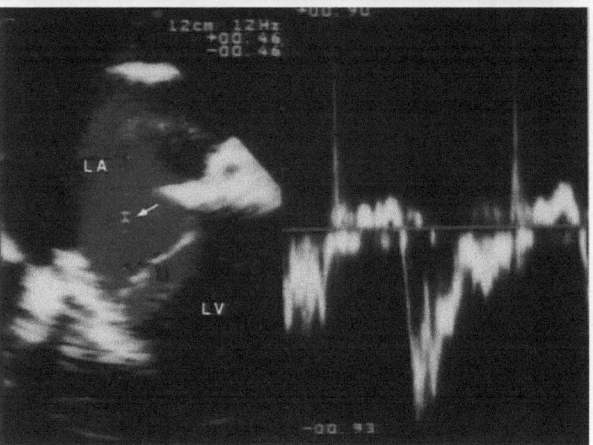

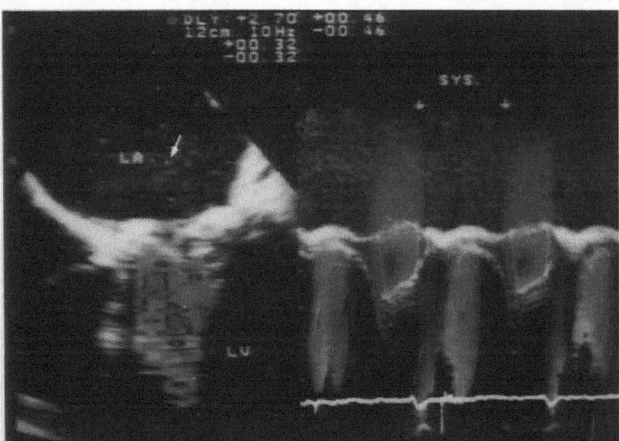

Mitral Valve Prolapse

The most frequent etiology of mitral valve prolapse is myxomatous degeneration of the leaflets and tendinous chordae. Other conditions such as rheumatic endocarditis, chordal rupture due to myocardial ischemia, bacterial endocarditis, trauma, and heritable disorders of connective tissue may also cause prolapse of the mitral valve.

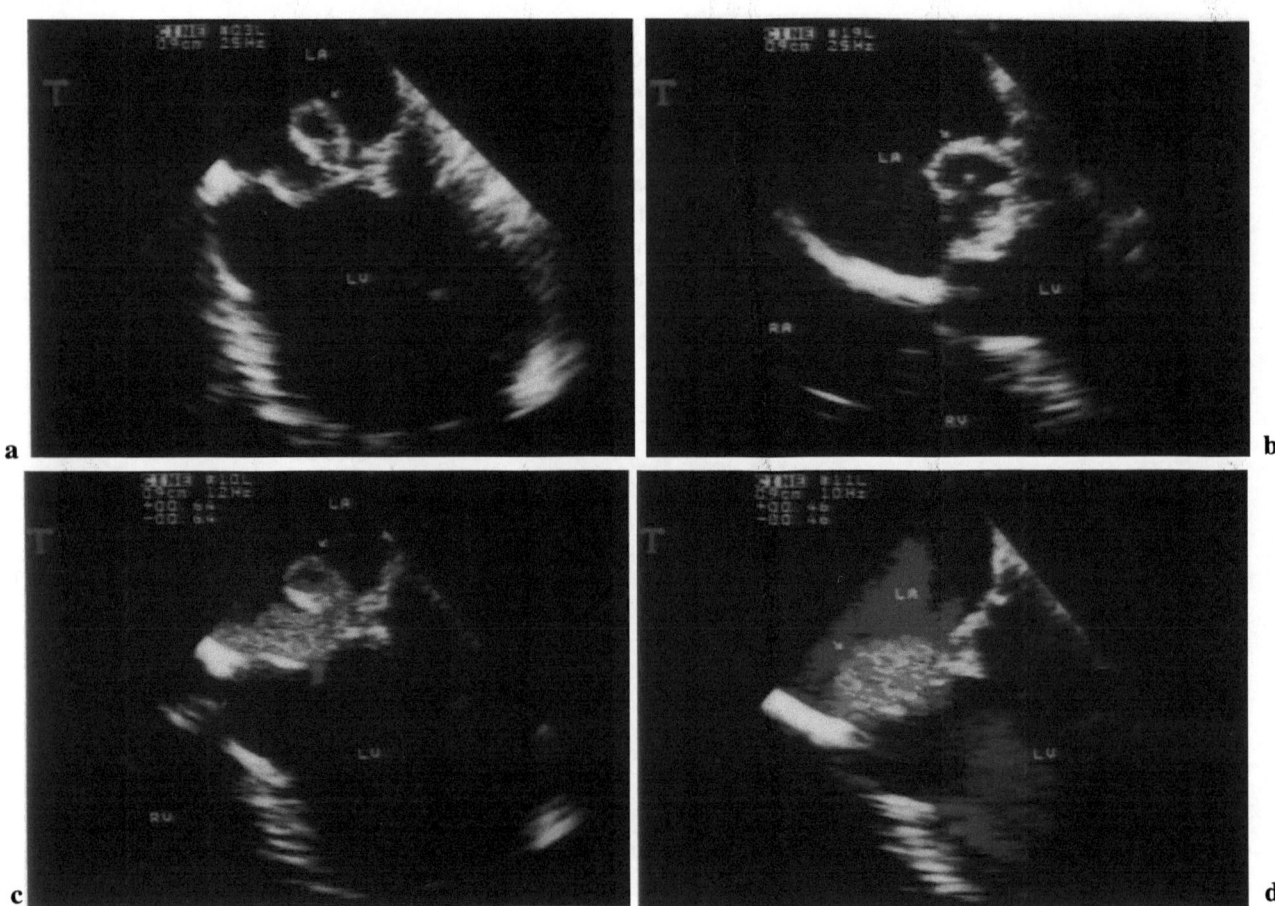

Fig. 2.5 a–d. Mitral valve prolapse, TEE before valvuloplasty. **a, b** Two-dimensional TEE, four-chamber views shows a massive systolic prolapse of the posterior mitral leaflet (*arrow*) in the left atrium. **c, d** Corresponding views as above (**a, b**) show color Doppler flow imaging. A regurgitant jet directed away from the prolapsing leaflet can be observed.

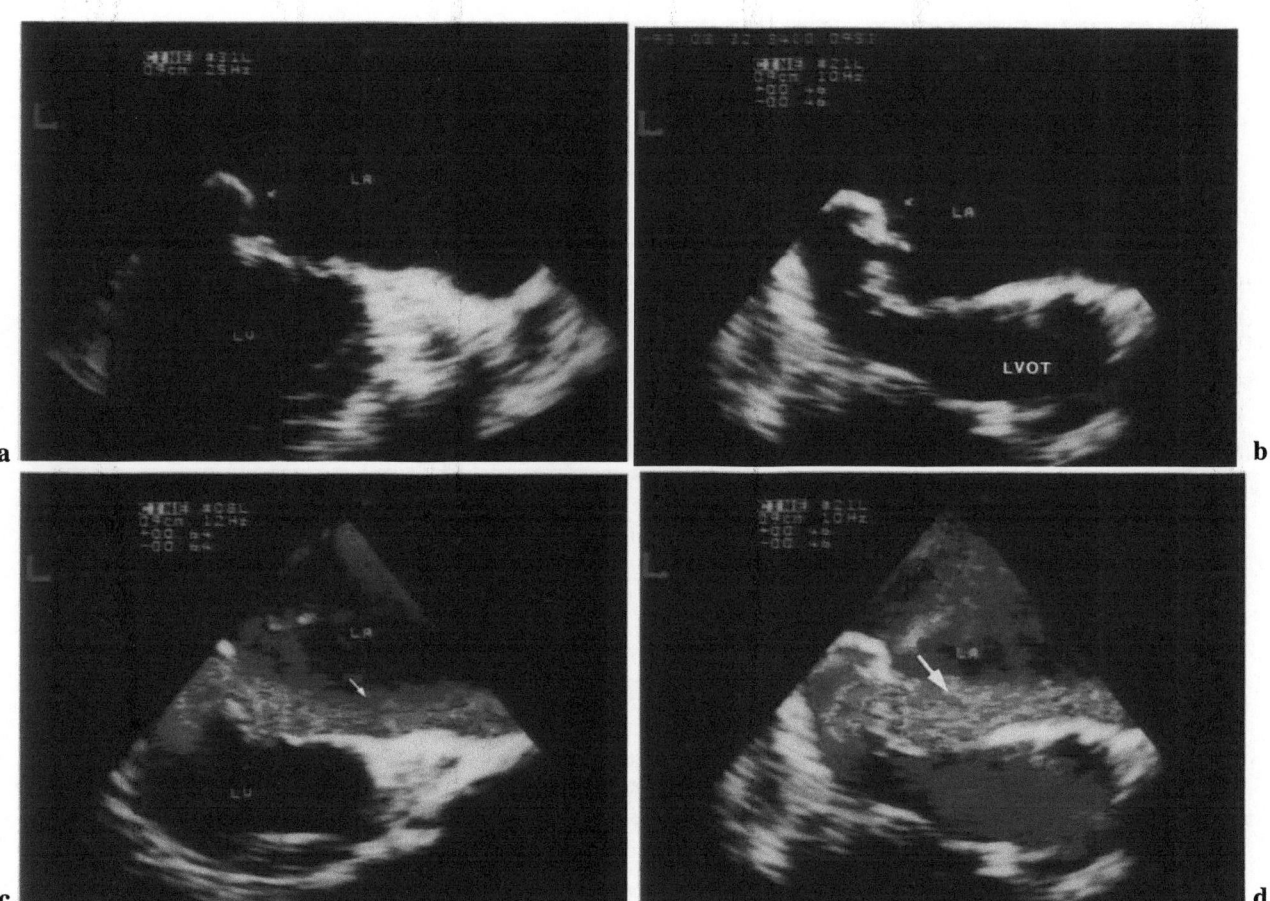

Fig. 2.6a–d. Mitral valve prolapse, TEE before valvuloplasty; same patient as in Fig. 2.5. **a, b** Two-dimensional TEE, longitudinal LV-LA views, show prolapse of the posterior mitral leaflet (*arrow*) in the left atrium. **c, d** Corresponding views as above (**a, b**) show color Doppler flow imaging. The regurgitant jet (*arrows*) is directed into the pulmonary veins, away from the prolapsing leaflet.

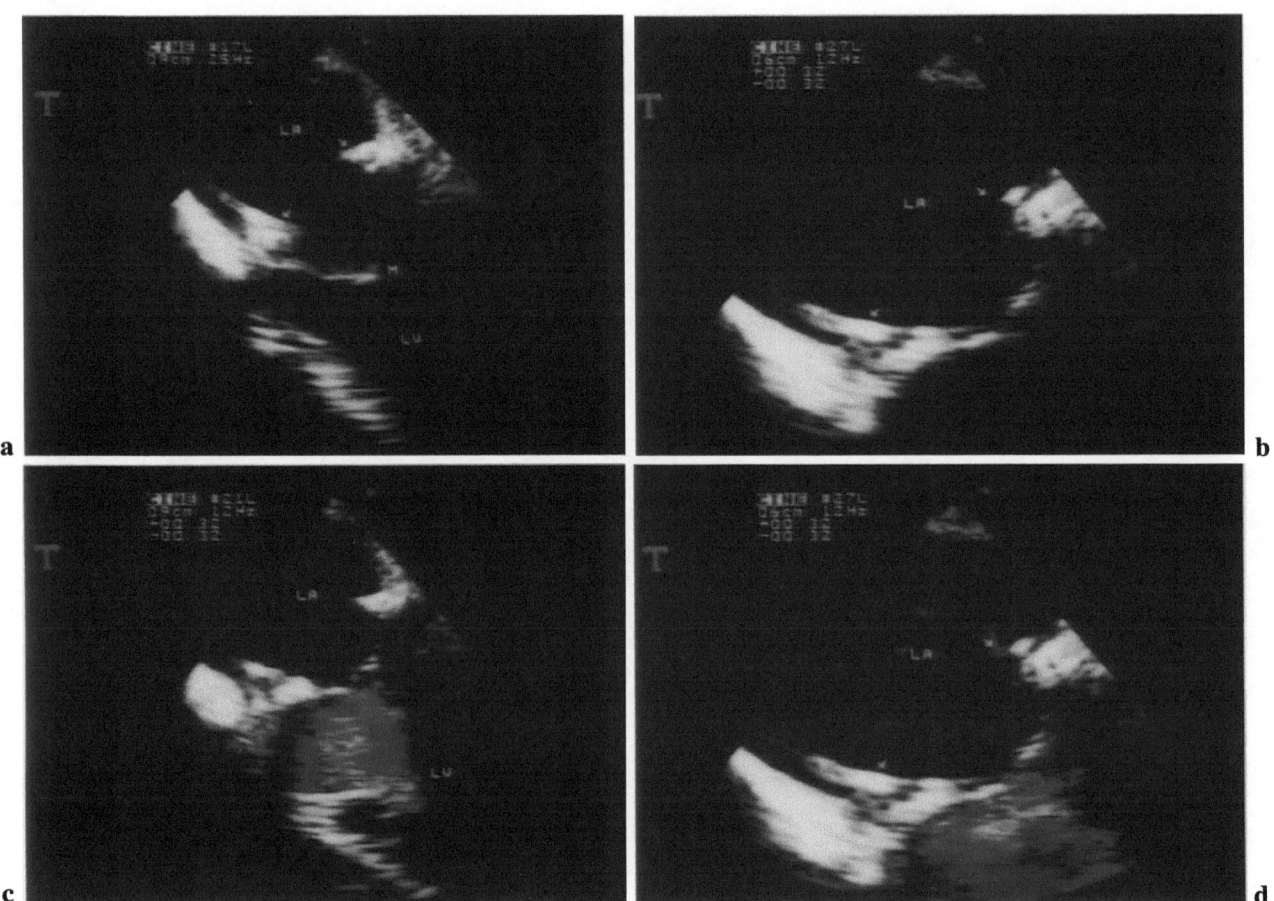

Fig. 2.7 a–d. After mitral valvuloplasty, same patient as in Figs. 2.5, 2.6. Quadrangular resection of the posterior leaflet and implantation of a flexible ring were performed. **a, b** Two-dimensional TEE, four-chamber views. Magnification of the left atrium showing the position of the prosthetic ring (*arrows*). **c, d** Corresponding views as above (**a, b**) showing color Doppler flow imaging. No residual regurgitant jet could be detected in the left atrium in systole. *Red*, systolic ejection flow in the LVOT.

Contrast Echocardiography

Injection of contrast agents into the cardiac chambers can be used to detect intracardiac shunts and valve regurgitation. The contrast effect derives from suspended micro bubbles in the injected fluid.

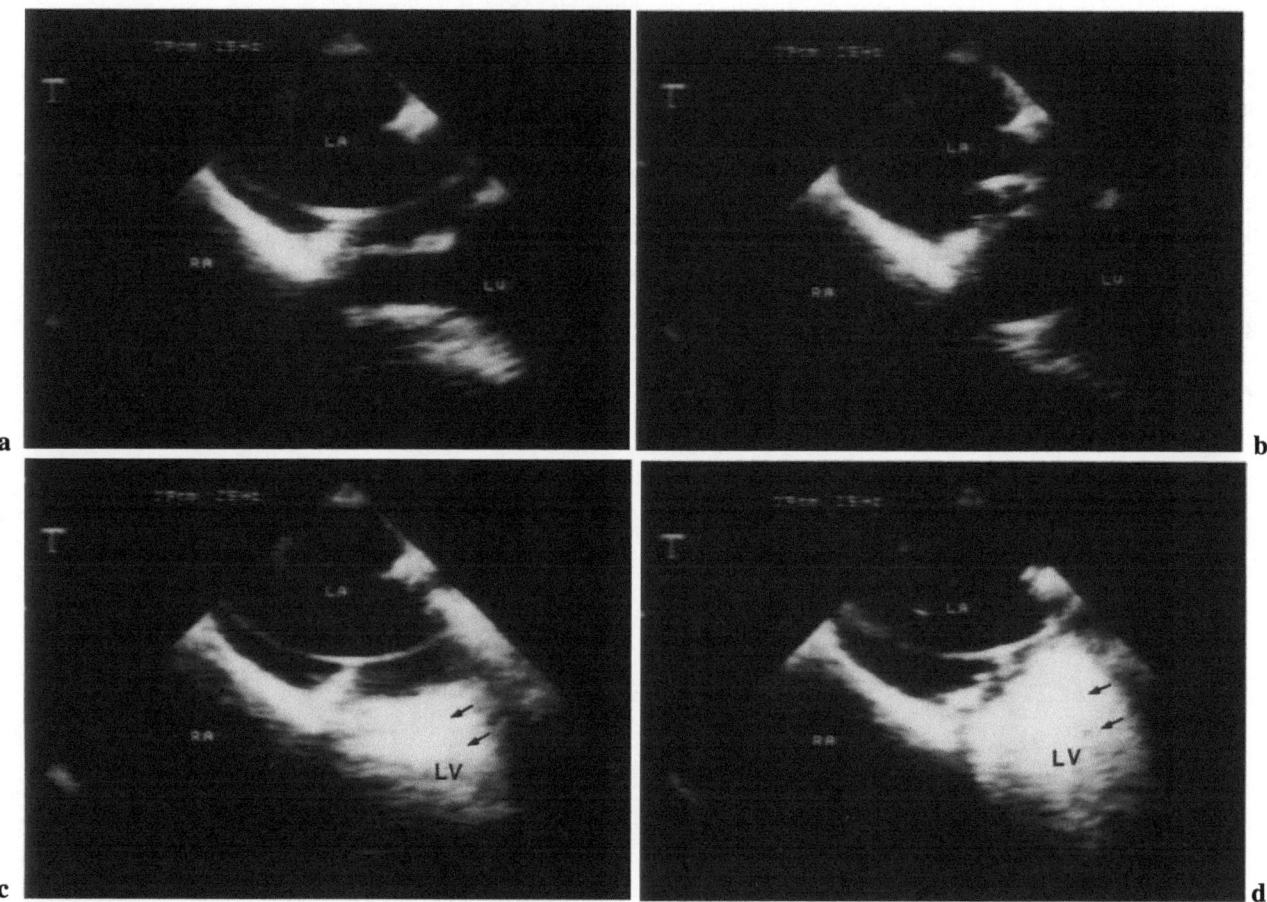

Fig. 2.8a–d. Contrast echocardiography, after mitral valvuloplasty; same patient as in Figs 2.5–2.7. **a, b** Two-dimensional TEE, four-chamber view, in diastole (**a**) and systole (**b**) without contrast. **c, d** After contrast injection into the left ventricle (*black arrows*) no contrast can be detected in the left atrium.

Mitral Regurgitation

Residual mitral regurgitation may occur after valve repair, requiring further surgery or valve replacement. Current clinical color Doppler grading of mitral regurgitation is based on the planimetry of the regurgitant jet area or on the ratio between the regurgitant jet and the cross-sectional area of the left atrium. Color Doppler criteria for assessing valve regurgitation are based on the assumption that the distribution of flow velocities of the regurgitant jet reflects the regurgitant flow volume. However, the regurgitant jet area is only a two-dimensional view of a three-dimensional jet. Other limitations may also influence the value of color Doppler for estimating valve regurgitation as well as jet geometry, temporal variation during systole, driving pressure, and gain setting. Color Doppler estimation of mitral valve insufficiency shows good correlation with the traditional angiographic evaluation. Color Doppler TEE can be considered the most adequate diagnostic method for assessing valve repair intraoperatively.

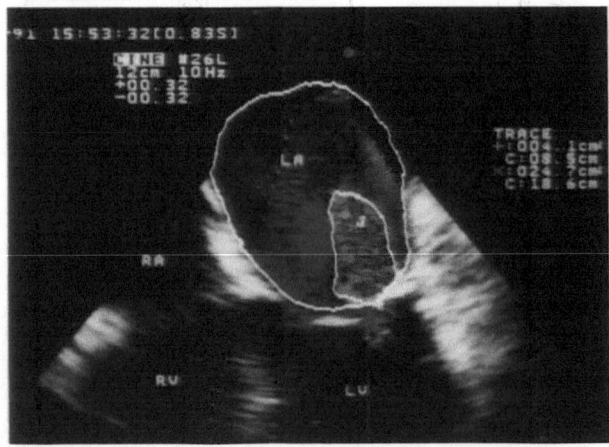

Fig. 2.9. Regurgitant jet area. Planimetry of mitral regurgitant jet (*J*) and the ratio between jet area and left atrial area provide useful clinical parameters for assessing the severity of mitral valve regurgitation.

Fig. 2.11a, b. Residual mitral regurgitation after repair. **a** Intraoperative TEE shows the persistence of severe mitral regurgitation after quadrangular leaflet resection and Carpentier-Edwards ring implantation. Part of the regurgitant jet is not visualized because of the narrow color flow area. Mitral valve replacement was performed during the same operation. **b** Persistence of two regurgitant jets. This patient showed two regurgitant jets after mitral valvuloplasty.

a b c d

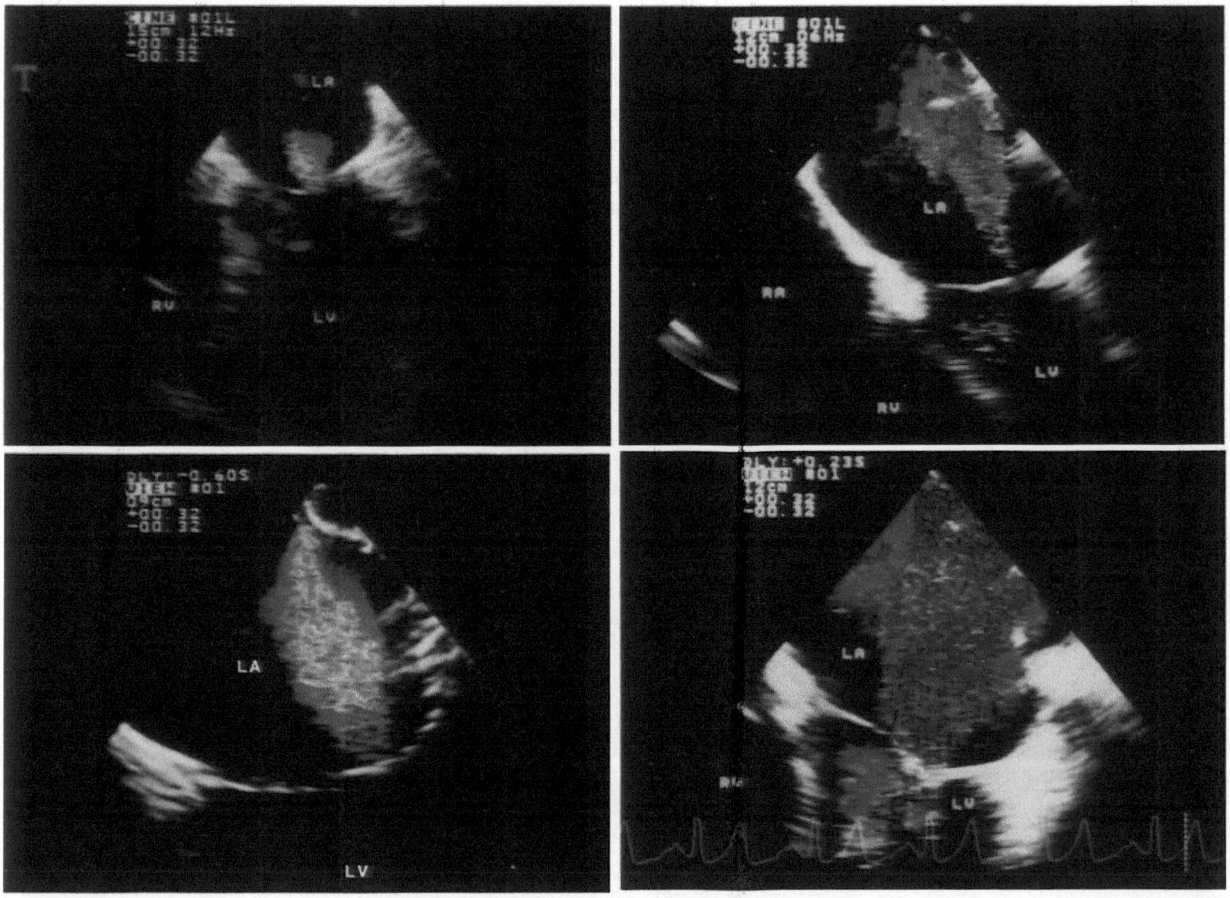

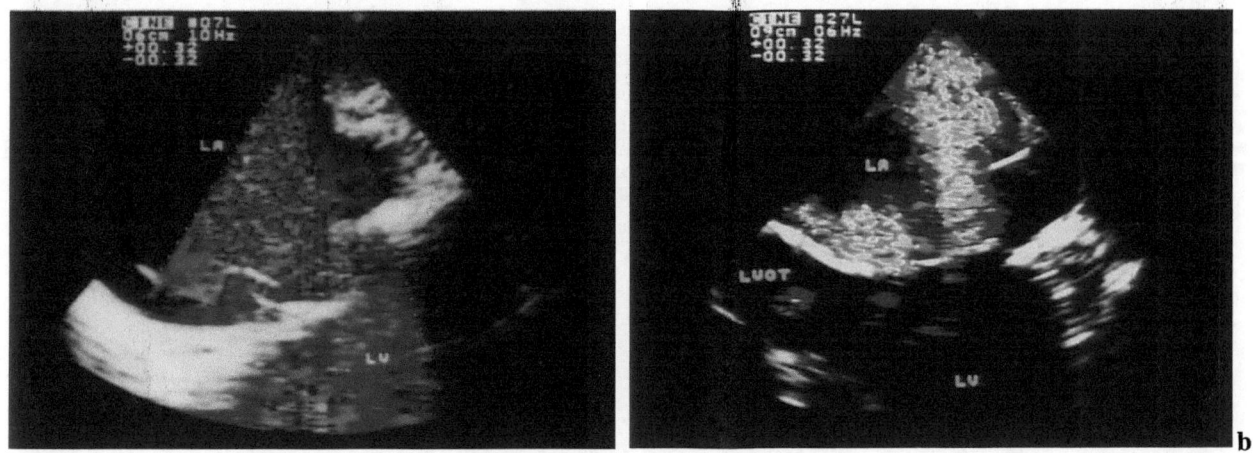

Fig. 2.10a–d. Mitral valve regurgitation, color Doppler. Examples show various degrees of mitral valve regurgitation: mild (**a**), moderate (**b, c**), and severe (**d**).

a b

Regurgitant Jets

The degree of mitral valve insufficiency may be incorrectly evaluated when regurgitant jets are asymmetrical. If the regurgitant jet does not lie on the same viewing plane as the two-dimensional echocardiography, the severity of regurgitation may be un-

derestimated. Multiple viewing by biplanar or multiplanar transducers can overcome this limitation. Conversely, the direction of regurgitant jet may provide helpful information on the etiology and pathophysiology of the regurgitant lesions. In patients with mitral valve prolapse the regurgitat jet is almost always directed away from the prolapsed leaflet.

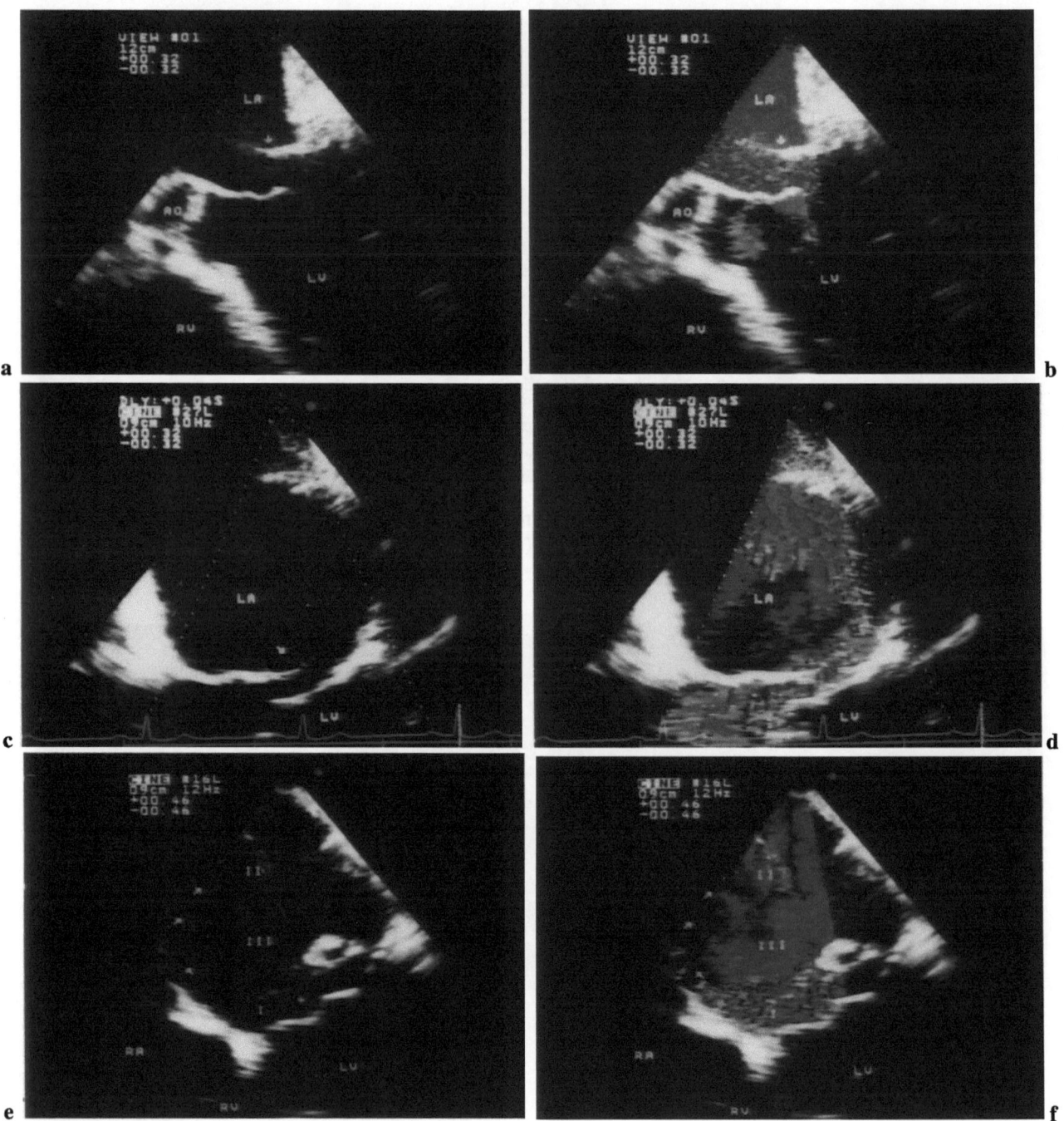

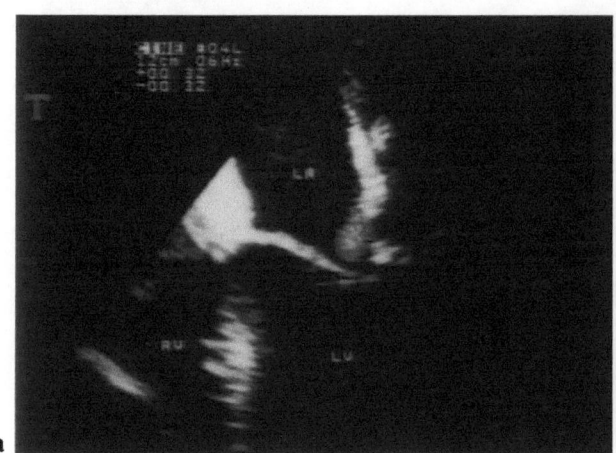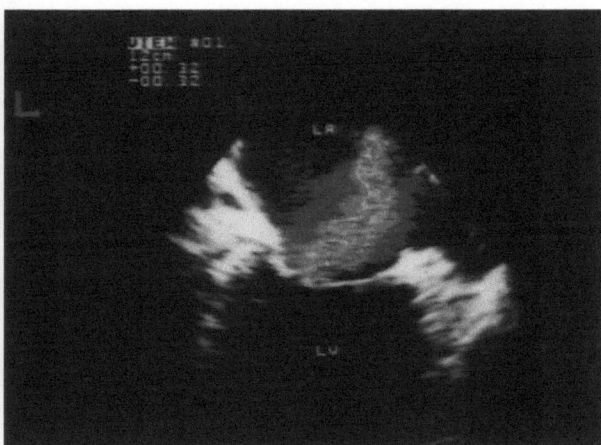

a

b

Fig. 2.13a, b. Biplanar imaging of regurgitant jet. The impact of biplanar TEE on assessment of mitral valve regurgitation is demonstrated. **a** Transverse plane, four-chamber view, shows a trivial mitral valve regurgitation. **b** The corresponding long-axis view reveals a moderate degree of mitral valve regurgitation.

Fig. 2.12a–f. Mitral valve prolapse, asymmetrical regurgitant jets. This series shows that the regurgitant jets due to mitral prolapse are asymmetrical and are directed in the opposite direction as the affected leaflet. **a** Prolapse of the posterior mitral leaflet (*arrow*). **b** The regurgitant jet is directed anteriorly. **c** Prolapse of the anterior mitral leaflet (*arrow*). **d** The regurgitant jet is directed posteriorly. **e** Prolapse of posterior mitral leaflet. **f** "Swirling" of the regurgitant jet into the left atrium. Three zones with different flow patterns can be observed in the left atrium: *I*, High-velocity turbulent flow (*mosaic*); *II*, displacement flow directed toward the transducer (*red*); *III*, displacement flow directed toward the mitral valve orifice (*blue*).

Regurgitation and Cardiac Pacing

Ventricular pacing affects the synchrony of myocardial contraction, resulting in significant changes in the degree of mitral valve regurgitation. Special attention must be paid when assessing the degree of mitral regurgitation upon ventricular pacing.

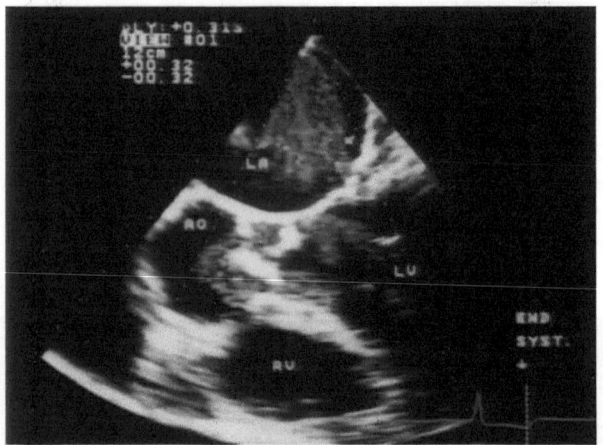

a

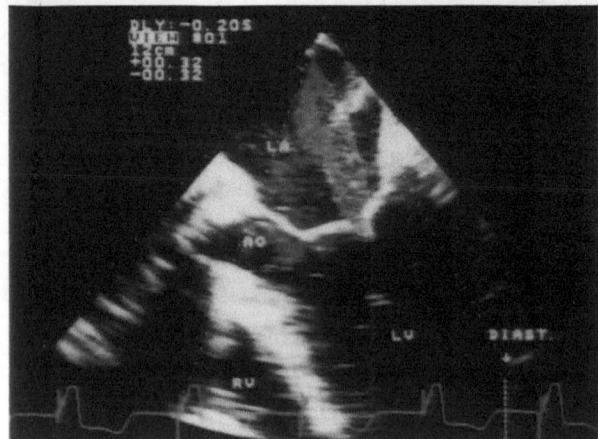

b

Fig. 2.14a, b. Mitral valve regurgitation during cardiac pacing. **a** Sinus rhythm. Mitral valve regurgitation is limited to ventricular systole. **b** The same patient during ventricular stimulation. Mitral valve regurgitation can be detected until early diastole (*arrows* on the ECG).

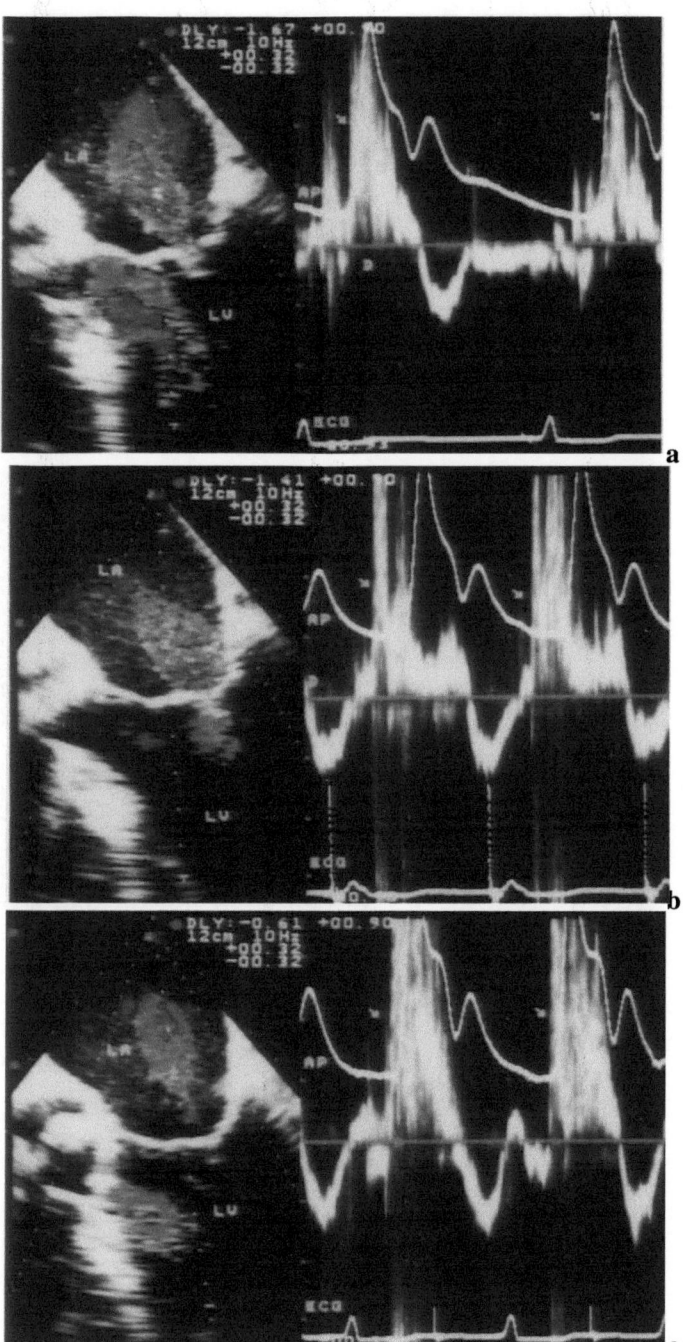

Fig. 2.15 a–c. Mitral regurgitation during cardiac pacing. Simultaneous recording of pulsed Doppler and arterial pressure pulse. The onset of mitral valve regurgitation varies with the different pacing modalities. **a** Sinus rhythm. Mitral valve regurgitation oc-

curs at the onset of arterial pulse (*arrow*). **b** Ventricular pacing. Mitral regurgitation occurs prior to the onset of the arterial pulse. **c** Atrial pacing. Mitral regurgitation occurs at the onset of the pulse (*arrow*).

Mitral Valve Stenosis

Valve opening area and leaflet separation, as well as the occurrence of mitral valve regurgitation, can be evaluated by transesophageal and epicardial echocardiography intraoperatively.

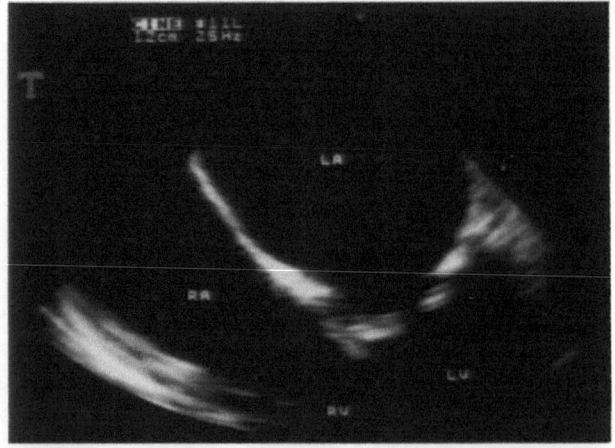

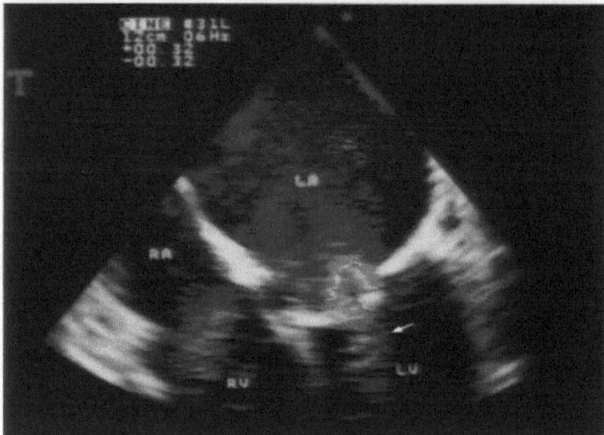

Fig. 2.16a, b. Mitral valve stenosis, four-chamber view (magnification). **a** Two-dimensional echocardiography. Diastolic opening of the mitral leaflets is highly impaired. **b** Color Doppler shows turbulent diastolic flow across the reduced opening of the mitral leaflets.

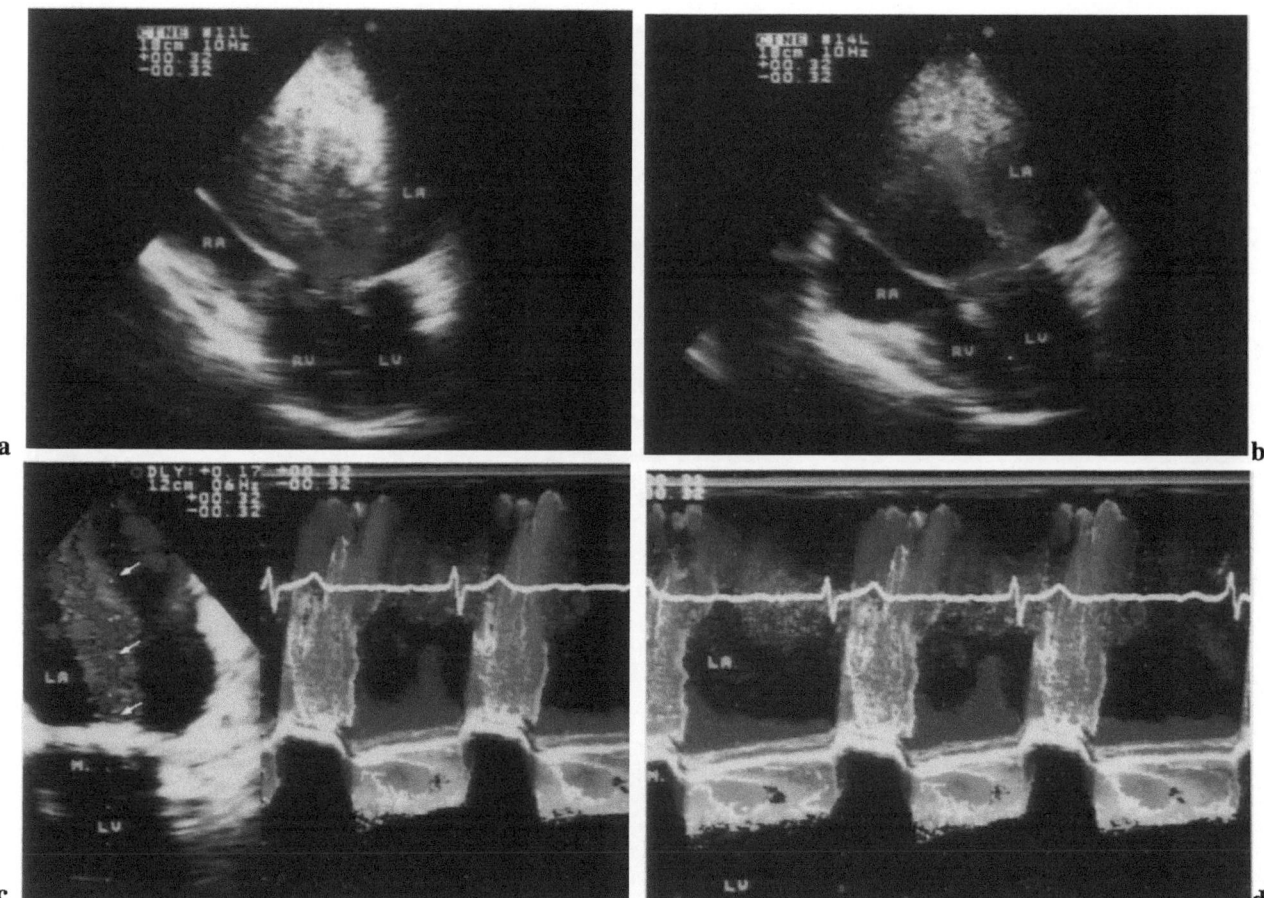

Fig. 2.17a–d. Combined mitral stenosis-insufficiency, color Doppler TEE. **a** Turbulent flow across the narrow mitral valve opening. Giant left atrium with spontaneous echo contrast (due to reduced blood flow velocity). **b** Mild mitral valve regurgitation. **c, d** Color M-mode. *Left,* the M-mode line is placed across the mitral valve (*arrows*); *right,* turbulent flow in diastole and in systole, due to stenosis and insufficiency.

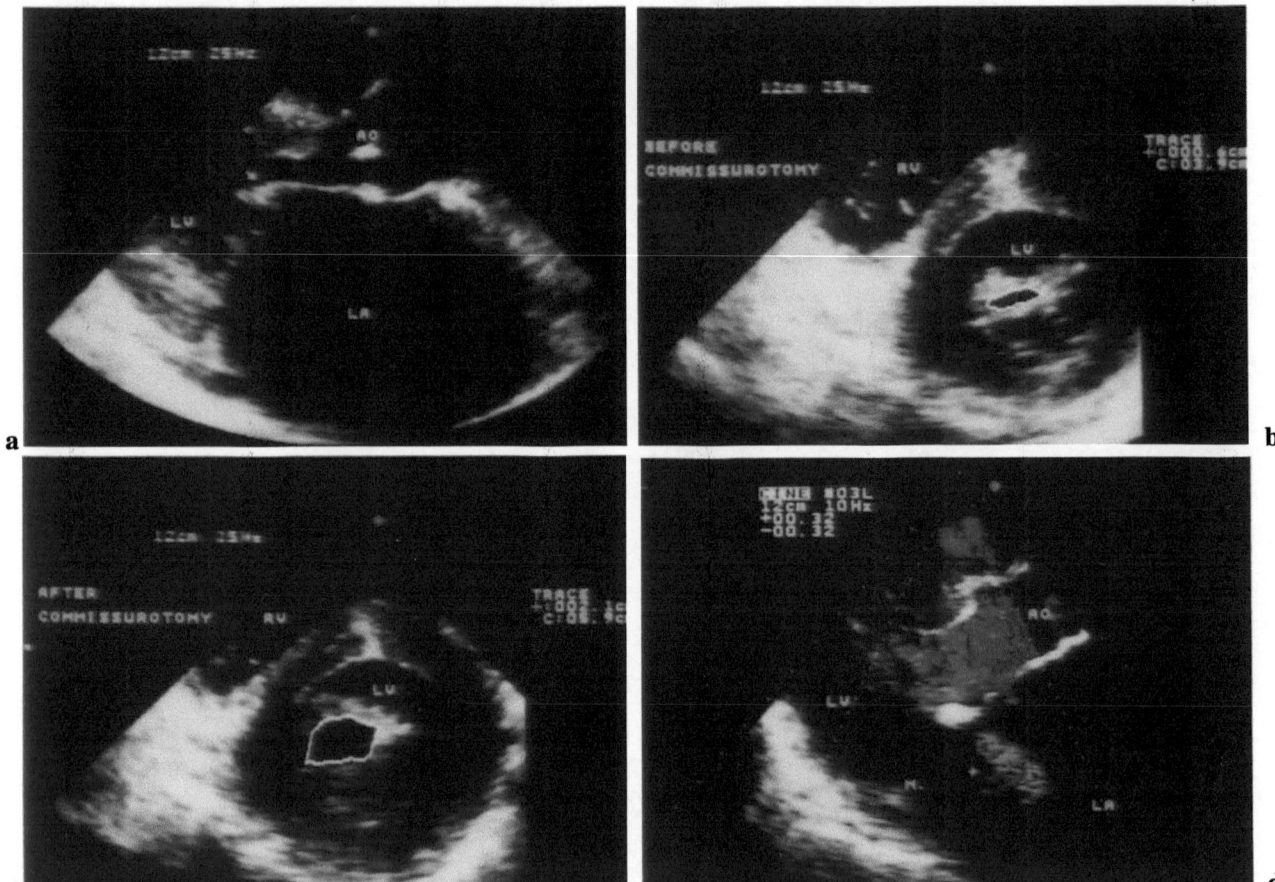

Fig. 2.18a–d. Mitral valve commissurotomy, intraoperative epicardial echocardiography. **a** Parasternal equivalent long-axis view, mitral stenosis. The arrow shows the diastolic "doming" of the anterior mitral leaflet, a typical sign of valve stenosis. Enlarged left atrium. **b** Short-axis view. The cross-sectional planimetry of mitral opening area before the commissurotomy is 0.6 cm². **c** After mitral valve commissurotomy. The planimetry of cross-sectional mitral opening area is now 2.1 cm². **d** Trivial residual mitral regurgitation (*arrow*) can be detected in the left atrium after the procedure.

Aortic Valve

TEE allows direct visualization of the aortic valve and the flow imaging in the left ventricular outflow tract (LVOT). Systolic separation of the aortic leaflets can be assessed by basal short-axis views. Regurgitant jet flows from incompetent aortic valves can be assessed by LVOT views.

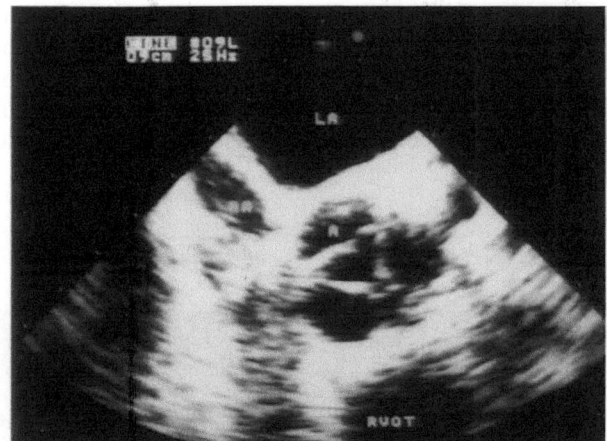

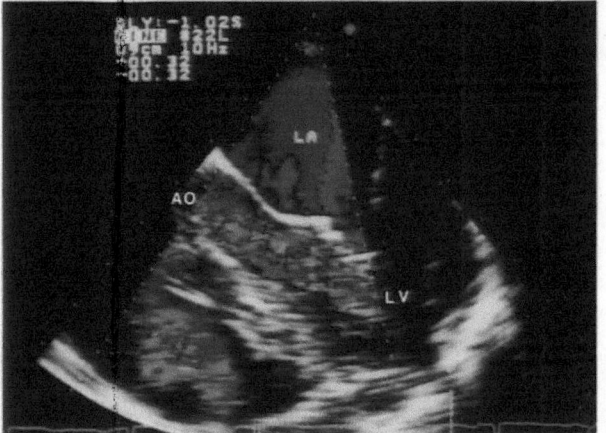

Fig. 2.19a, b. Aortic valve disease. **a** Basal short-axis view, aortic valve stenosis. Impaired systolic separation of the aortic cusps. **b** LVOT view, aortic valve insufficiency. A regurgitant jet spreads into the LVOT in diastole.

Aortic Stenosis

Assessment of systolic motion and the thickening or calcification of the aortic cusps is useful for the diagnosis of aortic valve stenosis. Direct measurement of the systolic aortic orifice area allows evaluation of the severity of the stenosis. Tricuspid, bicuspid, and unicuspid valves can be recognized in congenital aortic valve stenosis.

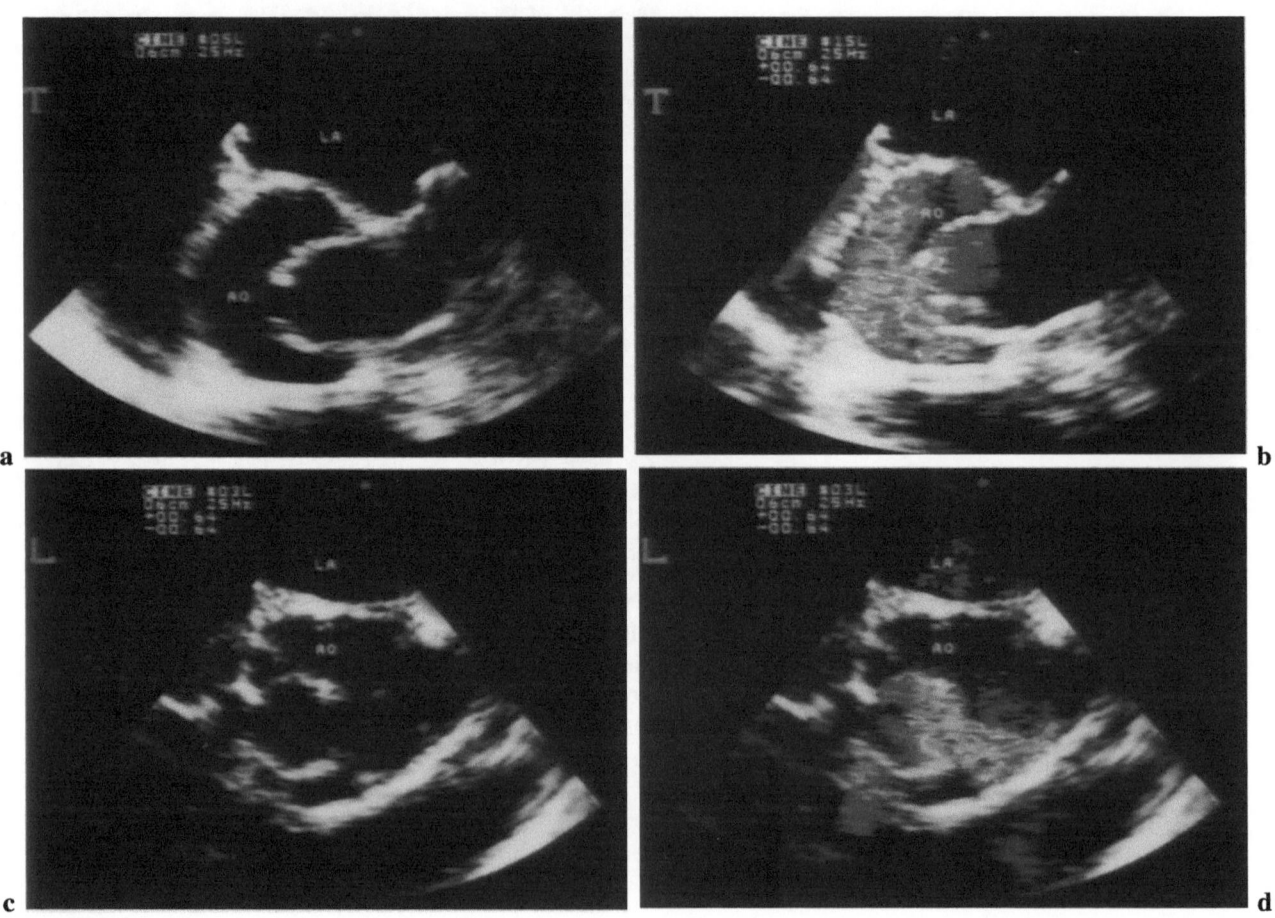

Fig. 2.20a–d. Aortic stenosis. **a** Two-dimensional echocardiography, basal short-axis view, shows reduced systolic opening of the aortic leaflets. **b** Color Doppler shows systolic turbulent flow beyond the stenotic valve. **c, d** Longitudinal basal views show the reduced leaflet opening and the poststenotic turbulent flow.

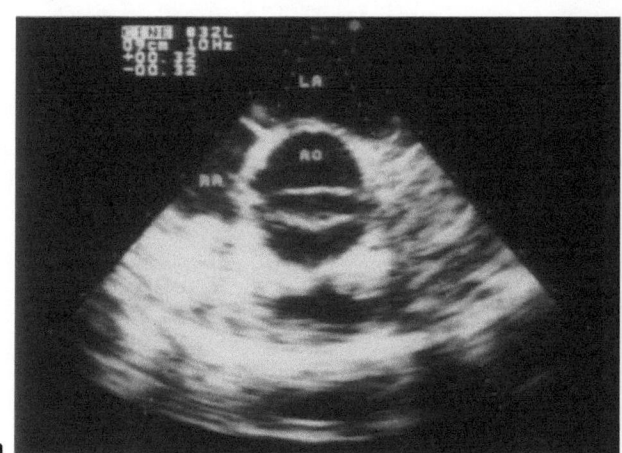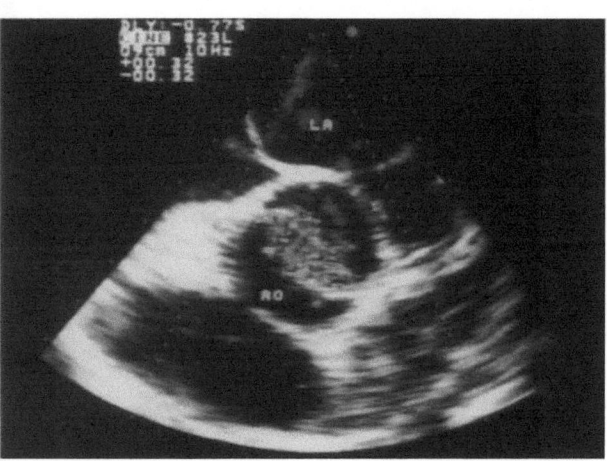

Fig. 2.21a, b. Bicuspid aortic valve, intraoperative TEE. **a** Two-dimensional echocardiography, basal short-axis view, shows impaired systolic separation of the two aortic leaflets. **b** Color Doppler shows systolic turbulent flow across the opening area of the aortic valve.

Aortic Commissurotomy

Intraoperative echocardiography represents the only diagnostic technique available for assessing the adequacy of aortic valve repair. Systolic opening area and residual aortic regurgitation can be measured immediately after repair. Aortic insufficiency can be evaluated by the length and area of a regurgitant jet into the LVOT.

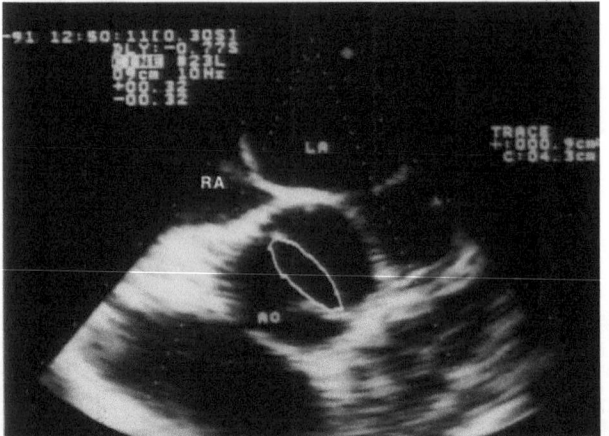

a

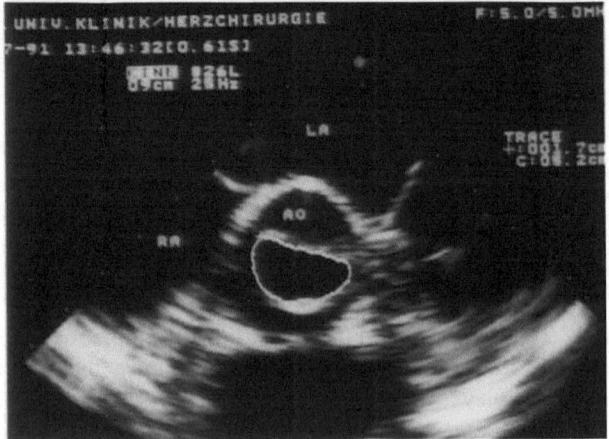

b

Fig. 2.22a, b. Aortic commissurotomy, planimetry of systolic aortic opening area. **a** Before commissurotomy the systolic opening area is 0.9 cm². **b** After commissurotomy the systolic opening area is 1.7 cm².

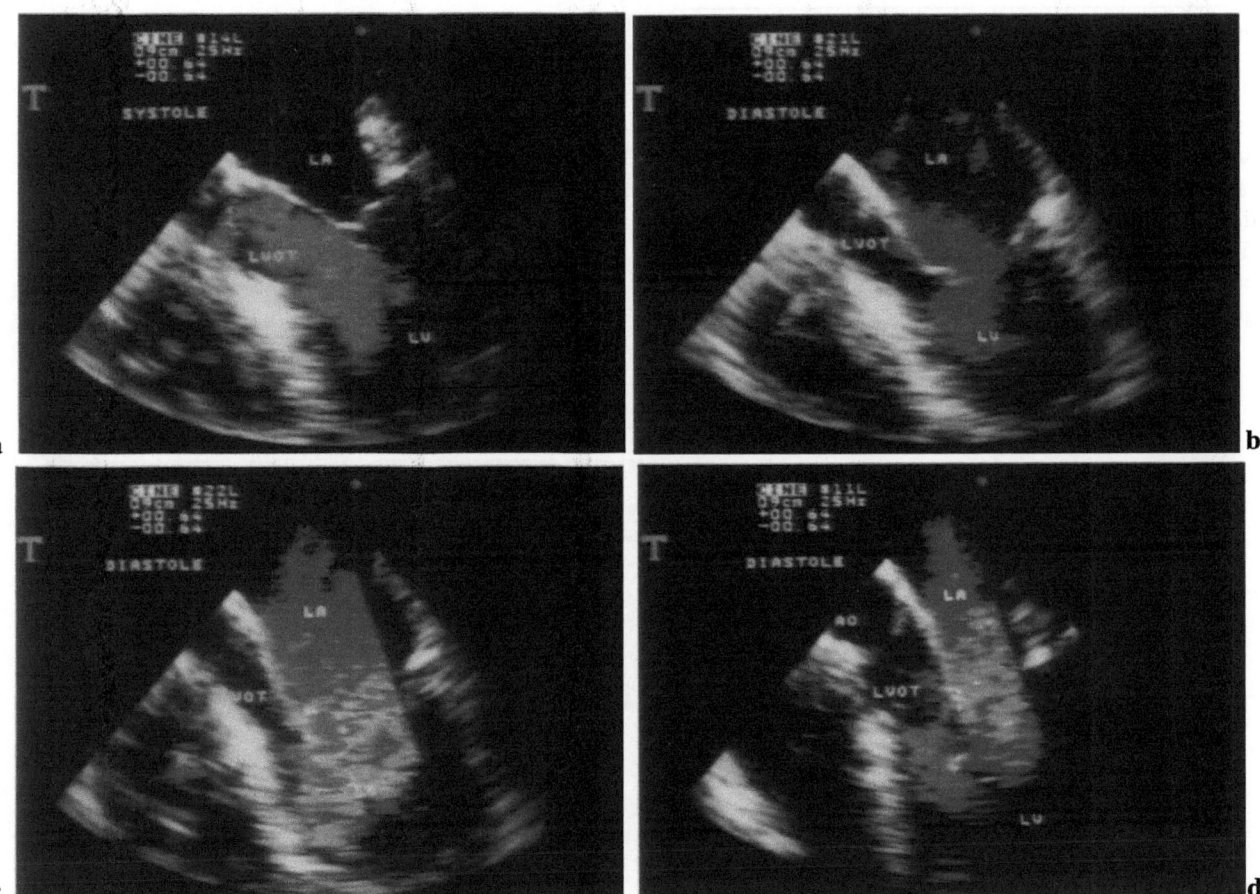

Fig. 2.23a–d. Aortic commissurotomy, assessment of aortic regurgitation. LVOT view. This sequence shows the absence of aortic regurgitation in the LVOT during various phases of the cardiac cycle. **a** Systolic ejection flow can be observed in the LVOT. **b–d** This sequence shows early, middle, and late diastole, respectively. No aortic regurgitation can be observed in the LVOT.

Aortic Regurgitation

Echocardiographic assessment of the degree of aortic regurgitation is still controversial. The length and width of the regurgitant jet have been proposed as parameters for evaluating the degree of aortic regurgitation. The extent to which left ventricular diastolic filling is hindered by the regurgitant jet is a useful parameter for evaluating the severity of aortic regurgitation.

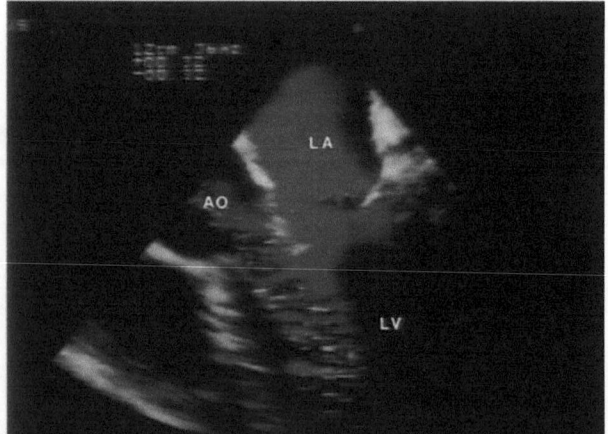

a

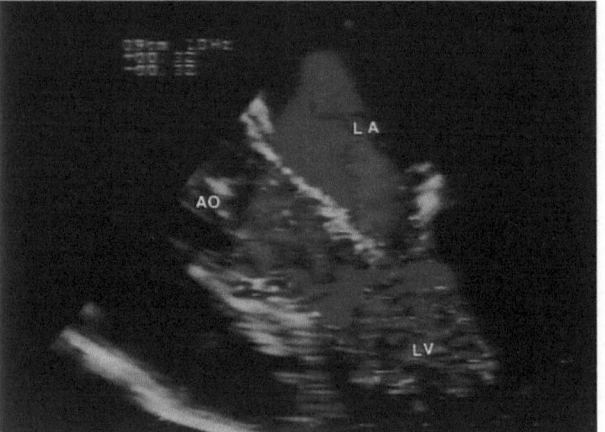

b

Fig. 2.24a, b. Aortic valve regurgitation, LVOT view. Different degree of regurgitation. **a** Moderate aortic regurgitation. The regurgitant jet is thin and does not hinder left ventricular diastolic inflow (*blue*). **b** Severe regurgitation. A large regurgitant jet hinders the diastolic left ventricular inflow, causing functional mitral stenosis (*mosaic effect* across the mitral valve).

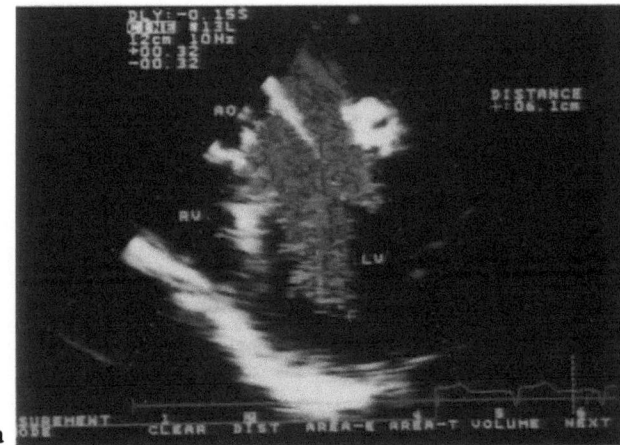

a

b

Fig. 2.25a, b. Residual aortic regurgitation after commissurotomy. Intraoperative color Doppler TEE, LVOT view. Severe aortic regurgitation detected by intraoperative color Doppler TEE. After aortic commissurotomy a large regurgitant jet hinders the diastolic left ventricular inflow, causing functional mitral stenosis (*mosaic effect* across the mitral valve). The regurgitant jet can be viewed up to the apex. The aortic valve was replaced during the same operation. In this case the regurgitant jet was directed toward the ventricular septum, and the surgeon could not palpate the thrill on the free wall of left ventricle.

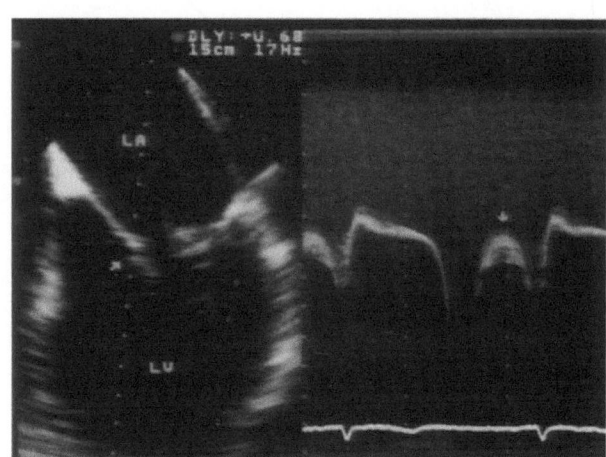

Fig. 2.26. Aortic regurgitation. M-mode TEE. Diastolic "fluttering" of the anterior mitral leaflet (*arrow*) is a useful echocardiographic sign of aortic regurgitation.

Tricuspid Valve

Tricuspid valve function can be easily evaluated by color Doppler TEE. An adjustable tricuspid suture annuloplasty guided by TEE has been developed at our institution.

Annuloplasty

Tricuspid suture annuloplasty is performed according to the technique described by De Vega. The free ends of the suture are brought through the right atrial wall and then passed through a rubber tourniquet. After cardiopulmonary bypass, with the heart beating, the reduction of the tricuspid annulus can be performed by adjusting the tension on the tourniquet (Fig. 2.27). The diameter of the tricuspid annulus can be reduced until the regurgitant jet disappears or, at least, until obtaining a major reduction of regurgitation. Tricuspid valve stenosis can be avoided since the diastolic inflow velocity and the gradient across the tricuspid valve are measured throughout the procedure. This technique allows substantial reduction of residual tricuspid regurgitation without creating valve stenosis. In most cases the systolic competence of the tricuspid valve can be achieved by this technique.

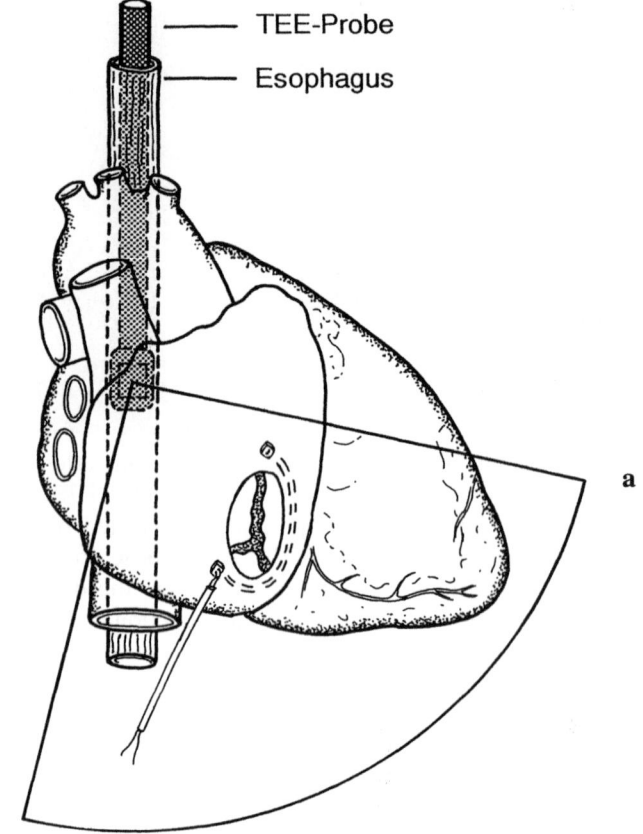

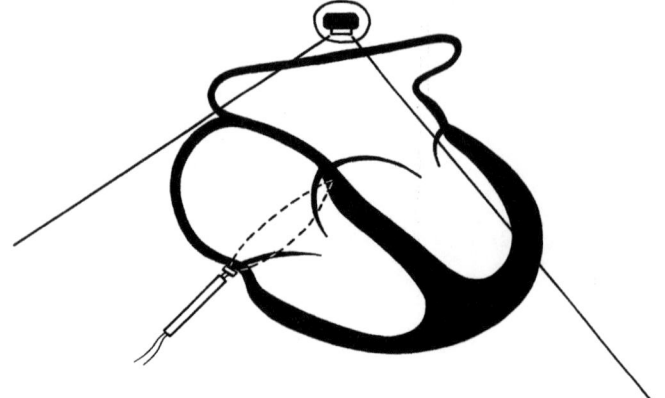

Fig. 2.27 a, b. Tricuspid suture annuloplasty guided by TEE. **a** The extent of annulus reduction can be regulated by adjusting the tension on the tourniquet, with the heart beating, until color Doppler shows the most adequate reduction of regurgitation without causing stenosis. **b** Schematic diagram of the four-chamber view for assessing tricuspid annuloplasty. (From De Simone R et al. (1993) Adjustable tricuspid valve annuloplasty assisted by intraoperative transesophageal color Doppler echocardiography. Am J Cardiol 71:926–931).

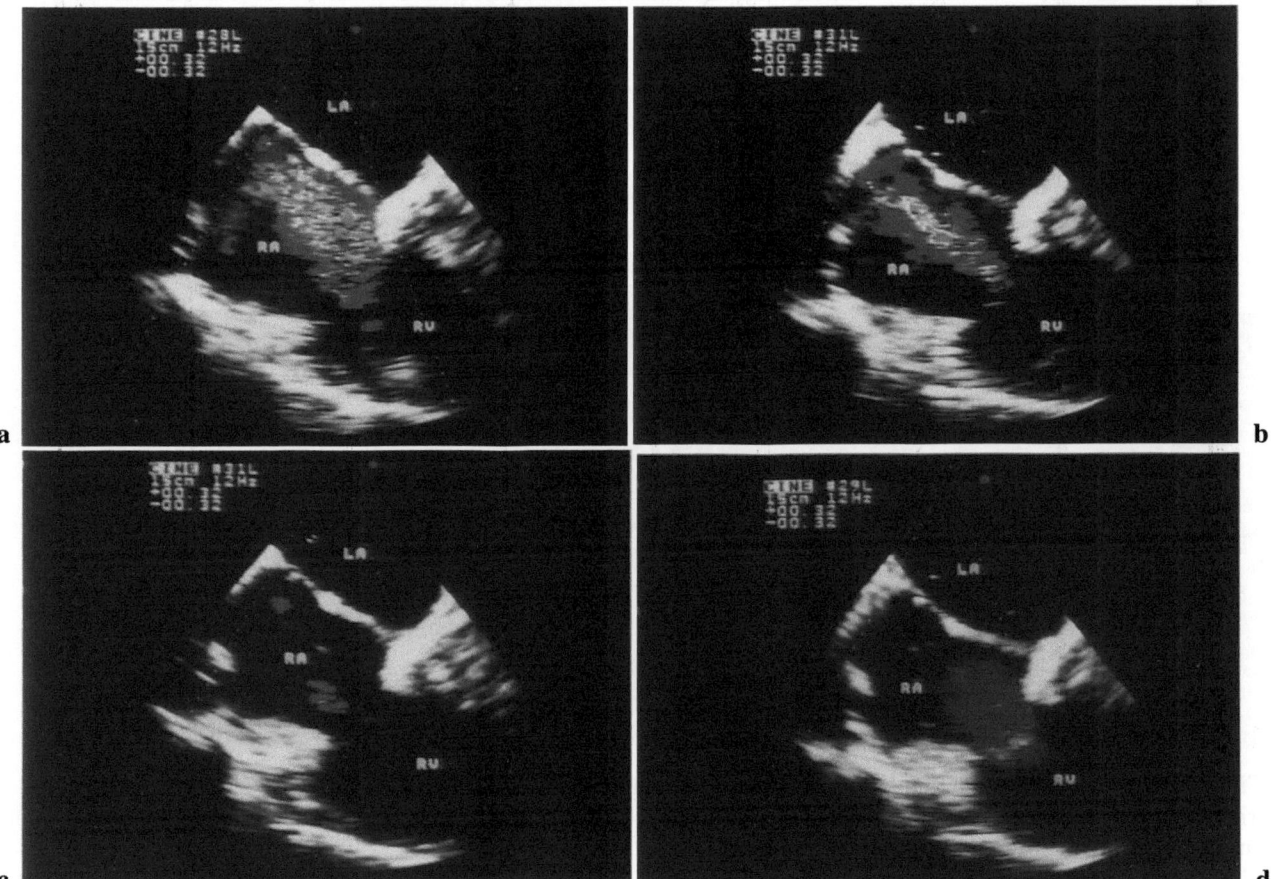

Fig. 2.28a–d. Tricuspid annuloplasty. Progressive reduction of tricuspid regurgitation during the adjustment of tricuspid annuloplasty, four-chamber view. **a** Severe regurgitation before adjustment of the suture. **b** Moderate regurgitation after annulus reduction. **c**

Complete disappearance of tricuspid regurgitation by further adjustment of the annulus. **d** Color Doppler shows normal diastolic flow (*blue*) across the tricuspid valve.

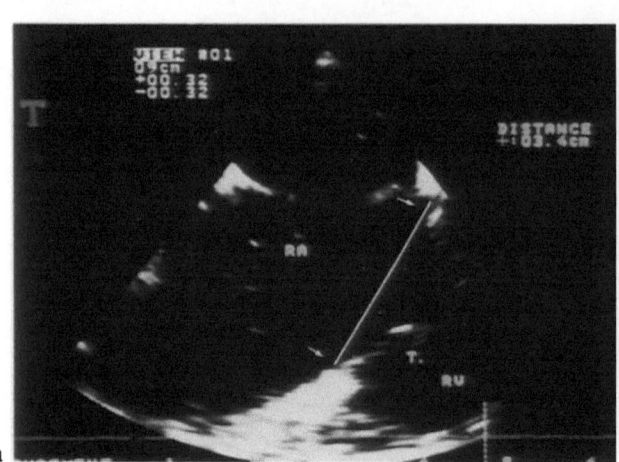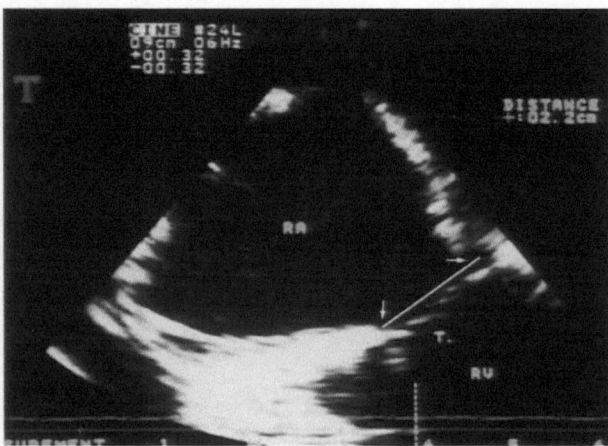

Fig. 2.29a, b. Tricuspid annuloplasty. Reduction of tricuspid valve annulus diameter (*arrows*). Before (**a**) and after (**b**) tricuspid valve annuloplasty. (From De Simone R et al. (1993) Adjustable tricuspid valve an- nuloplasty assisted by intraoperative transesophageal color Doppler echocardiography. Am J Cardiol 71:926–931).

Regurgitant Jet Area

The severity of tricuspid valve regurgitation can be assessed by color Doppler echocardiography by measuring the planimetry of the regurgitant jet.

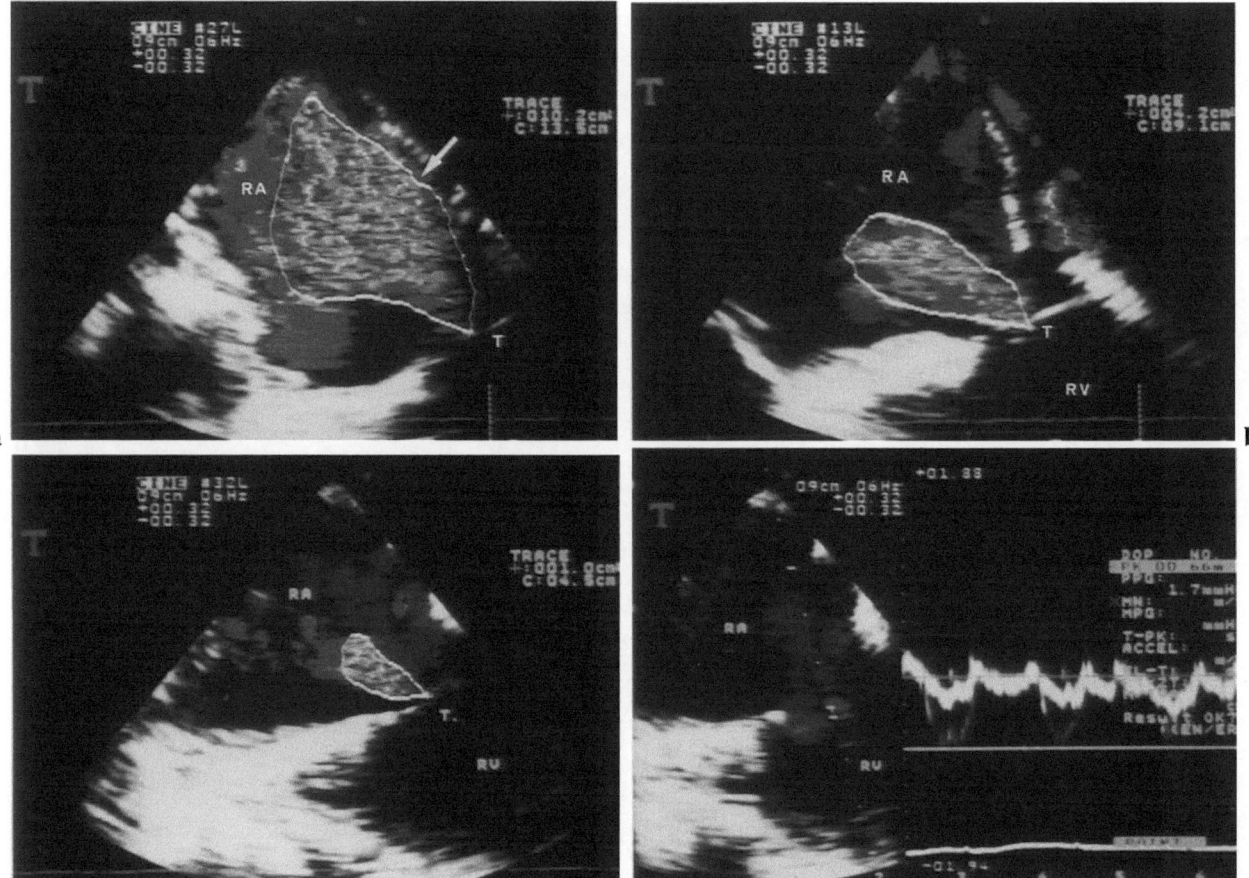

Fig. 2.30. Planimetry of the regurgitant jet area. This sequence shows the progressive reduction of tricuspid valve regurgitation (*arrows*) during adjustment of the suture annuloplasty. **a** Severe tricuspid regurgitation prior to the procedure (jet area, 10.2 cm^2). **b** Moderate regurgitation during the adjustment of the suture (jet area, 4.2 cm^2). **c** Further reduction of tricuspid regurgitation obtained by adjusting the suture un-der echocardiographic guidance (jet area, 1.0 cm^2). **d** Pulsed Doppler after tricuspid annuloplasty. Peak flow velocity across tricuspid valve is 0.66 m/s, showing no significant diastolic gradient (1.7 mmHg). (From De Simone R et al. (1993) Adjustable tricuspid valve annuloplasty assisted by intraoperative transesophageal color Doppler echocardiography. Am J Cardiol 71:926–931).

Tricuspid Valve Prolapse

Prolapse of the tricuspid valve leaflets is rare. It may result from myxomatous degeneration of the valve or from blunt chest trauma.

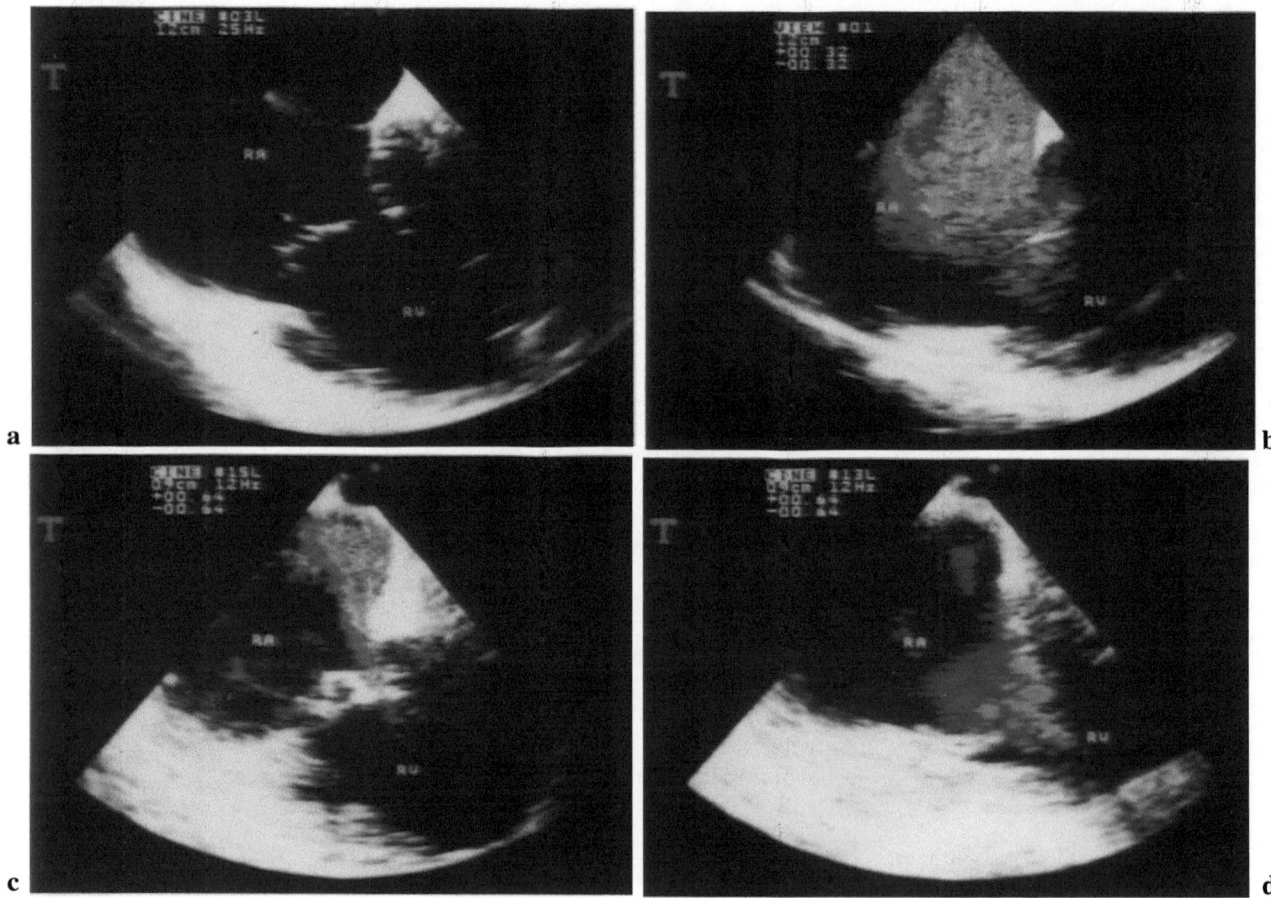

Fig. 2.31a–d. Prolapse of the tricuspid valve. A 36-year-old patient presented signs of right heart failure within weeks after a chest trauma. Echocardiographic examination showed a prolapse of the tricuspid valve. Intraoperative echocardiography. **a** Two-dimensional TEE. *Arrow*, prolapse of the posterior leaflet of the tricuspid valve. Right atrium and right ventricle are highly dilated. **b** Color Doppler shows severe tricuspid regurgitation. **c** After valvuloplasty. Reconstruction of the posterior leaflet with a pericardium patch was performed. Color Doppler shows a significant reduction of tricuspid regurgitation. **d** Normal diastolic flow across the tricuspid valve.

Pulmonary Valve

The pulmonary valve and the right ventricular out-flow tract (RVOT) may not be easily assessed by transesophageal transverse views. Monoplanar TEE can visualize flow in the main pulmonary artery, but not across the pulmonary valve. Biplanar TEE with longitudinal views provides direct visualization of the pulmonary valve and RVOT.

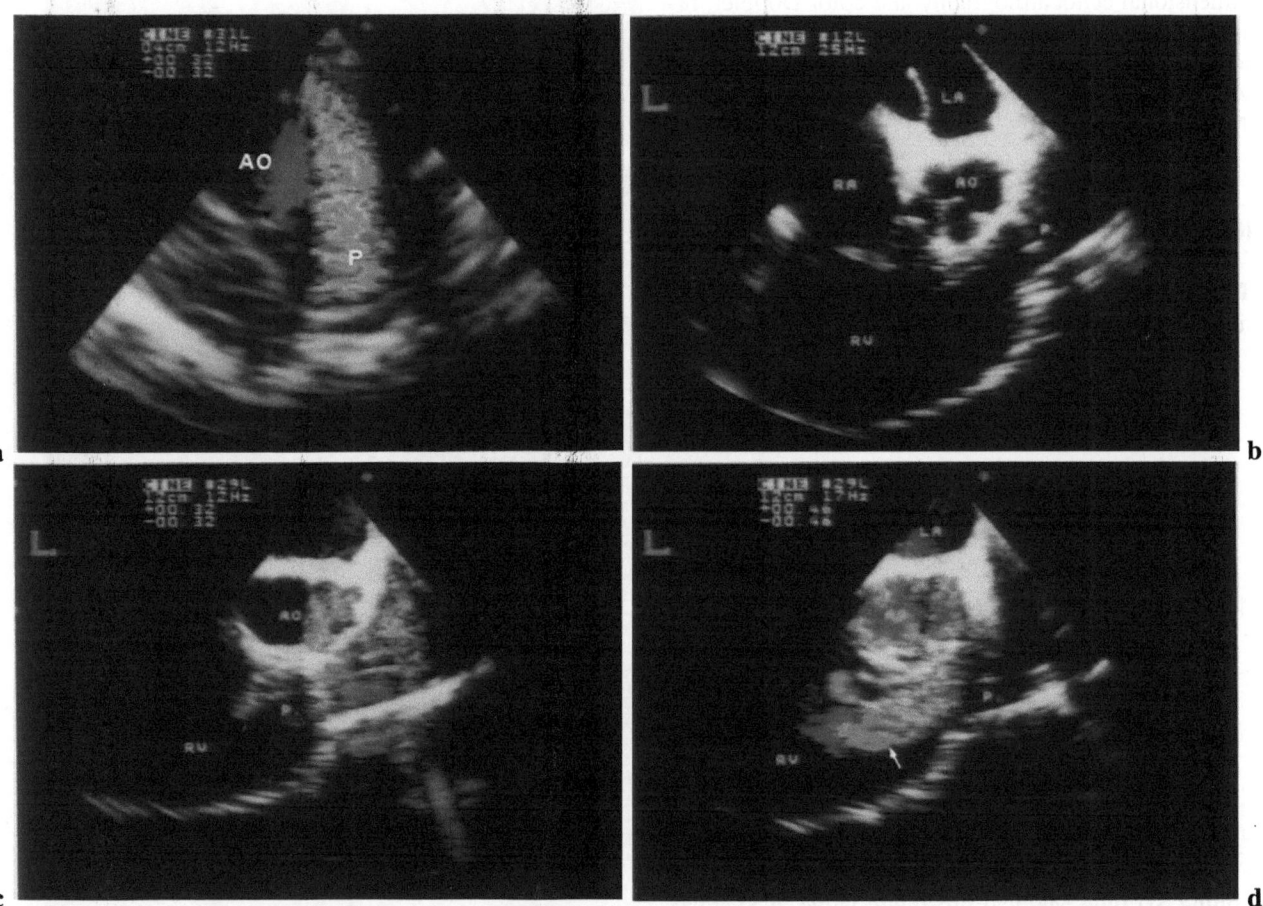

Fig. 2.32a–d. Stenosis and insufficiency of the pulmonary valve. **a** Basal short-axis view, color Doppler, shows turbulent poststenotic flow (*mosaic*) in the main pulmonary artery. **b** Two-dimensional TEE, RVOT long-axis view, shows stenosis of the pulmonary valve (*P*). **c** RVOT long-axis view. Color Doppler shows turbulent poststenotic flow in the main pulmonary artery immediately beyond the valve. **d** Color Doppler shows regurgitation of the pulmonary valve (*mosaic* in the RVOT).

Prosthetic Valves

TEE provides excellent visualization of prosthetic valves in the mitral position. The atrial approach overcomes the "shadowing" effect produced by the echo-reflective metallic parts of the valve. Mechanical function and prosthetic regurgitation can be assessed immediately after valve replacement by two-dimensional echocardiography and color Doppler, respectively. Early mechanical prosthetic dysfunction, which is a life-threatening complication of mitral valve replacement, can be detected by intraoperative TEE.

Normal Function

TEE allows the visualization and assessment of the motion of prosthetic valve leaflets.

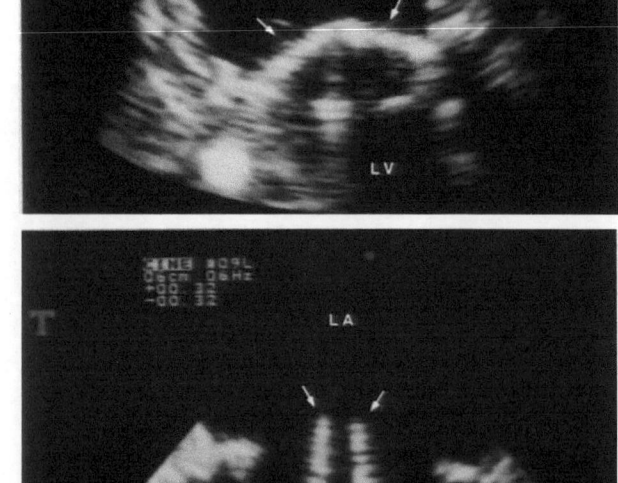

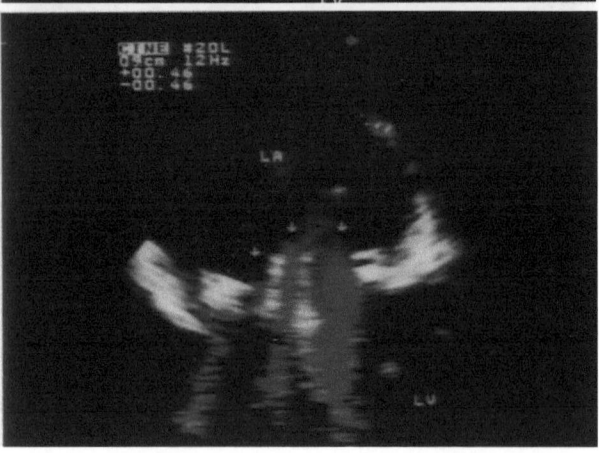

Fig. 2.33a–c. Prosthetic mitral valve, normally functioning St. Jude Medical prosthetic valve. **a** Systole; the two leaflets are closed. **b** Diastole; the leaflets are opened. Three channels between the two leaflets are visible (*arrows*). **c** Color Doppler shows a normal diastolic flow pattern across the valve (*arrows*).

Dysfunction

TEE provides a readily available diagnostic tool for the recognition of acute mechanical prosthetic valve dysfunction.

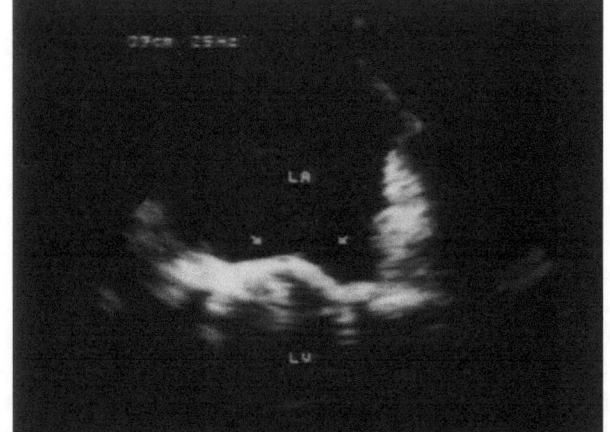

a

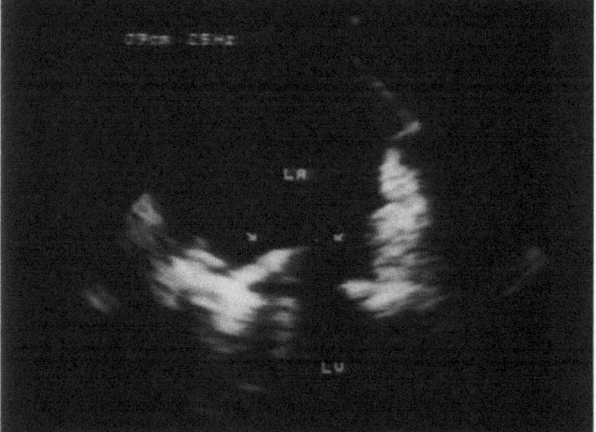

b

Fig. 2.34a–c. Prosthetic mitral valve. Mechanical dysfunction of the prosthesis was observed immediately after replacement. **a** St. Jude Medical mitral prosthetic valve in systole. *Arrows*, the two leaflets in closed position. **b** In diastole only one leaflet is open; the other is blocked in the closed position. **c** Color Doppler shows abnormal turbulent diastolic flow (*mosaic*) across the partially open valve. The patient could not be weaned off the cardiopulmonary bypass. Operative inspection of the prosthetic valve confirmed the echo finding. The prosthesis was replaced and the patient could easily be weaned off the bypass.

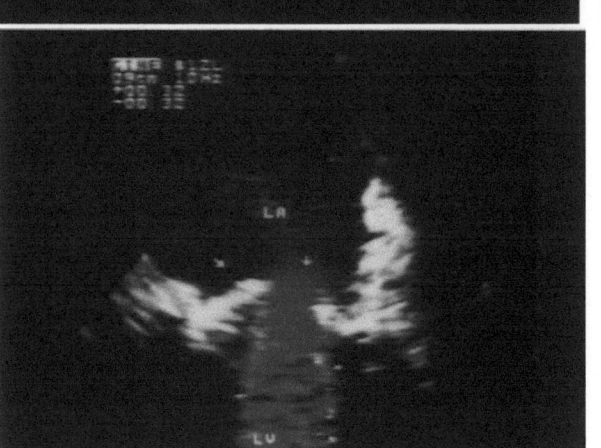

c

Prosthetic Regurgitation

Normally functioning mechanical prosthetic valves exhibit a "normal" regurgitation. The color Doppler characteristics of normal prosthetic valve regurgitation have not yet been well defined. In our series of patients two types of regurgitant jets can be distinguished: (a) central jets, originating from the prosthetic valve (normal prosthetic backflow), and (b) lateral jets, originating from the sewing cuff (paravalvular leaks). The echocardiographic pattern of normal prosthetic regurgitation should be recognized in each type of prosthesis to avoid replacement of normally functioning valves. The characteristics of normal regurgitant jets of two types of prosthetic valves in mitral position are shown in Table 2.1.

Table 2.1. Characteristics of normal prosthetic regurgitant jets.

	St. Jude Medical valve	Medtronic Hall valve
Origin	Central/from the gap between the leaflets and the ring	Central/from the gap between the leaflets and the ring
Duration	Early systolic	Holosystolic
Direction	Central	Central
Turbulence	Low	High (mosaic)

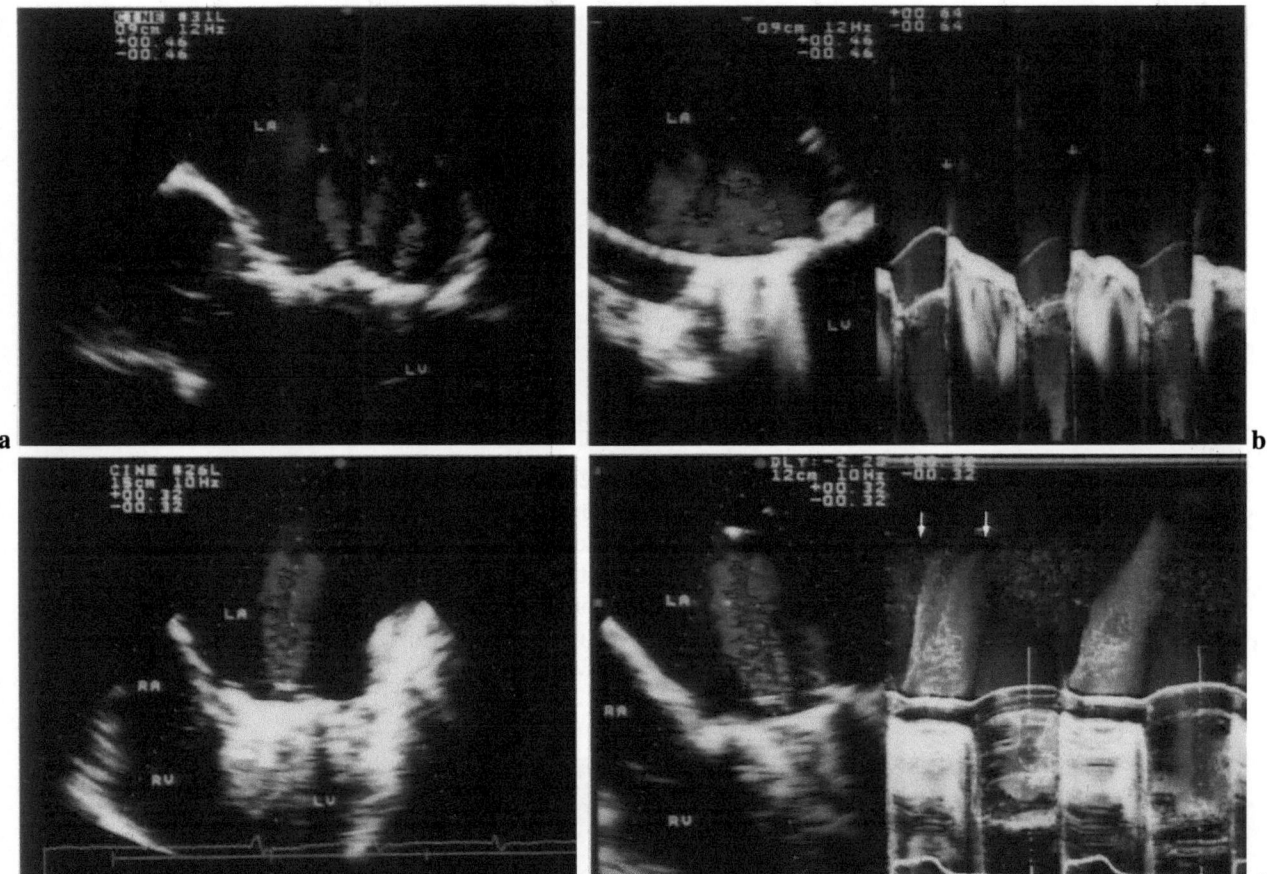

Fig. 2.35a–d. Normal prosthetic valve regurgitation. **a** Two-dimensional TEE, color Doppler. Three regurgitant jets (*arrows*) originate from the central part of a St. Jude Medical prosthetic mitral valve. **b** Color M-mode of the same valve as in **a**. The M-mode line is placed across the central part of the prosthesis. *Arrows*, a thin regurgitant jet which lasts a few millisec-onds. **c** Color Doppler. A large turbulent regurgitant jet (*mosaic*) originates from the central part of a Medtronic-Hall prosthetic valve in mitral position. **d** Color M-mode of the same valve as in **c**. The M-mode line is placed across the central part of the prosthesis. A regurgitant jet (*right*) lasts throughout systole (*arrows*).

Paravalvular Leak

The characteristics of abnormal prosthetic valve regurgitant jets as they appear in color Doppler echocardiography are presented in Table 2.2.

Table 2.2. Characteristics of prosthetic paravalvular reguritant jets.

	Paravalvular jets
Origin	From the sewing cuff
Duration	Early systolic
Direction	Central
Turbulence	High (mosaic)

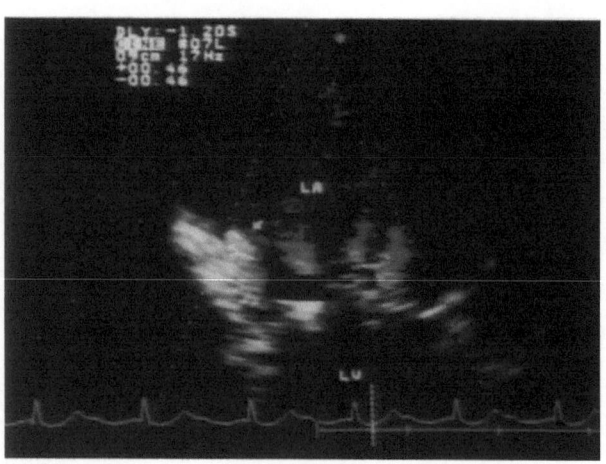

Fig. 2.36. Prosthetic valve regurgitation. Color Doppler shows two types of regurgitant jets of a St. Jude Medical prosthetic valve in mitral position. Three regurgitant jets (*red*) originate from the central part of the prosthetic valve (normal prosthetic backflow). *Arrow*, a lateral jet originating from the sewing cuff (paravalvular leak).

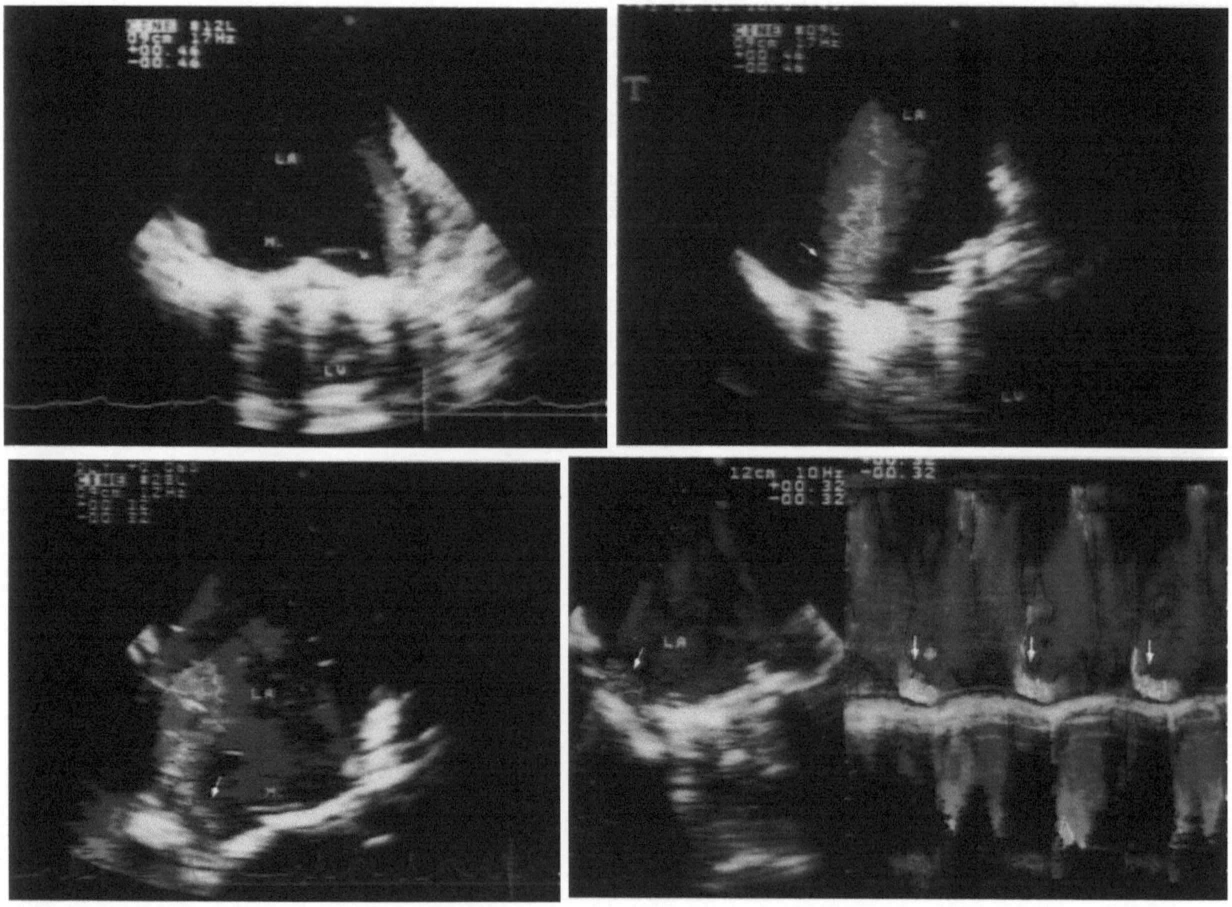

a

b

c

d

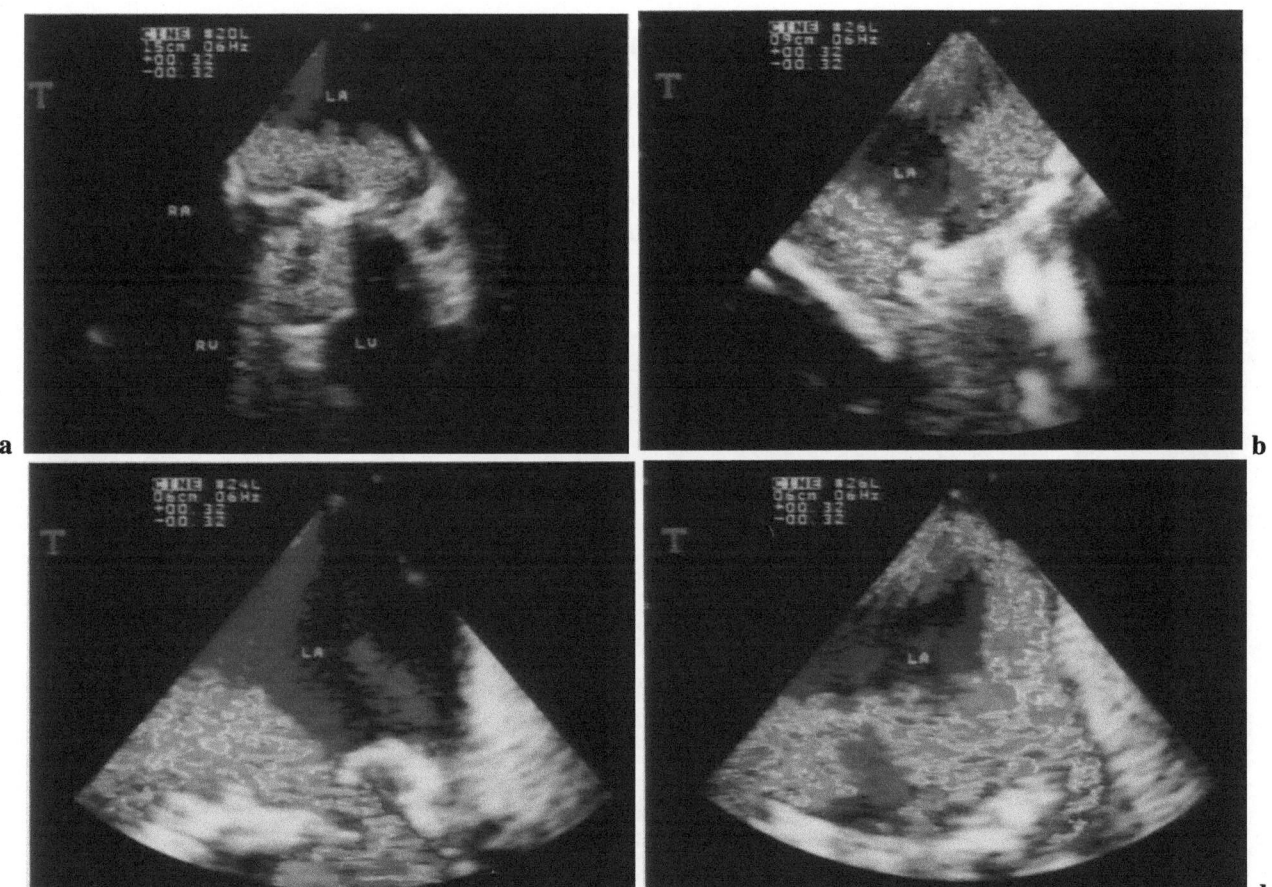

Fig. 2.38a–d. Paravalvular leakage, prosthetic valve endocarditis. Severe valve regurgitation originating from the mitral annulus. Intraoperative inspection of the valve showed suture dehiscence. Reconstruction of the mitral annulus with a patch and replacement of the prosthetic valve was performed.

Fig. 2.37a–d. Prosthetic paravalvular leakage. **a** Regurgitant jets (*arrow*) originating from the lateral part of the prosthetic valve. **b** Paravalvular regurgitant jet originating from the anterior portion of the annulus (*arrow*). **c** Paravalvular leak directed along the atrial septum. **d** Color M-mode echocardiography. *Left*, the M-mode line is placed across the regurgitant jet (*arrow*); *right*, the regurgitant jet persists throughout systole.

Endocarditis

TEE provides a very sensitive tool for the diagnosis of infective endocarditis. It allows direct visualization of floating vegetations and assessment of valve function.

Mitral Valve Endocarditis

The diagnosis of mitral valve endocarditis is based on direct visualization of floating vegetations attached to the leaflets or the chordae. Mitral valve regurgitation due to leaflet perforation or chordal rupture can be easily detected by Color Doppler.

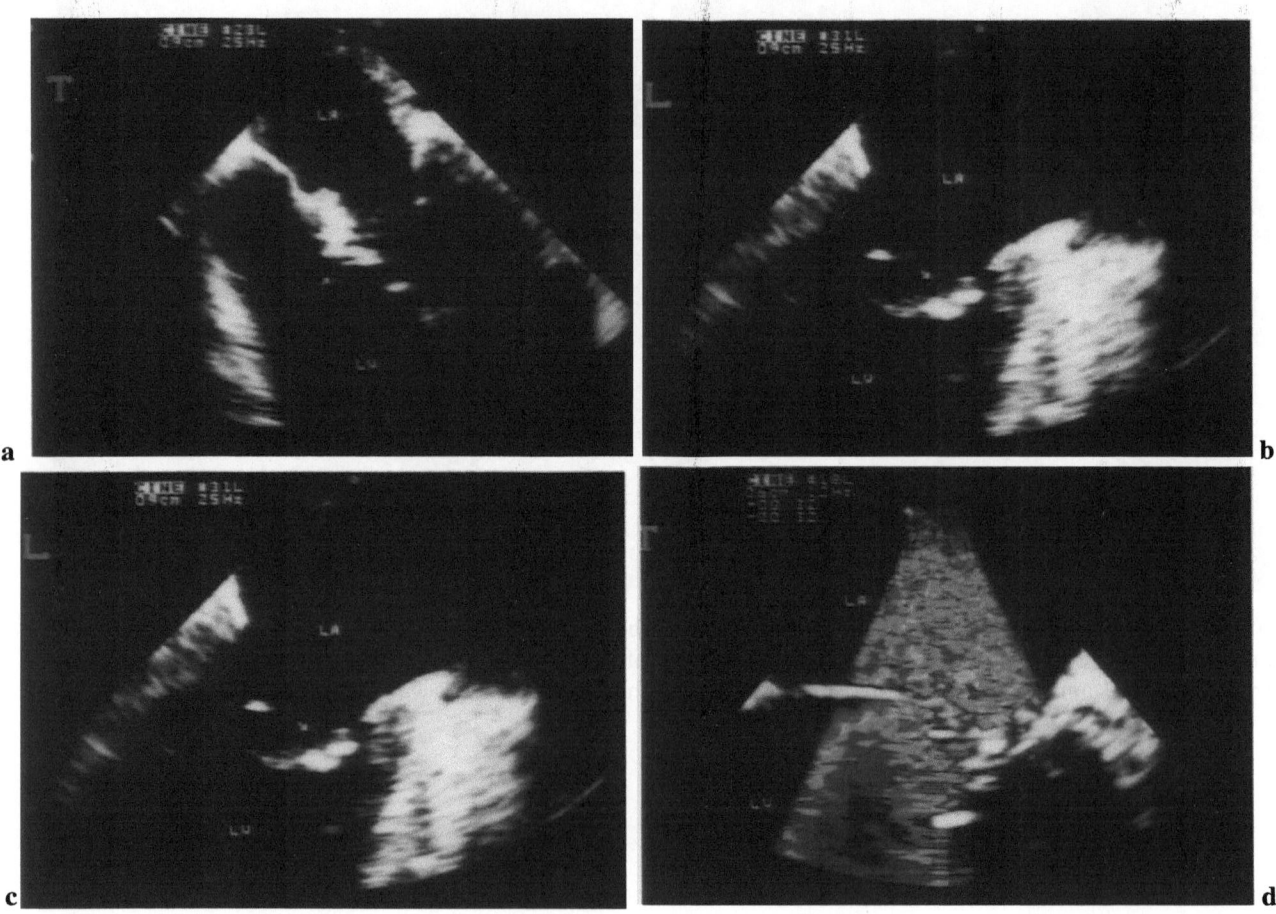

Fig. 2.39a–d. Mitral valve endocarditis. **a** Two-dimensional TEE, four-chamber view. Thickening of the anterior mitral valve leaflet due to infective vegetations (*arrow*). **b** Longitudinal four-chamber view; same patient as in **a**. Infective vegetation on the anterior mitral valve leaflet (*arrow*). **c** Prolapse of the anterior leaflet of the mitral valve due to rupture of the chordae tendineae. **d** Color Doppler shows a severe mitral regurgitation due to the prolapse of the anterior mitral valve leaflet.

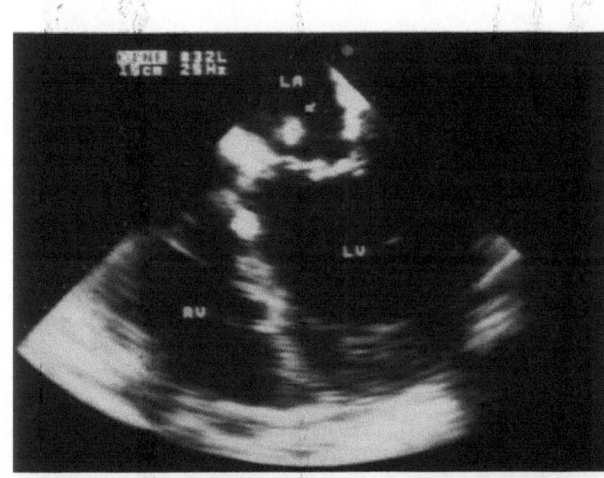

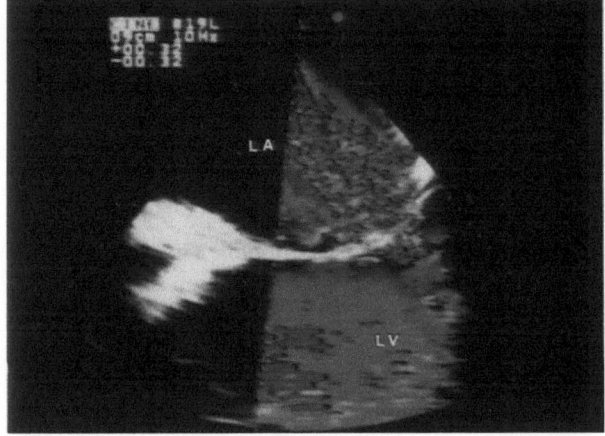

Fig. 2.40a, b. Endocarditis of the mitral valve. **a** Infective vegetation (*arrow*) on the atrial side of the mitral valve. **b** Color Doppler shows a large regurgitant jet (*mosaic*) in the left atrium consistent with severe mitral regurgitation.

Aortic Valve Endocarditis

Aortic valve endocarditis can be diagnosed by the visualization of infective vegetations on the aortic cusps or by the detection of abscess formations at the aortic annulus. Turbulent diastolic flow in the LVOT due to aortic valve regurgitation may be observed in patients with perforation of the cusps.

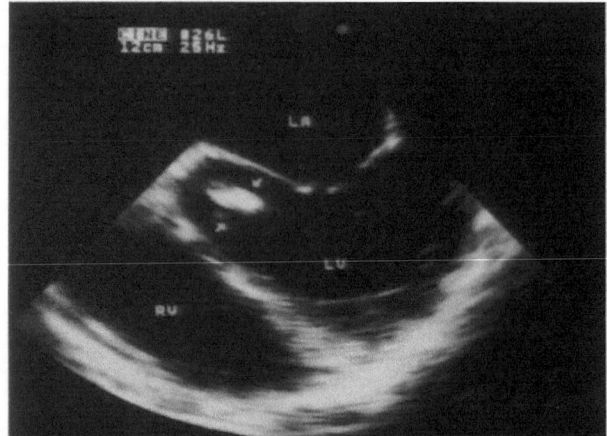

a

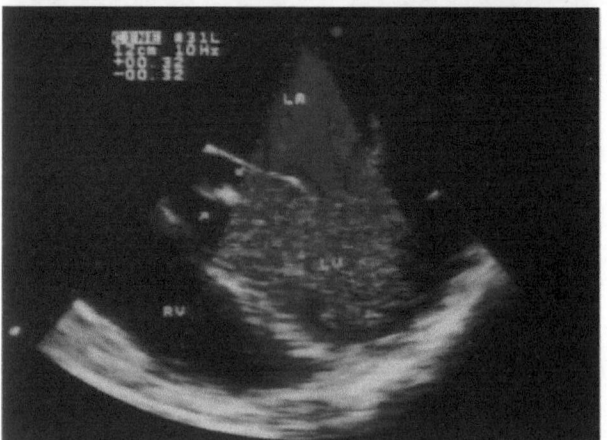

b

Fig. 2.41a, b. Aortic valve endocarditis. **a** Two-dimensional TEE shows a floating vegetation protruding into the LVOT in diastole. **b** Severe aortic regurgitation is detected by color Doppler. The regurgitant jet (*mosaic*) spreads into the LVOT up to the apex.

Tricuspid Valve Endocarditis

Infective endocarditis of the tricuspid valve is rare. Drug abusing patients have a relatively high incidence of tricuspid valve endocarditis. Leaflet perforation, rupture of chordae, and valve prolapse may lead to severe tricuspid valve regurgitation.

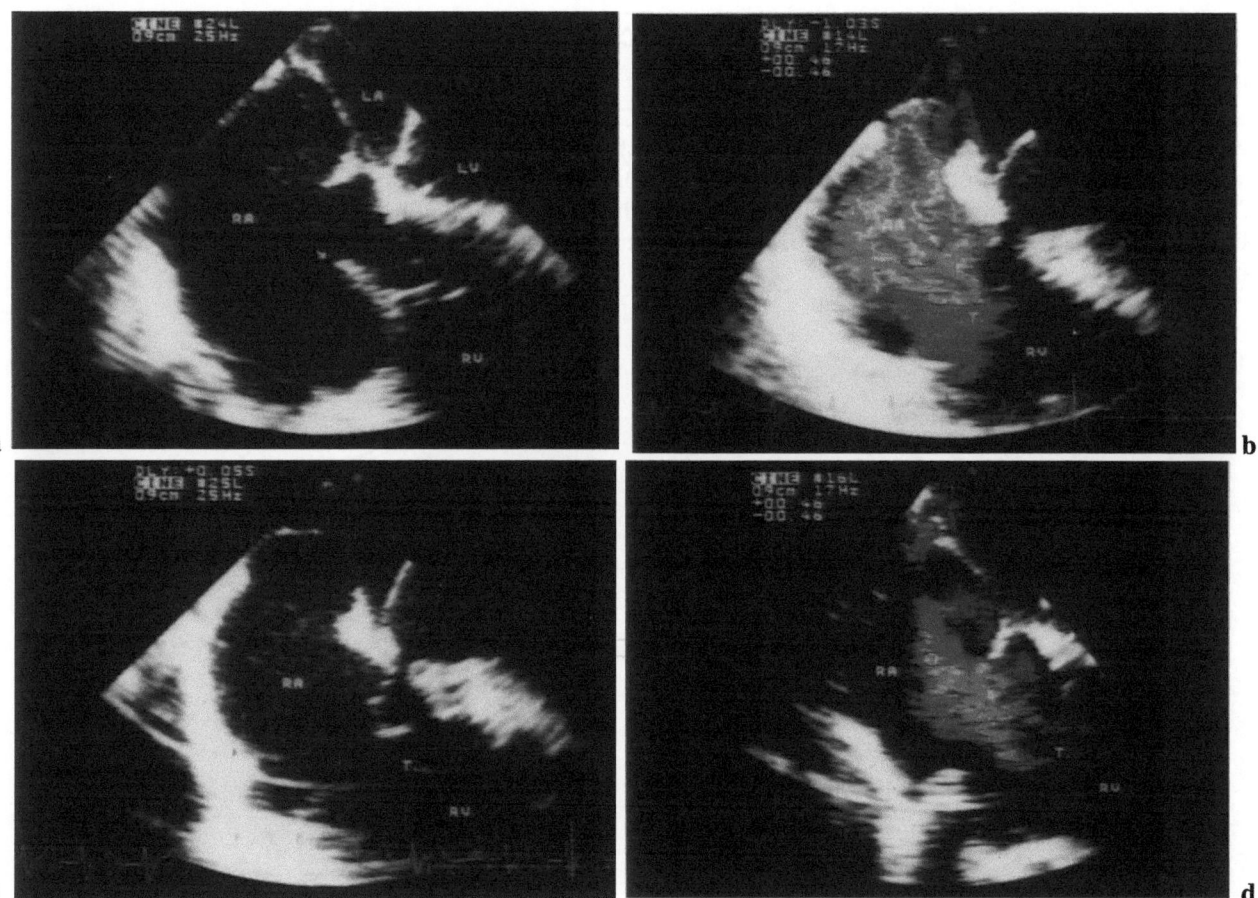

Fig. 2.42a–d. Tricuspid valve endocarditis in a drug-addicted patient. **a** Floating vegetations of the tricuspid valve prolapse into the right atrium in systole. **b** Severe tricuspid regurgitation. **c** The patient underwent vegectomy and reconstruction of the tricuspid valve. **d** Residual tricuspid regurgitation after tricuspid valve bicuspidalization.

Coronary Artery Disease

TEE offers new perspectives for the diagnosis of coronary artery disease. Direct visualization of the coronary arteries is a promising diagnostic approach for assessing the patency of the proximal segments of left and right coronary arteries. Coronary blood flow can be measured by pulsed-wave or color Doppler. The study of regional wall motion due to coronary disease can be performed by a transgastric view of the left ventricle.

Coronary Arteries

Coronary artery stenosis can be detected by TEE. However, despite the initial optimism this method today represents only a supplementary technique for the diagnosis of coronary artery disease since the success rate of visualization is limited.

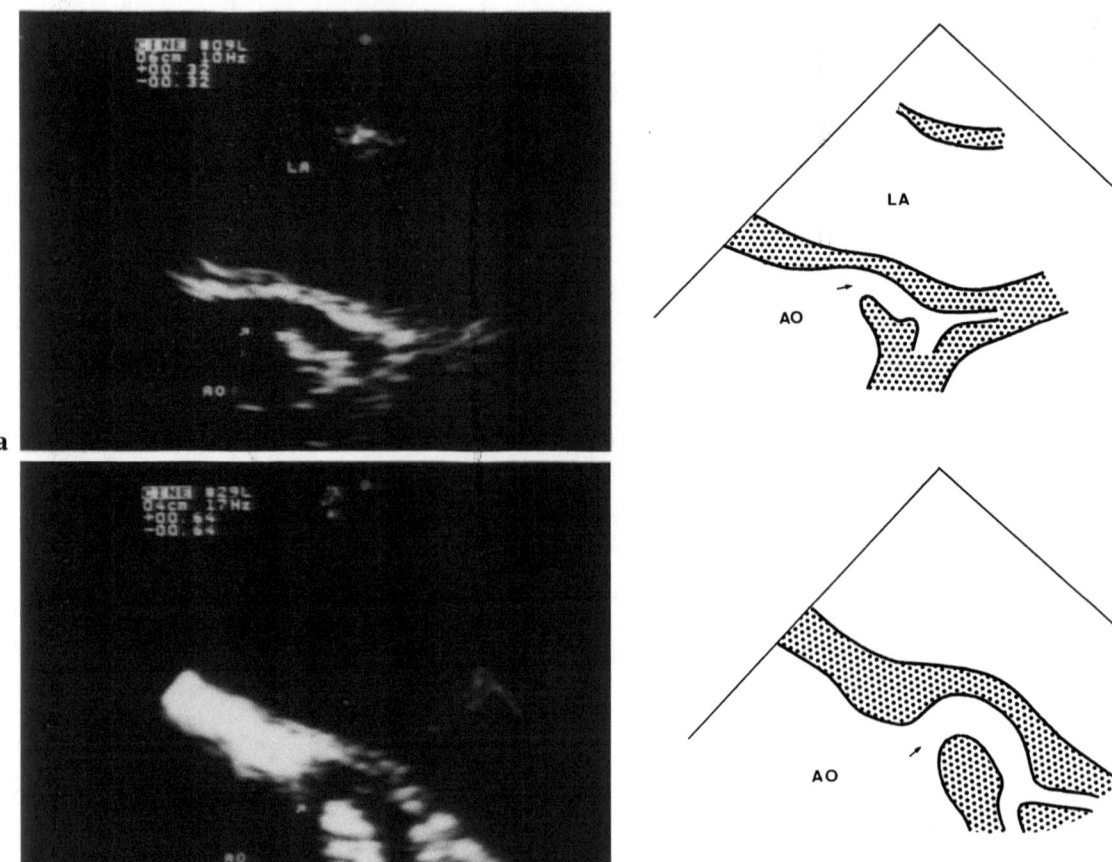

Fig. 2.43a–d. Left main coronary artery. Two-dimensional TEE shows the left coronary artery (*arrow*) up to the bifurcation.

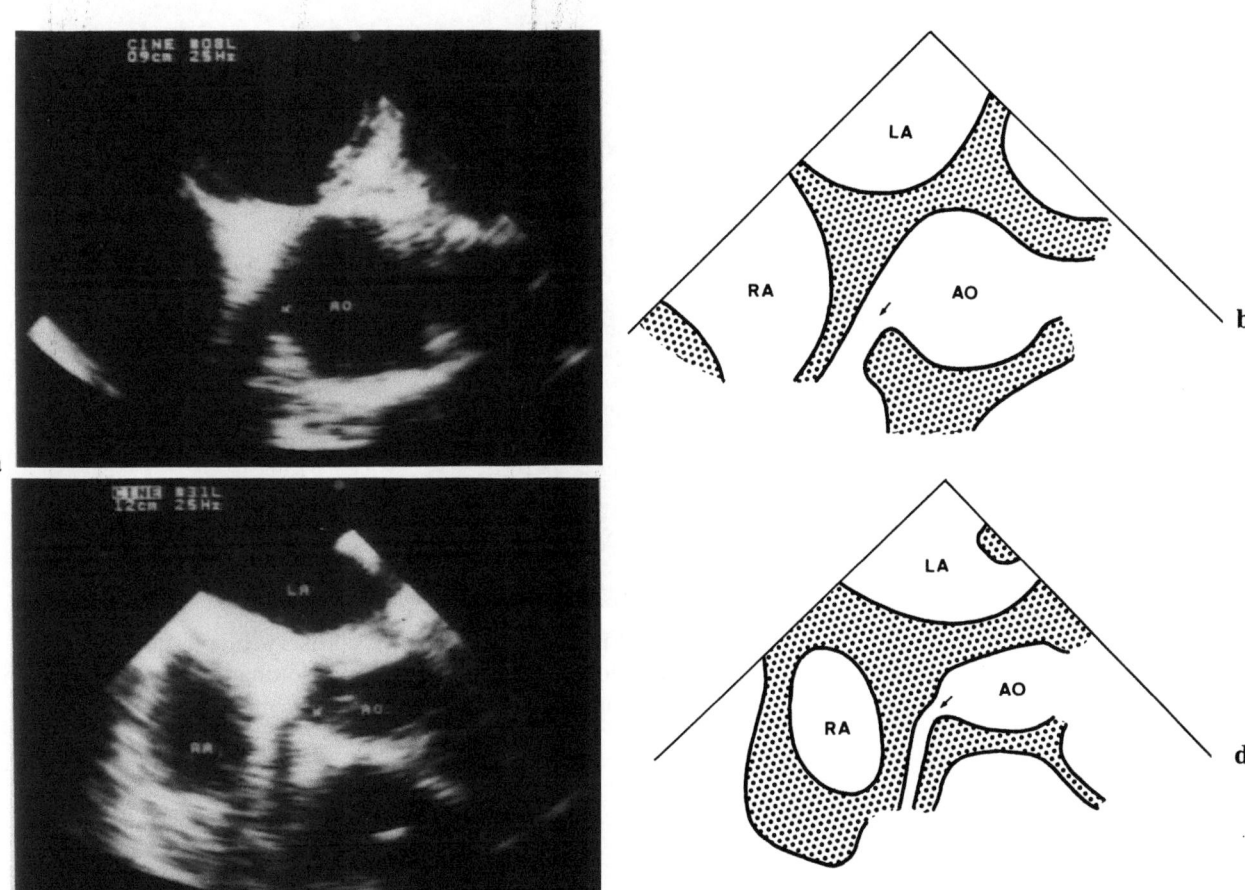

Fig. 2.44a–d. Right coronary artery. Two-dimensional TEE shows the proximal tract of the right coronary artery (*arrow*).

Coronary Blood Flow

Coronary blood flow can be assessed by color Doppler flow imaging. A number of studies reported the utility of pulsed-wave Doppler for quantitative assessment of coronary flow.

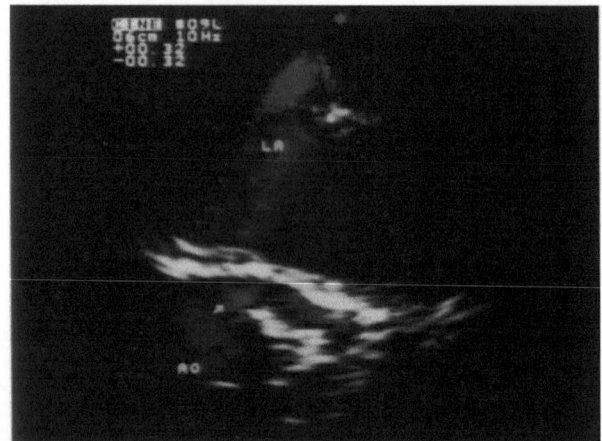

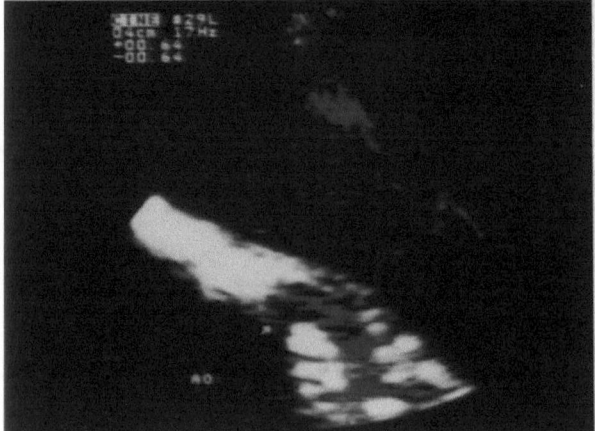

Fig. 2.45a, b. Normal coronary blood flow. Color flow Doppler shows normal coronary flow in the left main coronary artery.

Regional Wall Motion

Regional disturbances of wall motion is the most sensitive sign of myocardial ischemia. Two-dimensional TEE allows assessment of segmental contraction of the heart. The transgastric short-axis view is the most useful for visualizing regional wall motion.

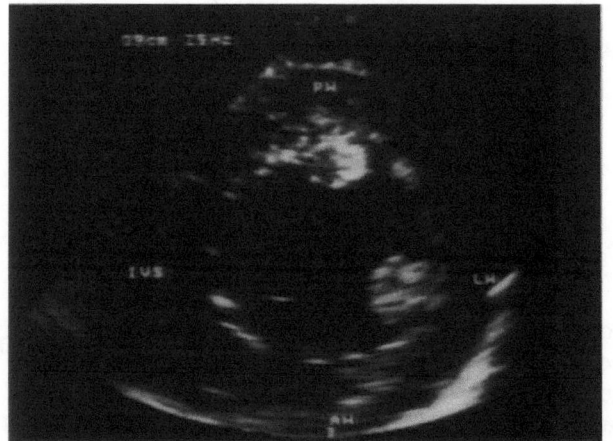

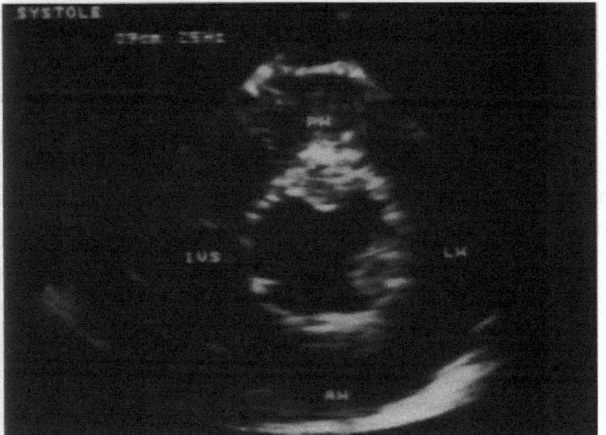

Fig. 2.46a, b. Regional wall motion of the left ventricle. Transgastric short-axis view of the left ventricle allows analysis of regional wall motion. **a** Diastole. **b** Systole. *PW*, Posterior wall; *LW*, lateral wall; *AW*, anterior wall; *IVS*, interventricular septum.

Aortic Dissection

Aortic dissection is characterized by detachment of the intima and by the entry of high-pressure flow into the disrupted media. Three types of aortic dissections can be distinguished, according to the classification of DeBakey. In type I the entry is in the ascending aorta, and the dissection extends to the descending aorta; in type II the dissection does not extend beyond the arch; in type III, the dissection is confined to the descending aorta. TEE represents a highly accurate method for the diagnosis of aortic dissections and for evaluating flow dynamics in the true and false lumen.

Dissecting Aneurysm

The degeneration of the aortic media, which is a prerequisite for the development of aortic dissection, is often associated with aneurysmatic enlargement of the vessel. The dilatation of the ascending aorta may extend to the aortic annulus, causing aortic regurgitation.

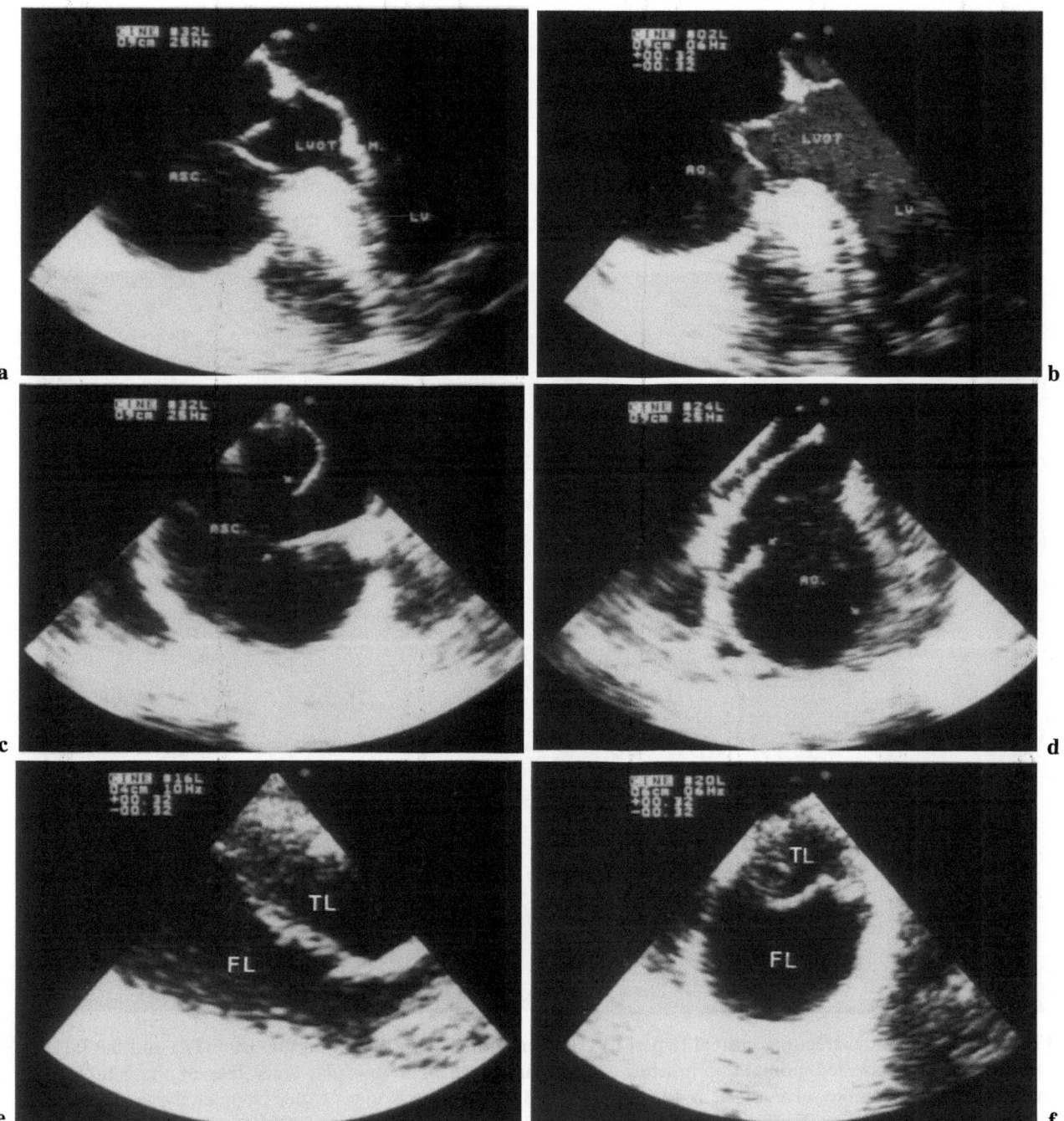

Fig. 2.47a–f. Dissecting aortic aneurysm. **a** LVOT view shows massive dilatation of the ascending aorta (*ASC*). **b** LVOT view, color Doppler shows turbulent diastolic flow in the LVOT due to aortic regurgitation. **c, d** Transverse view of the ascending aorta (*ASC, AO*). *Left, arrows,* aortic valve; *right, arrows,* intimal flaps. **e** Transverse view of the aortic arch showing the intimal flap. **f** Cross-sectional view of the descending aorta showing a small true lumen (*TL*) compressed by the false lumen (*FL*).

Intimal Flap

The echocardiographic diagnosis of aortic dissection is based primarily on visualizing an intimal flap and on distinguishing two lumina within the aorta.

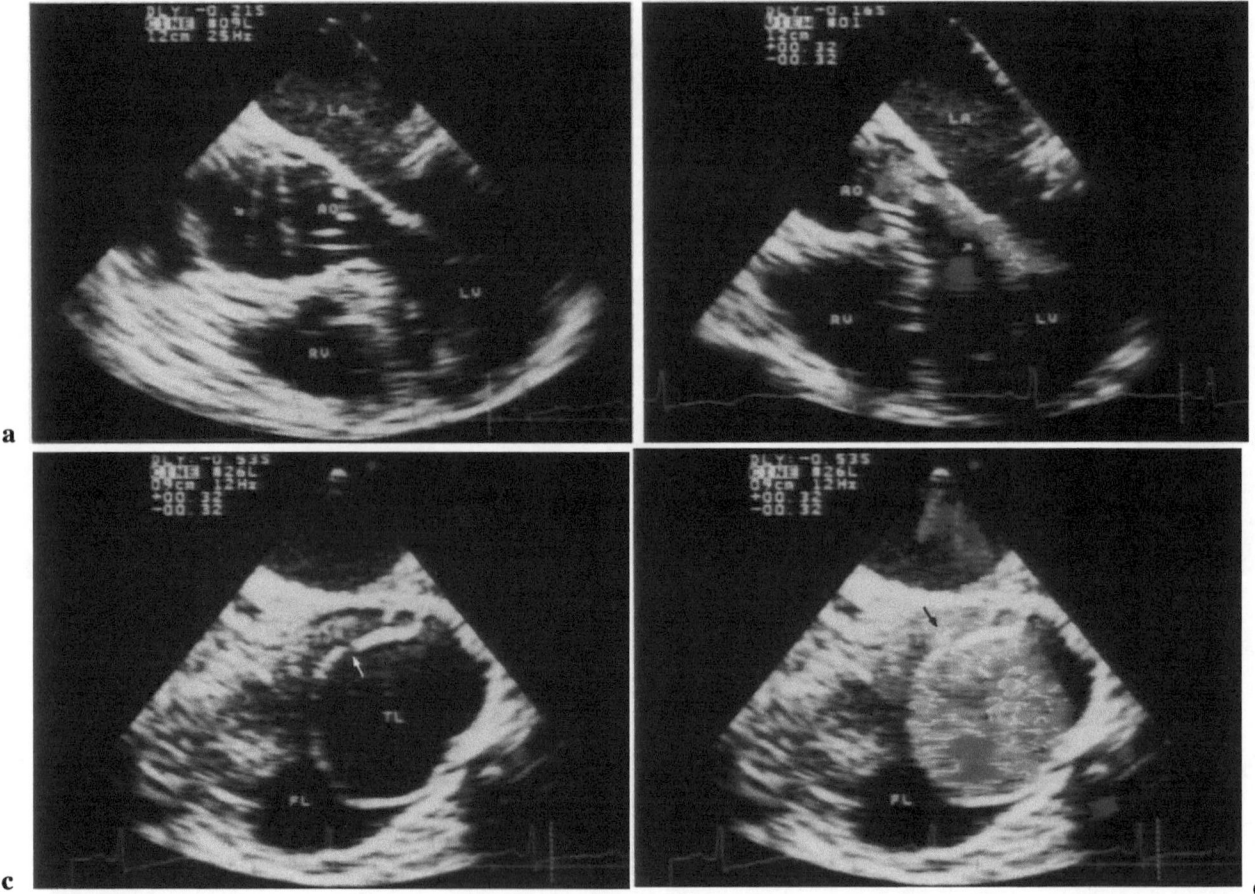

Fig. 2.48a–h. Aortic dissection, intimal flap. **a** LVOT view. *Arrow*, the dissected intimal flap just few centimeters above the aortic valve (*AO*). **b** LVOT view, color Doppler. Aortic insufficiency. *Arrow*, a regurgitant jet directed along the anterior leaflet of the mitral valve. **c** Basal short-axis view. Ascending aorta with an intimal flap separating the true (*TL*) and the false lumen (*FL*). *Arrow*, the entry tear of the intima. **d** Basal short-axis view. Color Doppler shows turbulent flow in the true lumen and the flow entering the false lumen (*arrow*).

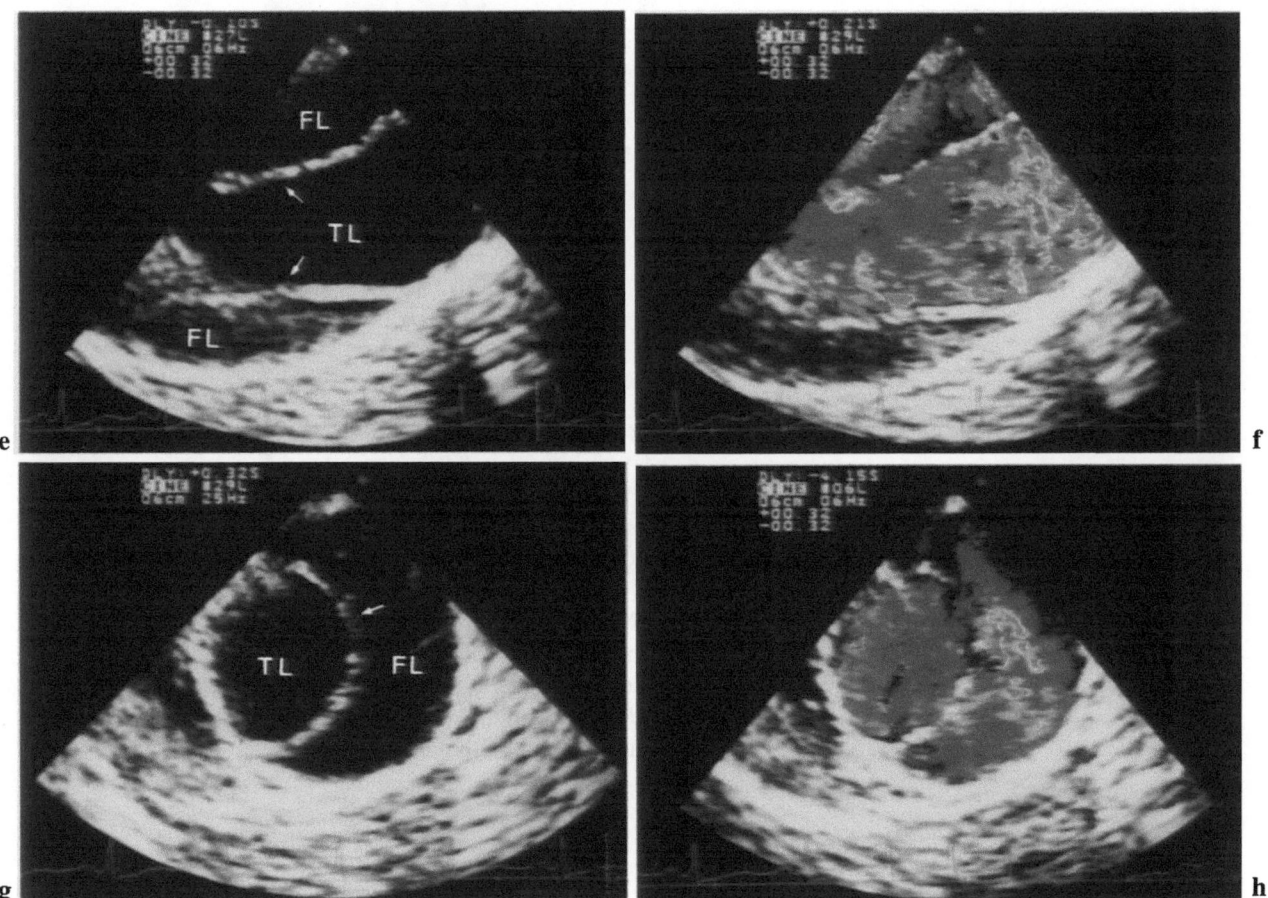

Fig. 2.48 e. Basal short-axis view of the aortic arch. The intimal flap (*arrows*) divides the true lumen (*TL*) from the false lumen (*FL*). The true lumen is almost completely surrounded by a tubular dissection. **f** Co-lor Doppler shows the flow in the true lumen. **g, h** Transverse view of the descending aorta showing the intimal flap (*arrow*) and the flow in the true and in the false lumen.

True and False Lumen

The echocardiographic criteria for differentiating the true from the false lumen are: (a) the true lumen shows systolic expansion and diastolic collapse, (b) systolic jets (entry) are directed away from the false lumen, and (c) the false lumen shows spontaneous echocardiographic contrast due to slow flow velocity.

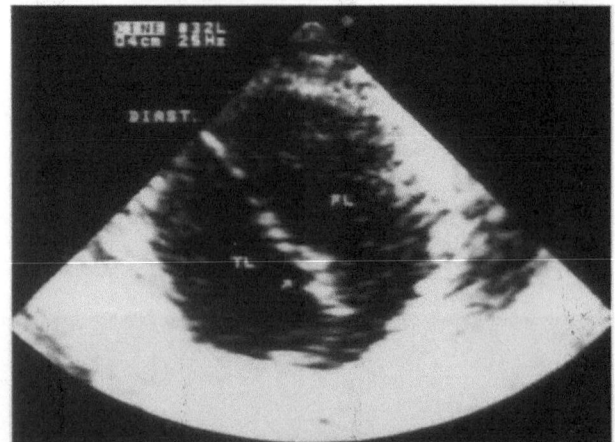

a

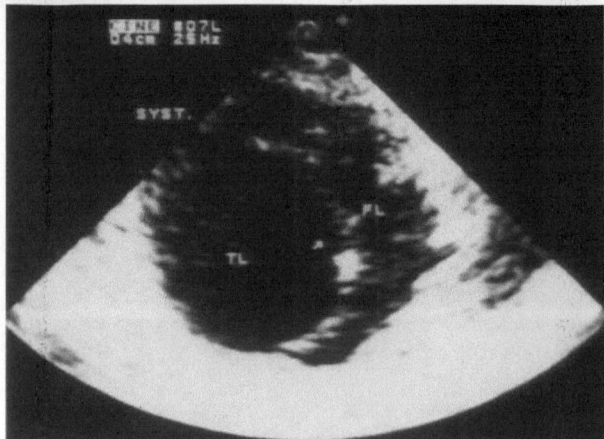

b

Fig. 2.49a, b. Differentiation between true and false lumen. Aortic dissection. Cross-sectional view of the descending aorta. **a** Expansion of the false lumen (*FL*) and compression of the true lumen (*TL*) in diastole. **b** Opposite motion in systole.

Fig. 2.50a–l. TEE and computed tomography, aortic dissection. **a** LVOT view shows a small aortic regurgitant jet (*arrow*). **b** An intimal flap (*arrow*) can be visualized 2 cm above the aortic valve. **c, d** *Left*, transverse view of the ascending aorta shows the true (*TL*) and the false lumen (*FL*); *right*, computed tomogaphy at the same level. *Arrows*, dissecting membrane. **e, f** *Left*, Transverse view of the aortic arch 22 cm from the incisors; *right*, computed tomography at the same level.

TEE and Computed Tomography

Computed tomography is another useful diagnostic technique for diagnosing dissection of the aorta. Adequate visualization of the dissecting membrane requires the injection of contrast.

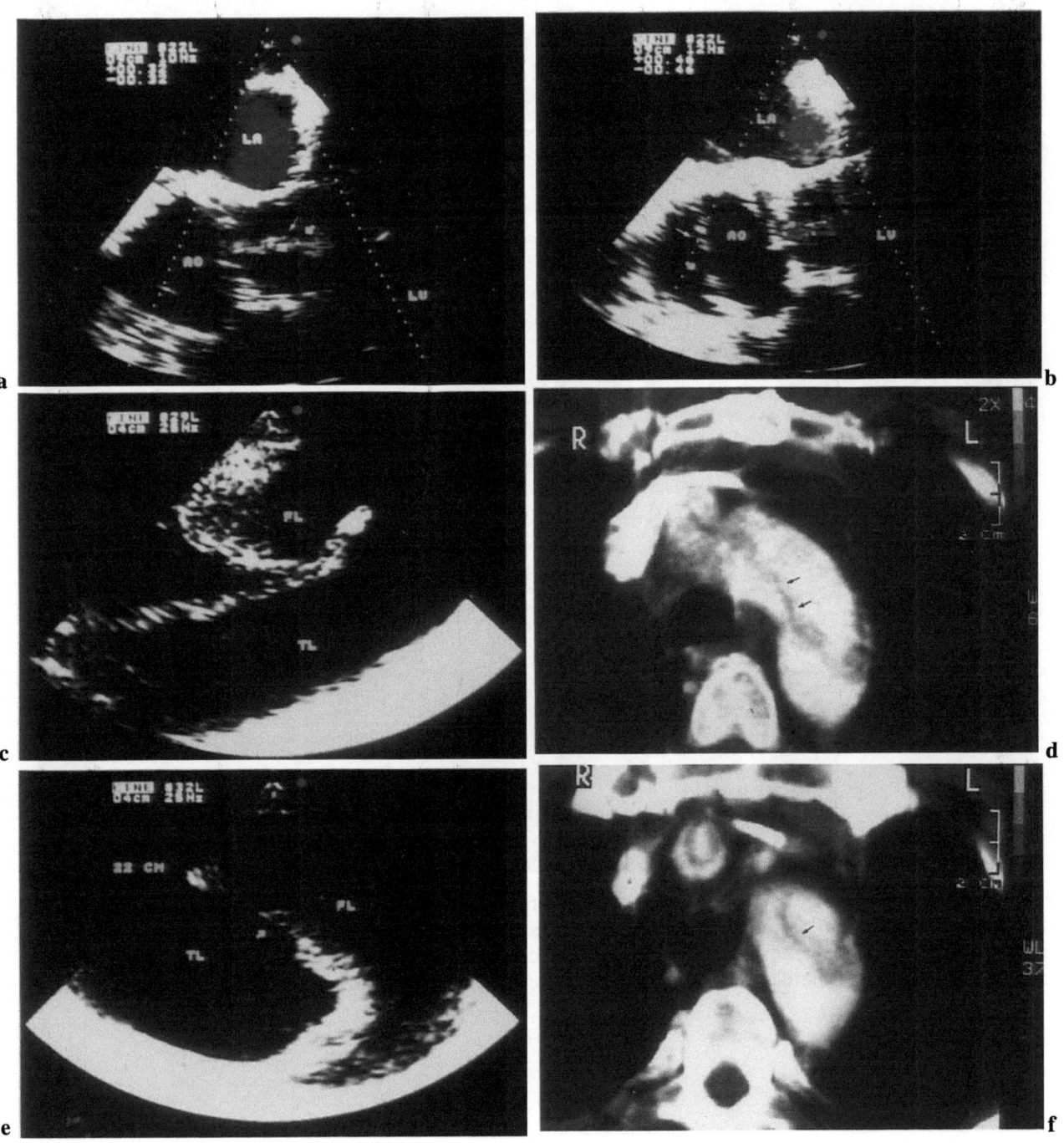

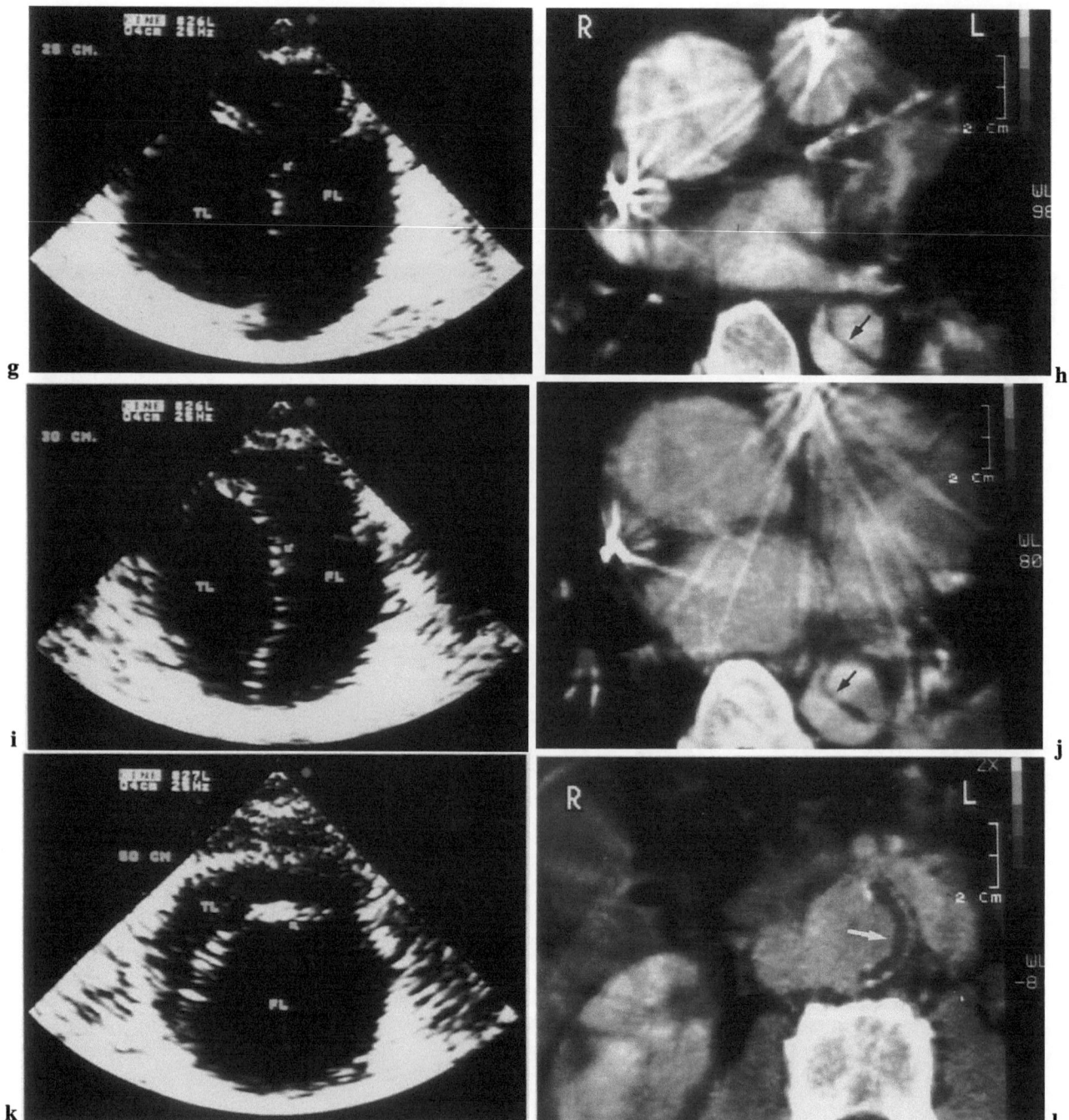

Fig. 2,50 g, h *Left*, TEE cross-sectional view of the descending aorta 25 cm from the incisors; *right*, computed tomography at the same level. **i, j** *Left*, cross-sectional view of the descending aorta 30 cm from the incisors; *right*, computed tomography at the same level. **k, l** *Left*, cross-sectional view of the descending aorta about 50 cm from the incisors; *right*, computed tomography at the same level.

Flow in the False Lumen

Surgery for aortic dissection replaces the ascending aorta with a tubular Dacron prosthesis at the level of the proximal entry tear so that the aortic flow is devi-ated into the true lumen. Persistence of false lumen is described in more than 90% of patients after surgery for of aortic dissection. If the false lumen extends to the descending aorta, the flow deviation causes obliteration of the distal dissection, provided that no distal entry is present.

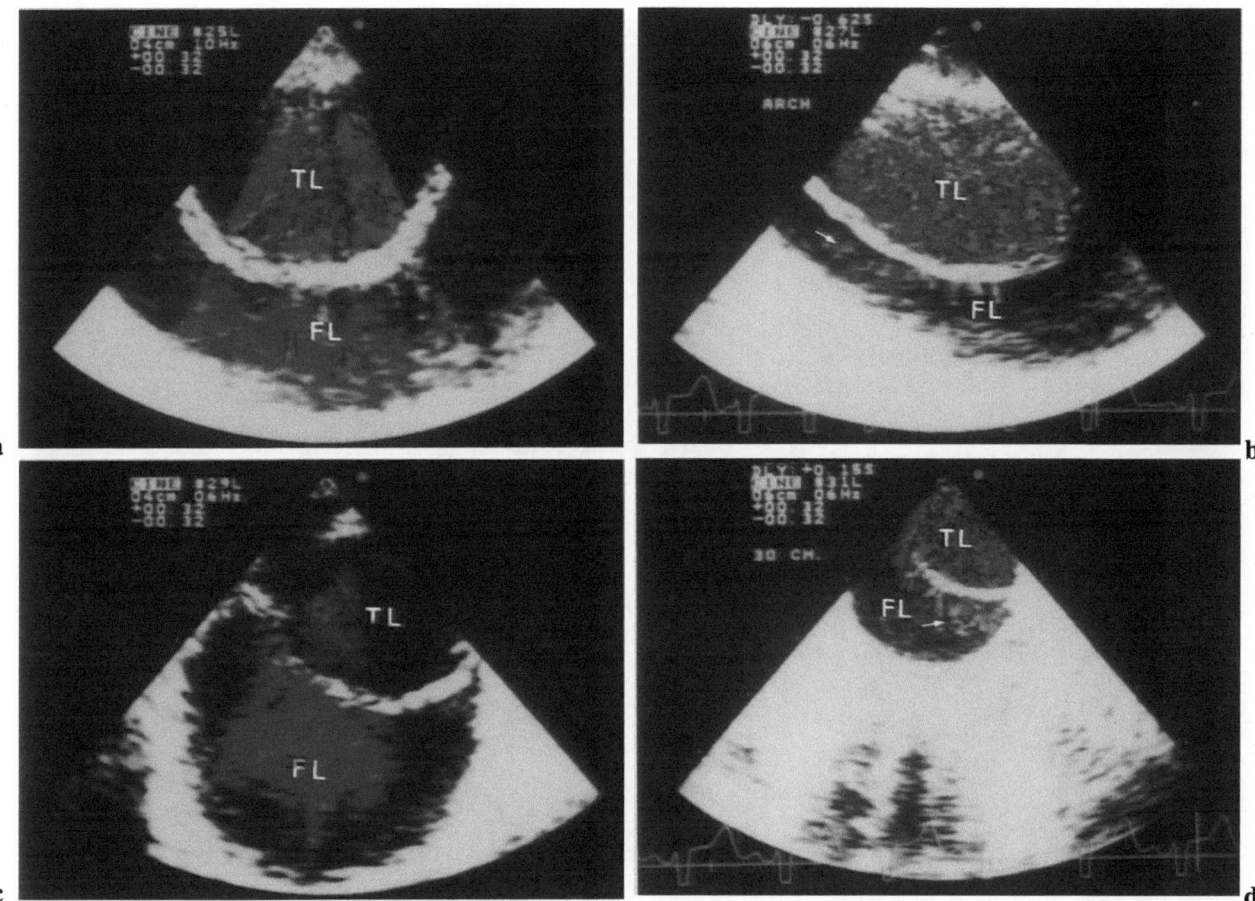

Fig. 2.51a–h. Flow in the false lumen after surgery, aortic dissection. *Left*, prior to surgery, color Doppler shows flow in the false lumen; *right*, after surgery the false lumen is reduced, and no flow can be detected (*arrows*, color reverberations due to excessive "gain" of the Doppler signal). **a, b** Transverse view of the aortic arch. **c, d** Cross-sectional view of the descending aorta 30 cm from the incisors.

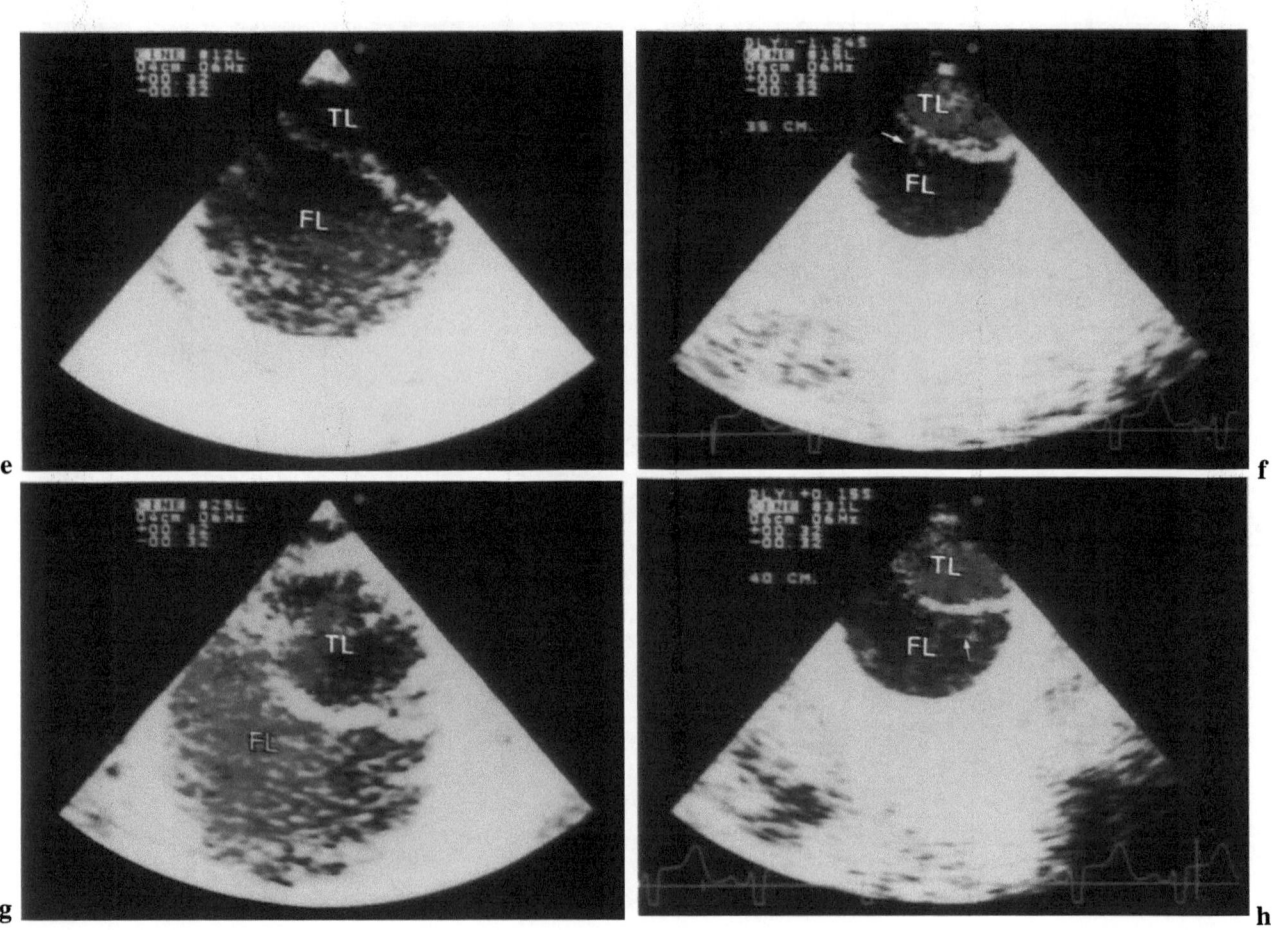

Fig. 2.51 e–h. *Left*, prior to surgery, color Doppler shows flow in the false lumen; *right*, after surgery the false lumen is reduced, and no flow can be detected (*arrows*, color reverberations due to excessive "gain" of the Doppler signal). **e, f** Cross-sectional view of the descending aorta at 35 cm. **g, h** Cross-sectional view of the descending aorta at 40 cm.

Thrombus Formation

Surgical deviation of aortic blood flow into the true lumen reduces blood flow velocity and allows thrombus formation in the false lumen. Obliteration of the false lumen by thrombus formation can be regarded as a favorable prognostic sign.

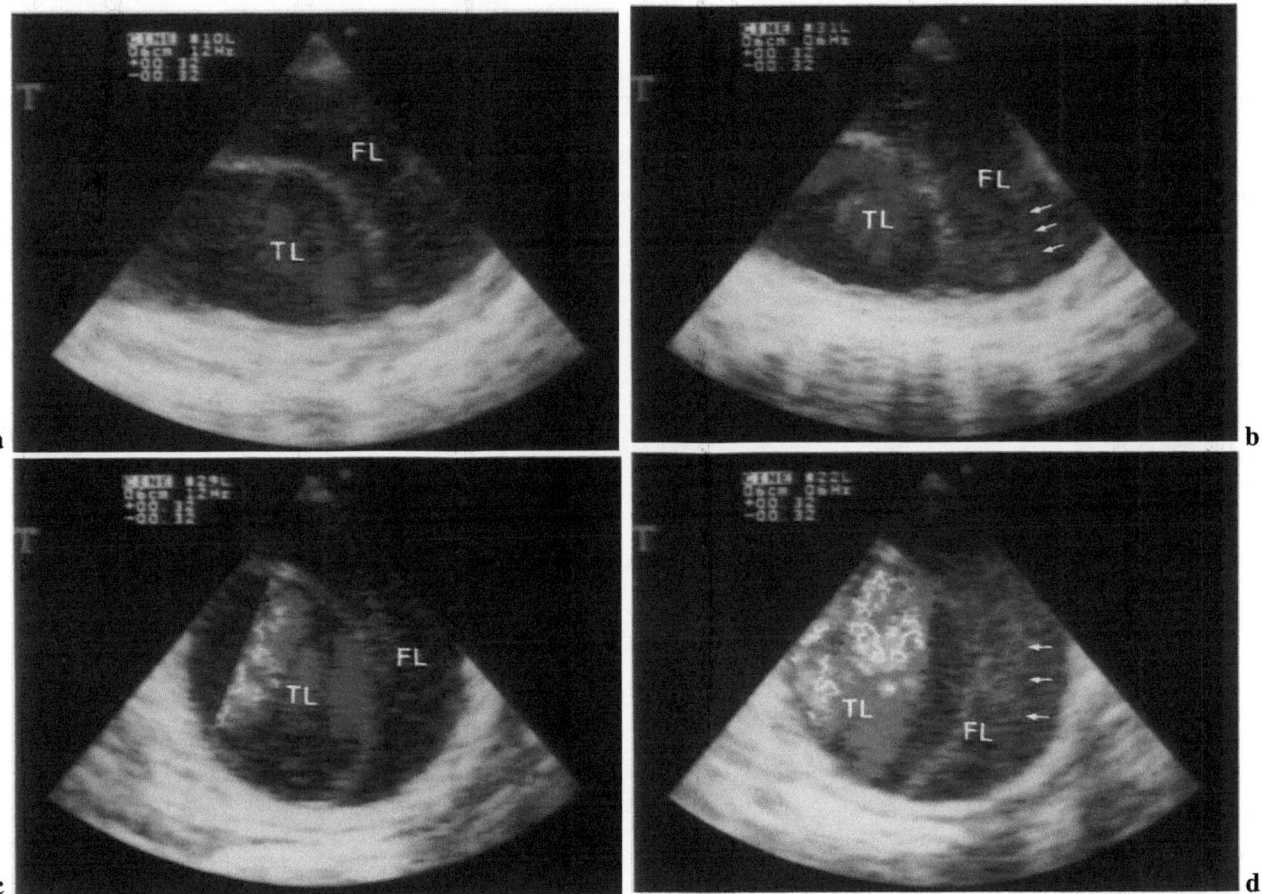

Fig. 2.52a–d. Thrombus formation in the false lumen after surgery, aortic dissection. The ascending aorta was replaced by a conduit that deviated the aortic flow into the true lumen. *Left*, immediately after surgery; *right*, 1 week after surgery the false lumen was partially occluded by thrombus formation (*arrows*). **a, b** Transverse view of the proximal tract of the descending aorta immediately distal to the aortic arch. **c, d** Transverse view of the descending aorta.

Reentry

TEE allows visualization of flow communication between true and false lumen (entry). The persistence
of flow in the false lumen after surgical repair of
proximal entry in the ascending aorta may be due to a
communication located distally in the descending
aorta (reentry).

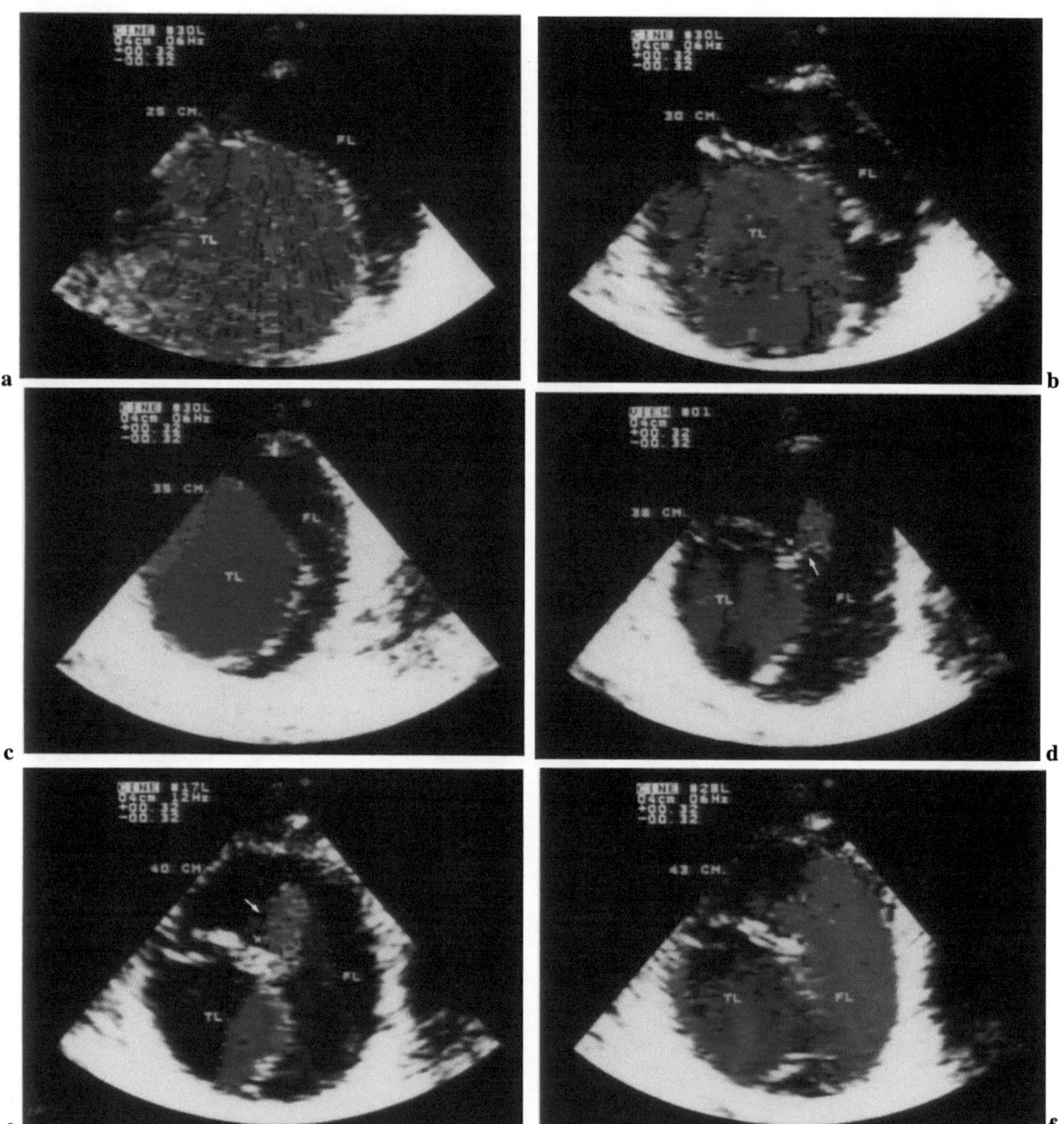

Valved Conduit

Surgical therapy of aortic dissection replaces the ascending aorta and/or the arch with or without the re- implantation of the coronary arteries and brachiocephalic vessels. The diseased segment of the aorta is replaced by a woven Dacron valved conduit that deviates the left ventricular ejection flow into the true lumen.

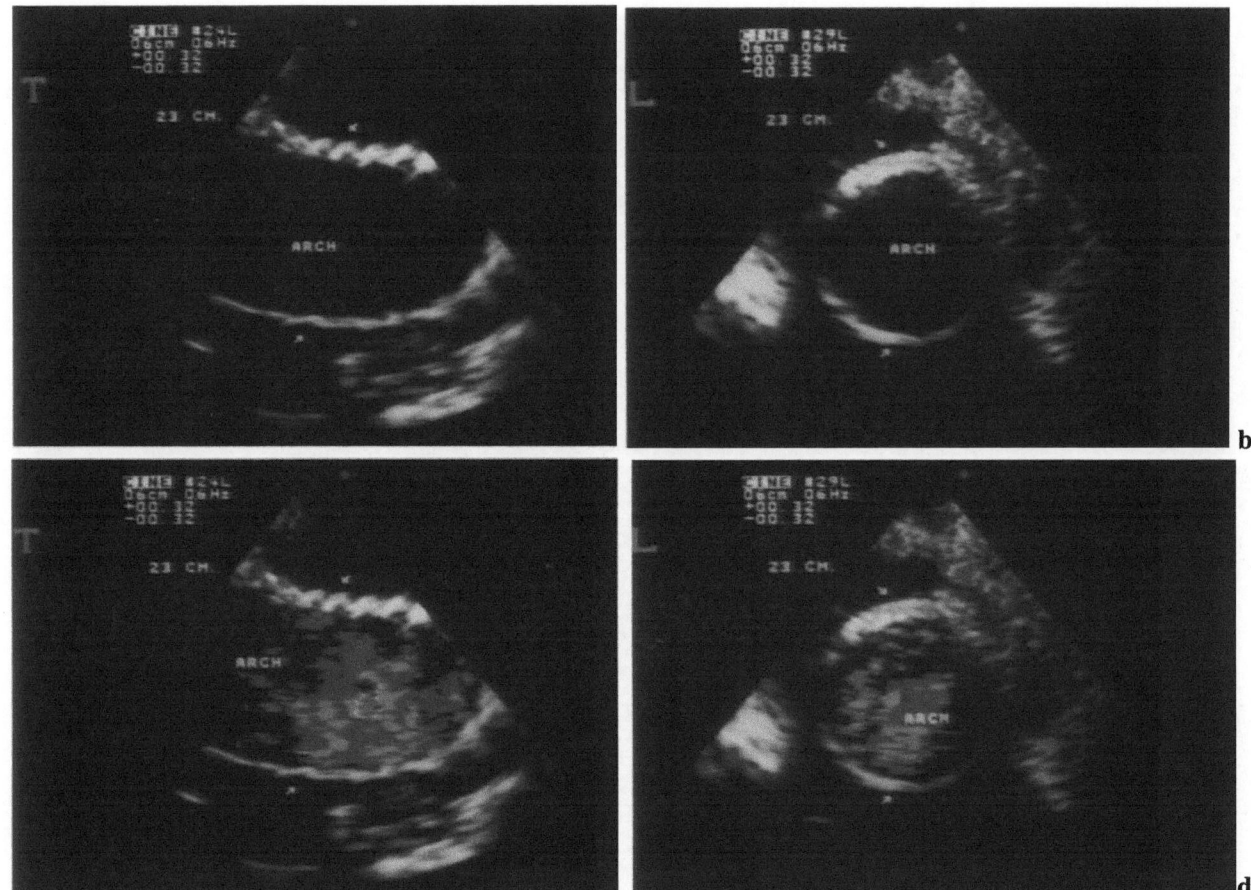

Fig. 2.54a–l. Valved conduit, aortic dissection. The patient underwent replacement of the aortic valve and ascending aorta with a valved Dacron conduit. **a, b** Transverse (left) and longitudinal (*right*) views of the conduit (*arrow*) at the level of the aortic arch. **c, d** Same frames as above, with color Doppler showing the flow in the prosthesis.

Fig. 2.53a–f. Reentry, aortic dissection. The patient underwent replacement of the ascending aorta with a valved conduit. A reentry with antegrade flow was found in the distal descending aorta 38–40 cm from the incisors. **a** Transverse view of the aortic arch just distal to the anastomosis. Turbulent flow in the true lumen (*TL*); absence of flow in the false lumen (*FL*). **b** Cross-sectional view of the descending aorta at 30 cm. Color Doppler shows flow in the true lumen and absence of flow in the false lumen. **c** Cross-sectional view of the descending aorta at 35 cm. Absence of flow in the false lumen. **d, e** Cross-sectional view of the descending aorta at 38 and 40 cm. *Arrows*, a reentry into the false lumen. **f** Cross-sectional view of the descending aorta at 43 cm. Presence of antegrade flow in the false lumen.

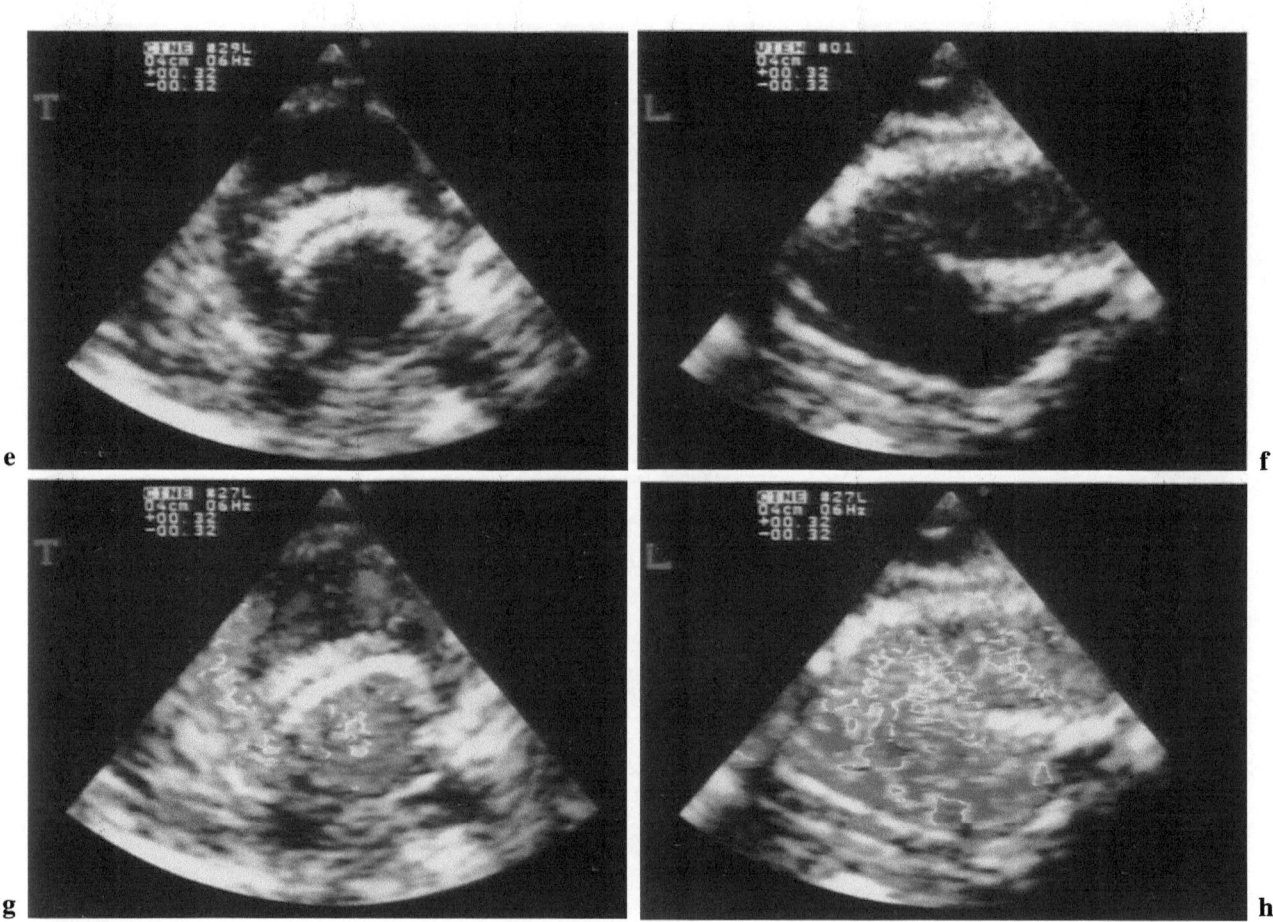

e

f

g

h

Fig. 2.54 e, f Transverse (*left*) and longitudinal (*right*) views of the conduit (*arrow*) at the level of the proximal descending branch of the aortic arch (depth, 26 cm). **g, h** Same frames as above, with color Doppler.

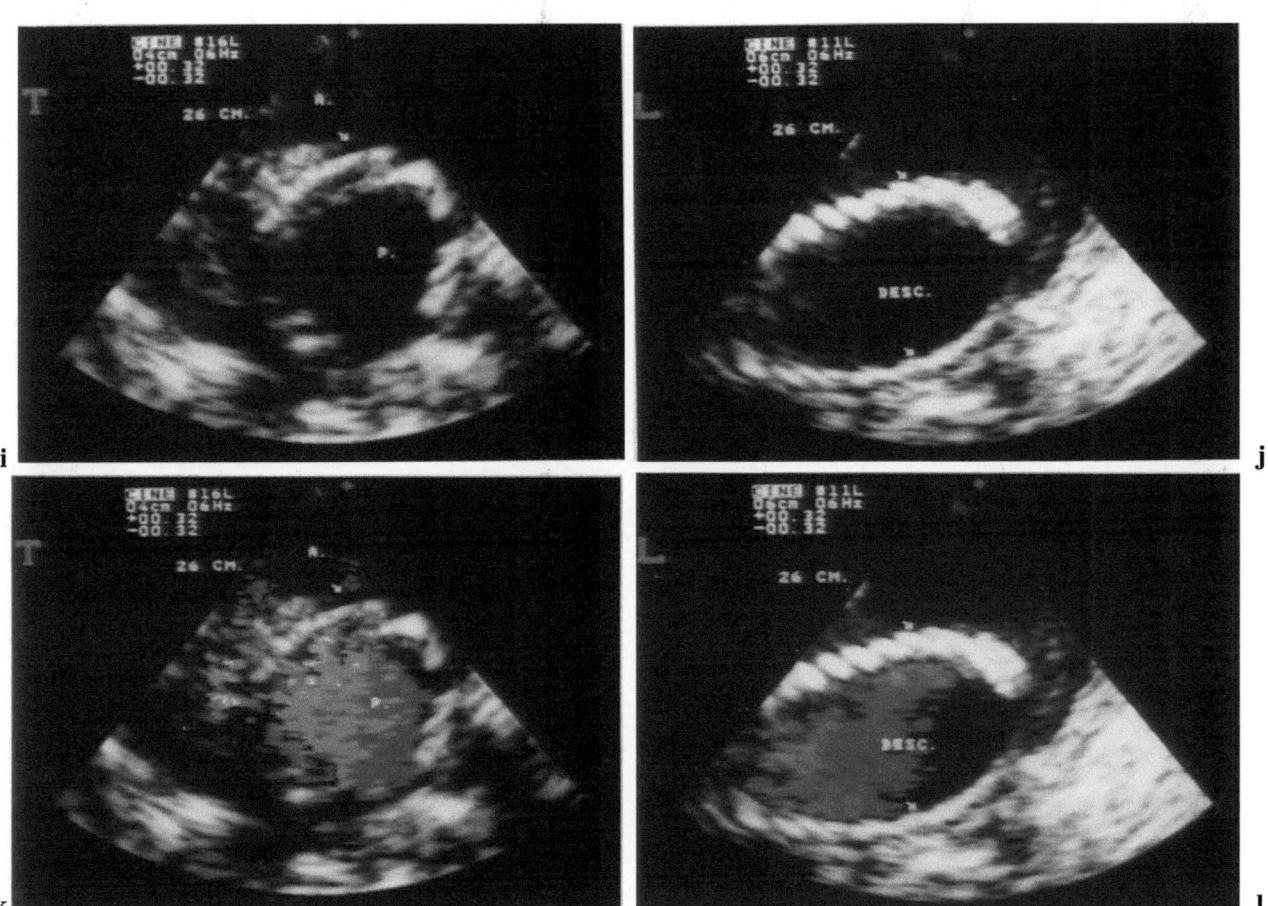

Fig. 2.54 i, j Transverse (left) and longitudinal (*right*) views of the distal end of the conduit at the level of the proximal descending aortic arch. **k, l** Same frames with color Doppler.

Cardiac Tumors

Intracardiac masses can be diagnosed and localized accurately by TEE. Benign tumors appear as pedunculated masses within the atria. Atrial myxomas are the most frequent finding. Malignant tumors may infiltrate the free walls of the ventricles. Tumor location and attachment and the visualization of the myocardial wall are important additional factors in the diagnosis of diverse tumor types.

Myxoma

Atrial myxomas are the most common tumors of the heart. The left atrium is the most frequent localization (75%). Right atrial myxomas are rare, and only occasional reports describe ventricular localization. Myxomas are generally pecunculated masses, attached to the area of the fossa ovalis. Clinical symptoms include systemic or pulmonary embolization and signs of mechanical obstruction to the left ventricular diastolic filling.

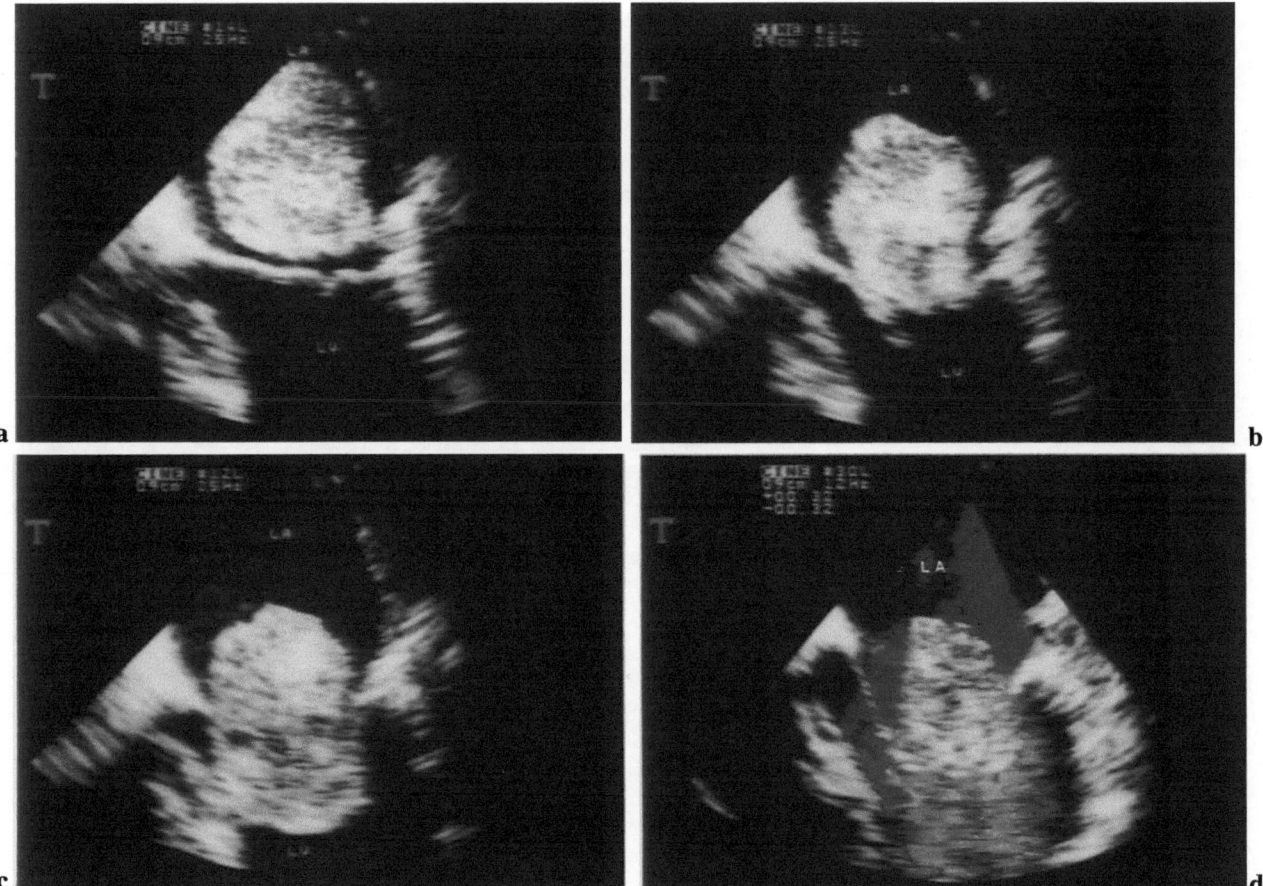

Fig. 2.55a–d. Myxoma of the left atrium. **a–c** Transesophageal four-chamber view. This sequence shows a pedunculated ovoid mass within the left atrium, protruding into the left ventricle in diastole. The tumor insertion could not be visualized by this imaging view. **d** Color Doppler. The tumor prolapses into the left ventricle through the mitral valve orifice, causing "functional" mitral stenosis (*turbulent flow*).

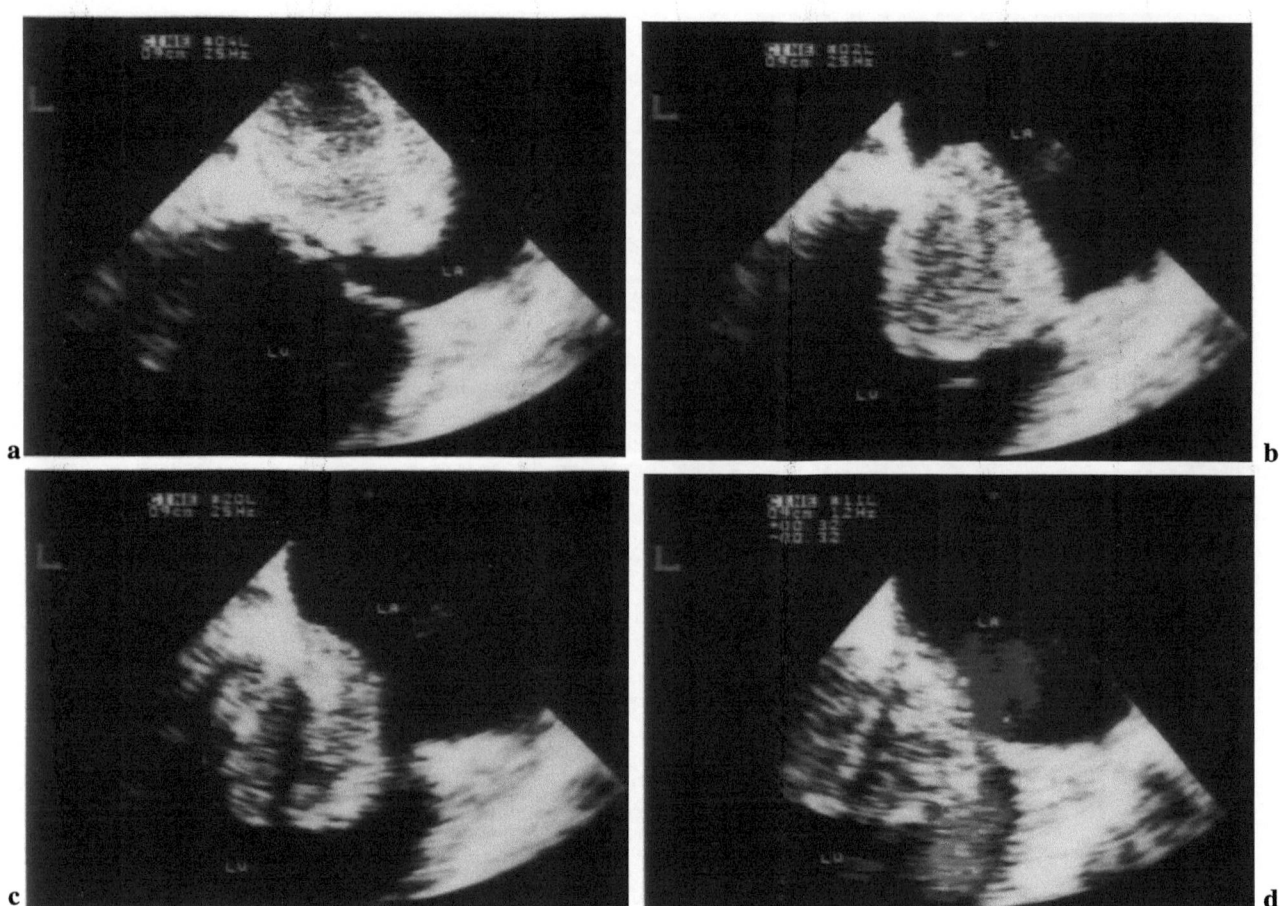

Fig. 2.56a–d. Myxoma of the left atrium. **a–c** LV-LA long-axis view. This sequence shows the tumor protruding into the left ventricle in diastole. The tumor attachment is localized at the posterior wall of the left atrium, close to the mitral valve annulus. **d** Color Doppler. The tumor prolapses into the left ventricle through the mitral valve orifice, causing obstruction to the diastolic filling of left ventricle (*turbulent flow*).

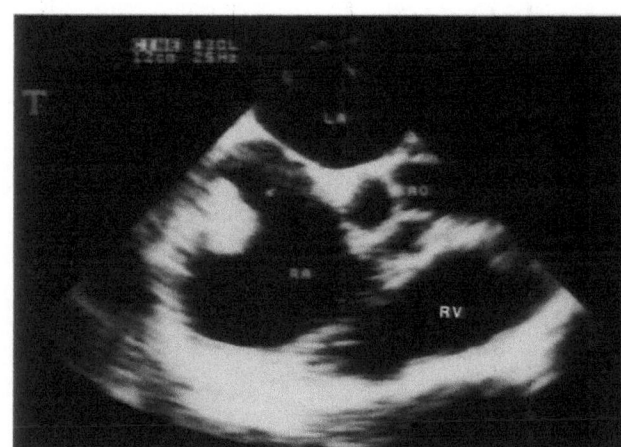
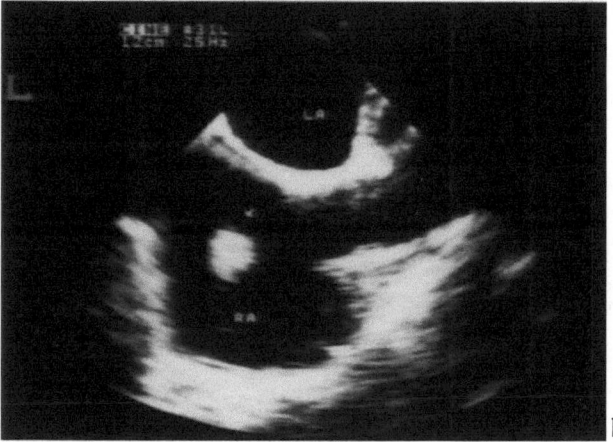

Fig. 2.57a, b. Right atrial myxoma, two-dimensional TEE. **a** *Arrow*, an ovoid mass within the right atrium consistent with myxoma. **b** Caval-atrial septal long-axis view. This longitudinal view shows the localization of the tumor insertion close to the orifice of the inferior vena cava.

Hemangioma

Hemangiomas are extremely rare benign vascular tumors of the heart. They may be localized in any part of the heart. Surgical removal may be difficult or impossible if massive infiltration of cardiac wall occurs.

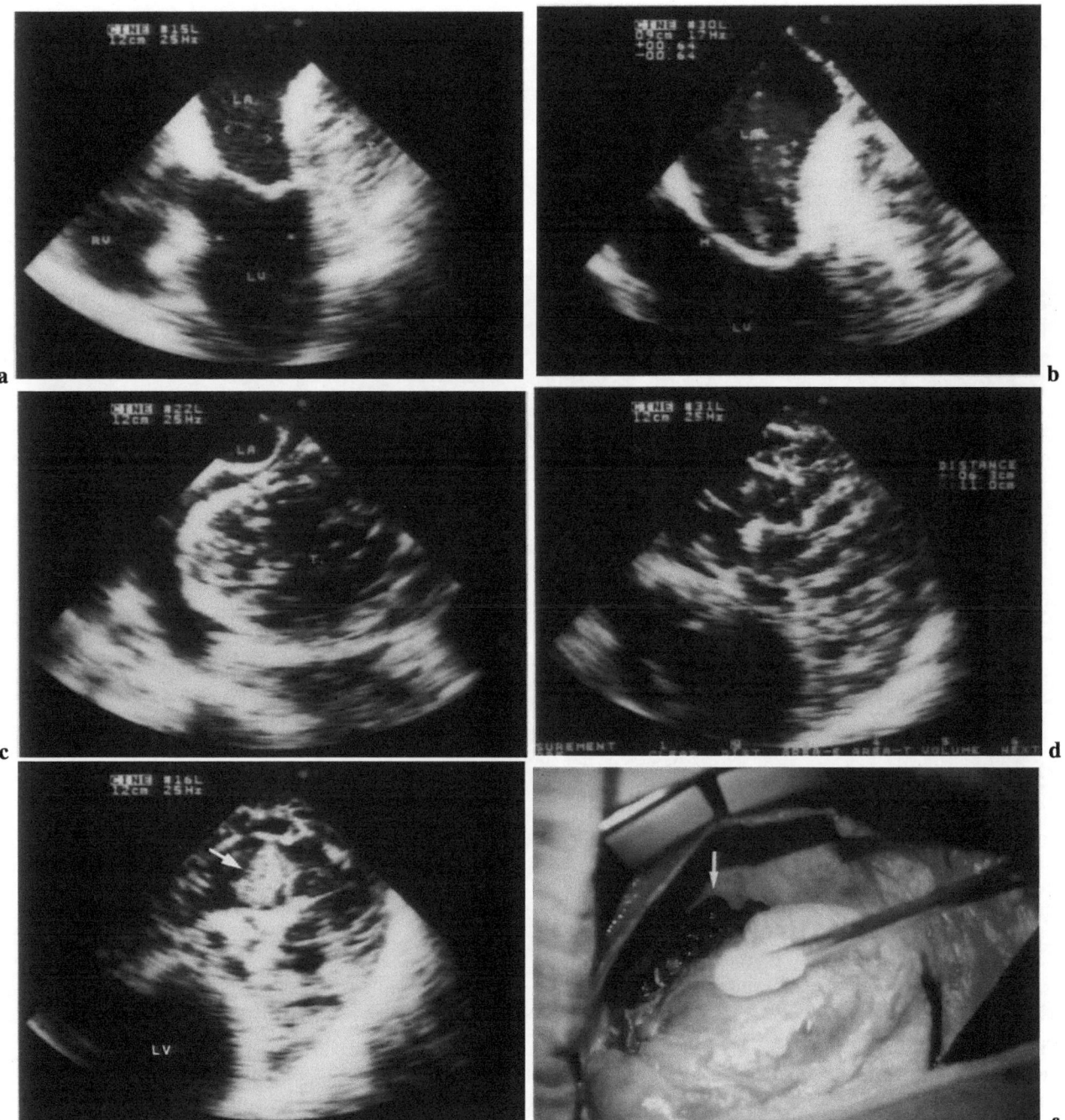

Fig. 2.58 a–f. Cardiac hemangioma. **a** Four-chamber view. A large extracardiac mass (*T*) compresses the left atrium and the left ventricle. The atrial (<) and the ventricular septum (*) appear thickened by infiltration. **b** Magnification of the left atrium. The arrows indicate the tumor compressing the left atrial wall. **c** The tumor can be visualized by rotating the transducer posteriorly. The tumor shows a cavernous appearance. **d, e** Transgastric short-axis views. *Arrow*, thrombus. It was not possible to remove the tumor because a large portion of the posterior wall and right ventricle were infiltrated. **f** Intraoperative view. Histological examination revealed a cavernous hemangioma.

Sarcoma

Sarcoma is the most common type of malignant tumor of the heart. It may proliferate intracavitarily or infiltrate the myocardial walls. Surgical removal is usually impossible. Pericardial invasion of the tumor produces pericardial effusion and tamponade.

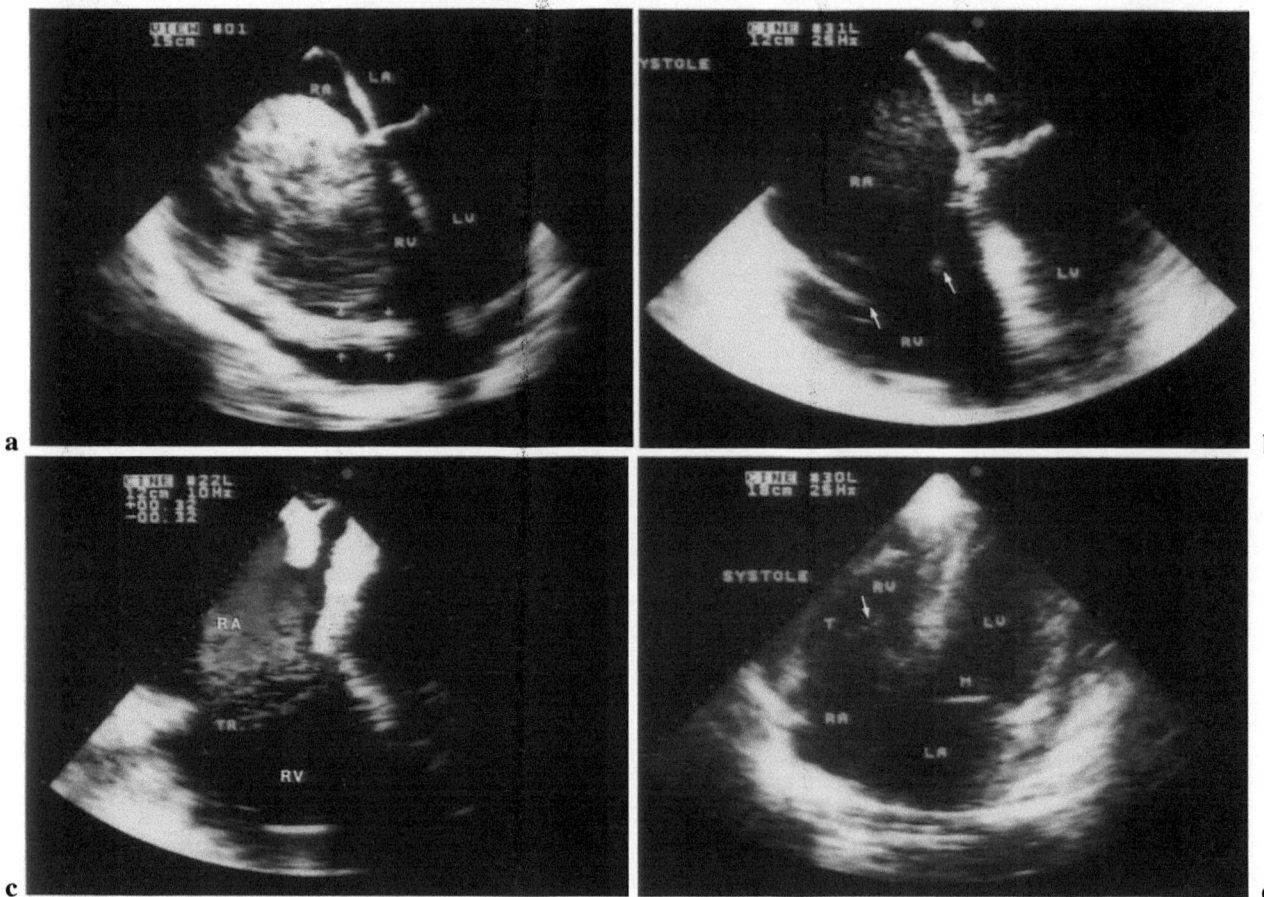

Fig. 2.59a–d. Cardiac sarcoma. **a** Four-chamber view shows a large mass occupying the right atrium and right ventricle. The abnormal thickening of the right ventricular wall (*arrows*) and the pericardial effusion are signs suggesting malignancy. Histological examination revealed a neurogenic sarcoma. **b** After the extirpation of the tumor incomplete systolic closure of the tricuspid valve occurred (*arrows*). Right atrium and ventricle are dilated. **c** Color Doppler shows severe tricuspid regurgitation. No surgical repair of the tricuspid valve was performed. **d** Transthoracic echocardiography. After 2 weeks the right atrium and right ventricle were reduced, and the tricuspid valve closed properly (*arrow*).

Extracardiac Tumors

Tumors originating elsewhere may invade the heart by infiltrating the walls, compressing the cavities or invading the cardiac chambers. Tumors of the kidney may invade the inferior vena cava and grow until protruding into the right atrium. A combined abdominal and thoracic surgical approach is necessary to remove the tumor.

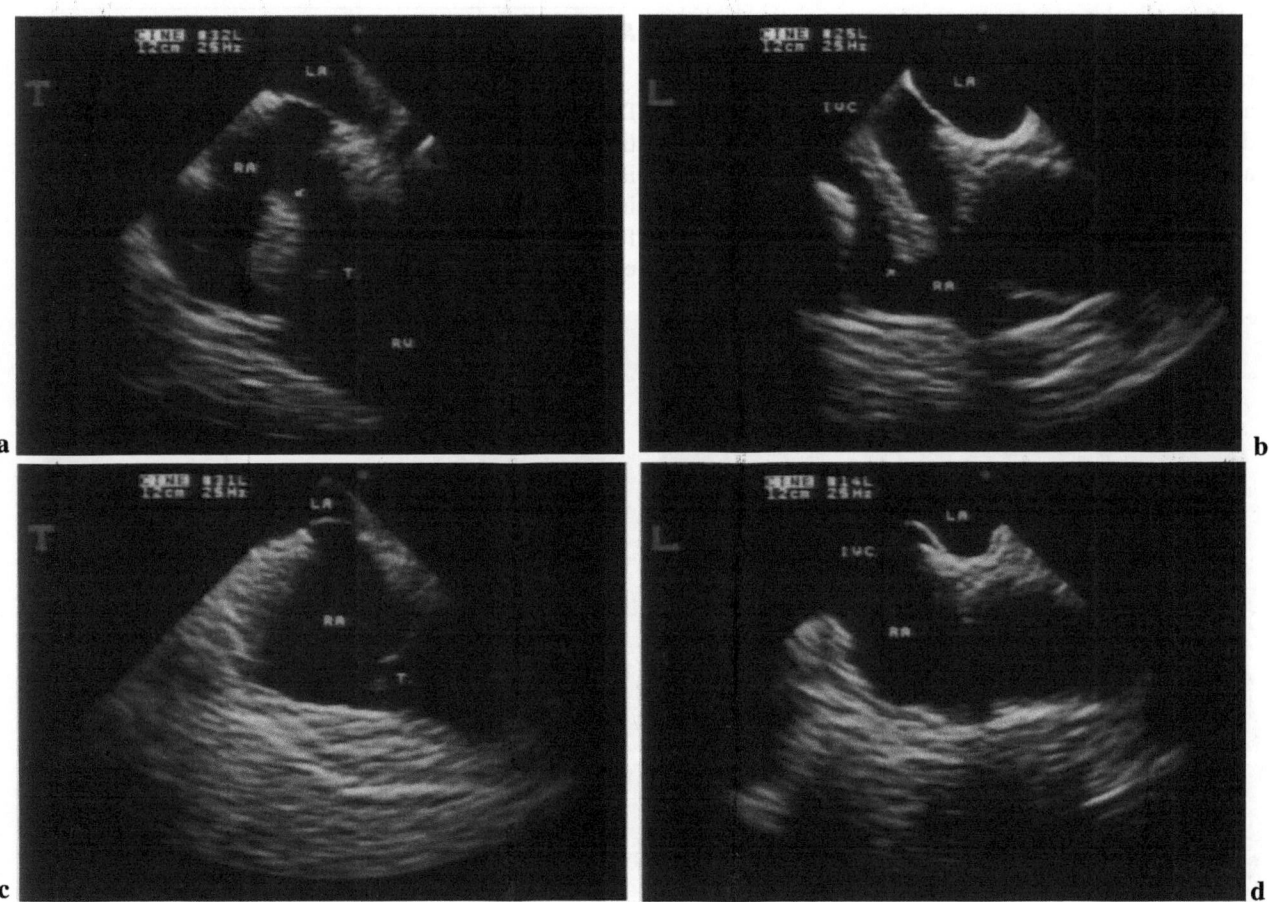

Fig. 2.60a–d. Extracardiac tumor, renal tumor protruding into the right atrium. **a** Transversal four-chamber view. *Arrow*, the extremity of the renal tumor protruding in the right atrium. **b** Longitudinal caval–atrial septal view shows the provenience of the finger like structure (tumor) from the inferior vena cava (*IVC*). **c, d** Transversal (*T*) and longitudinal (*L*) views after the extirpation of the tumor. Note: the tumor was removed by laparotomy in conjunction with thoracotomy and extracorporeal circulation.

Left Ventricular Aneurysm

Left ventricular aneurysm may occur in patients with coronary heart disease as a complication of transmural myocardial infarction. Rupture of the heart may arise acutely with cardiac tamponade and sudden death, or develop chronically, resulting in a "false" aneurysm.

Aneurysm

Diagnosing and quantifying the extent of aneurysmatic enlargement of the heart can be accomplished easily by two-dimensional TEE. Three-dimensional imaging of the myocardial wall may add further useful information on the extent and function of the aneurysm.

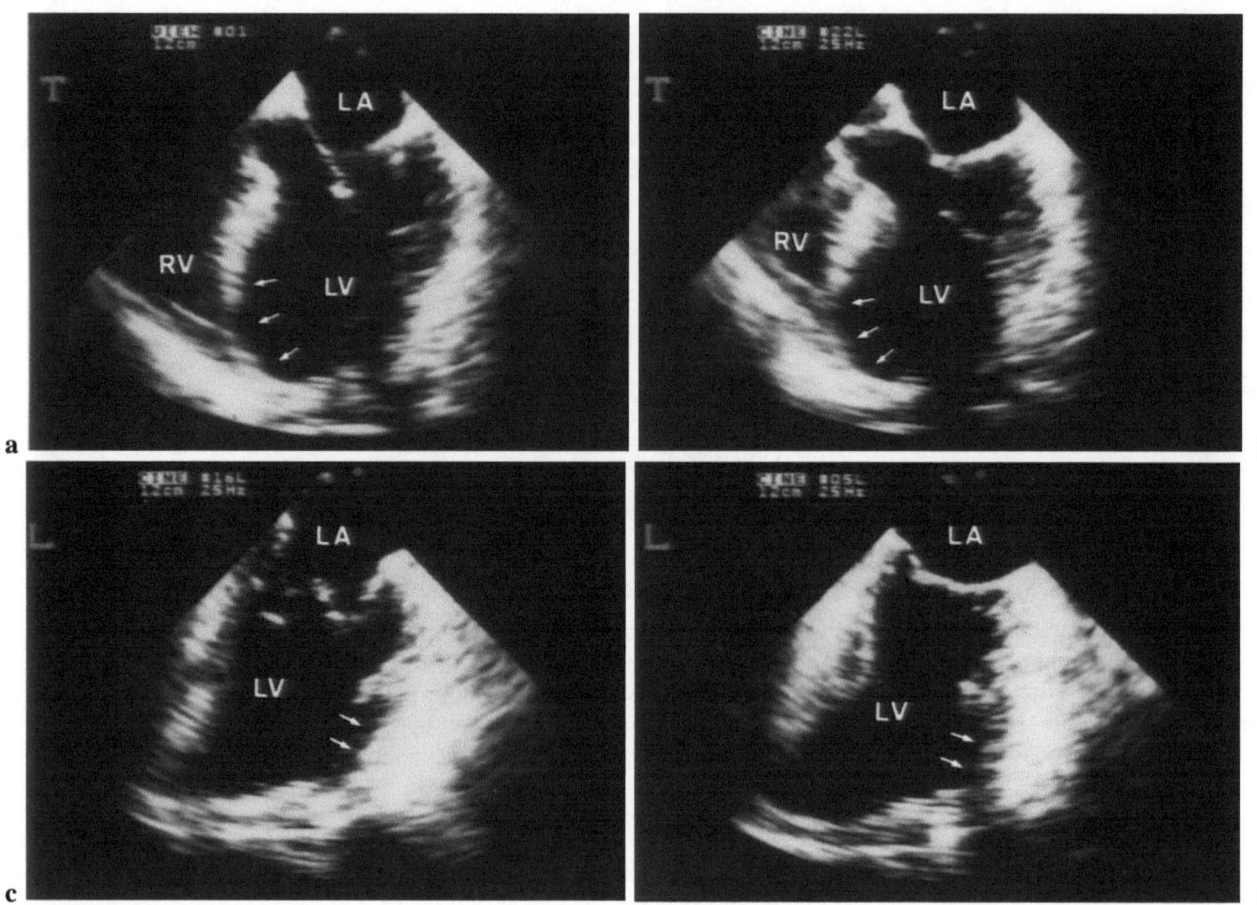

Fig. 2.61a–d. Left ventricular aneurysm. The patient had a large aneurysm involving the anterior wall of the left ventricle, the apex, and the apical portion of the ventricular septum. **a, b** Four-chamber view. *Arrows*, aneurysmatic dilatation of the apex and apical portion of the ventricular septum. **c, d** Corresponding longitudinal views. *Arrows*, aneurysm of the anterior wall. **a, c** Diastole. **b, d** Systole.

Pseudoaneurysm

Rupture of the heart and the formation of a "false aneurysm" of the heart is life threatening and may lead to sudden death.

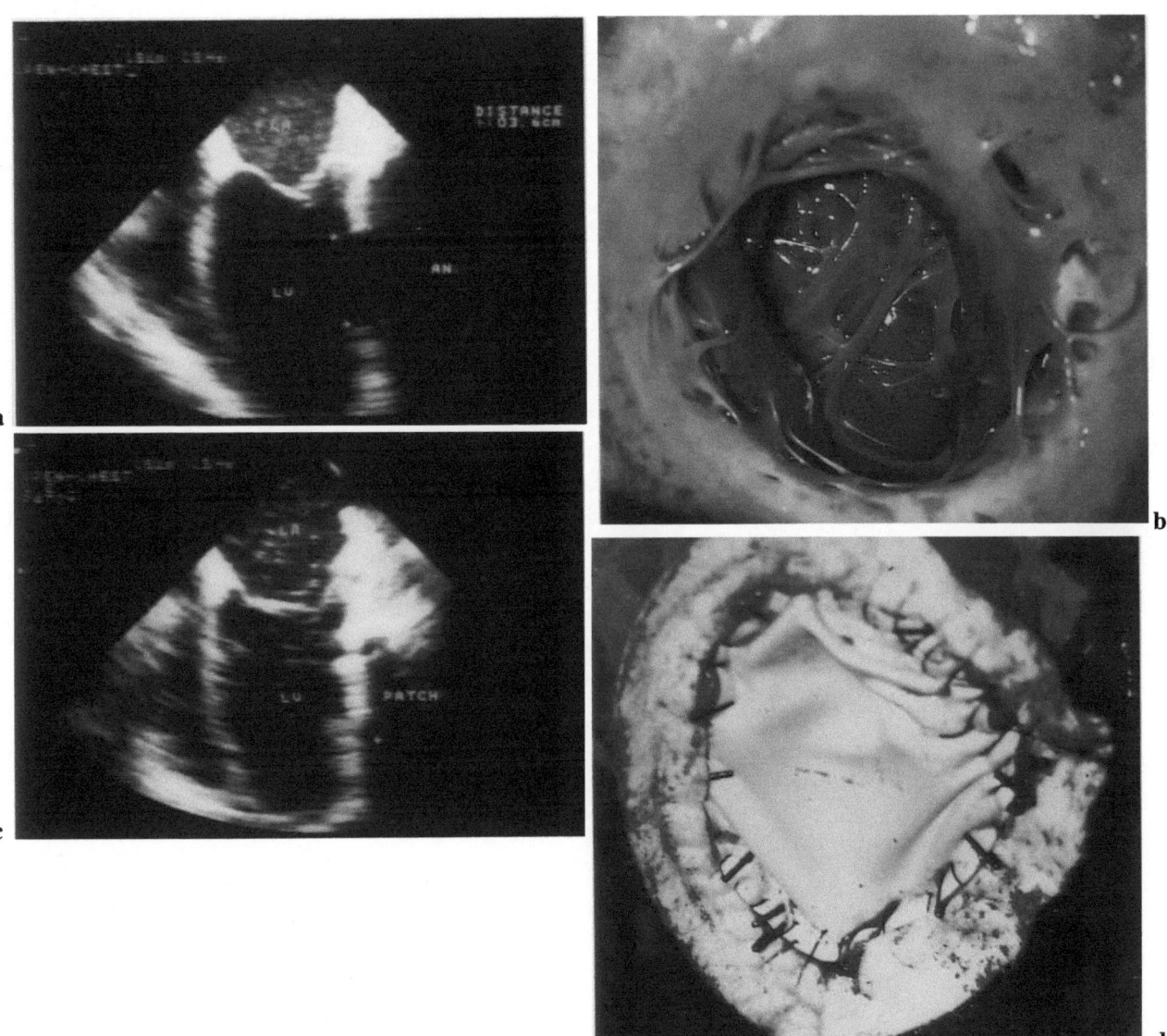

Fig. 2.62a–d. Pseudoaneurysm, left ventricular aneurysm with rupture. **a** Four-chamber view. *Arrows*, a large echo dropout of the posterolateral wall of the left ventricle. This was in communication with a large false aneurysm (*AN*) of the left ventricle. **b** Intraoperative view of the pseudoaneurysm. Border between fibrotic tissue and viable myocardium. **c** Four-chamber view after the resection of the aneurysm and closure of the defect with a patch. *Arrows*, patch. **d** Intraoperative view of the patch.

Cardiomyopathies

Cardiomyopathies are diseases affecting primarily the myocardium. The functional classification, based on the pathophysiological abnormality, includes three forms: dilated, hypertrophic, and restrictive.

Dilated Cardiomyopathy

Dilated (or congestive) cardiomyopathy is characterized by dilatation of cardiac chambers and poorly contracting left ventricle. The clinical manifestations of this disease are symptoms of congestive heart failure.

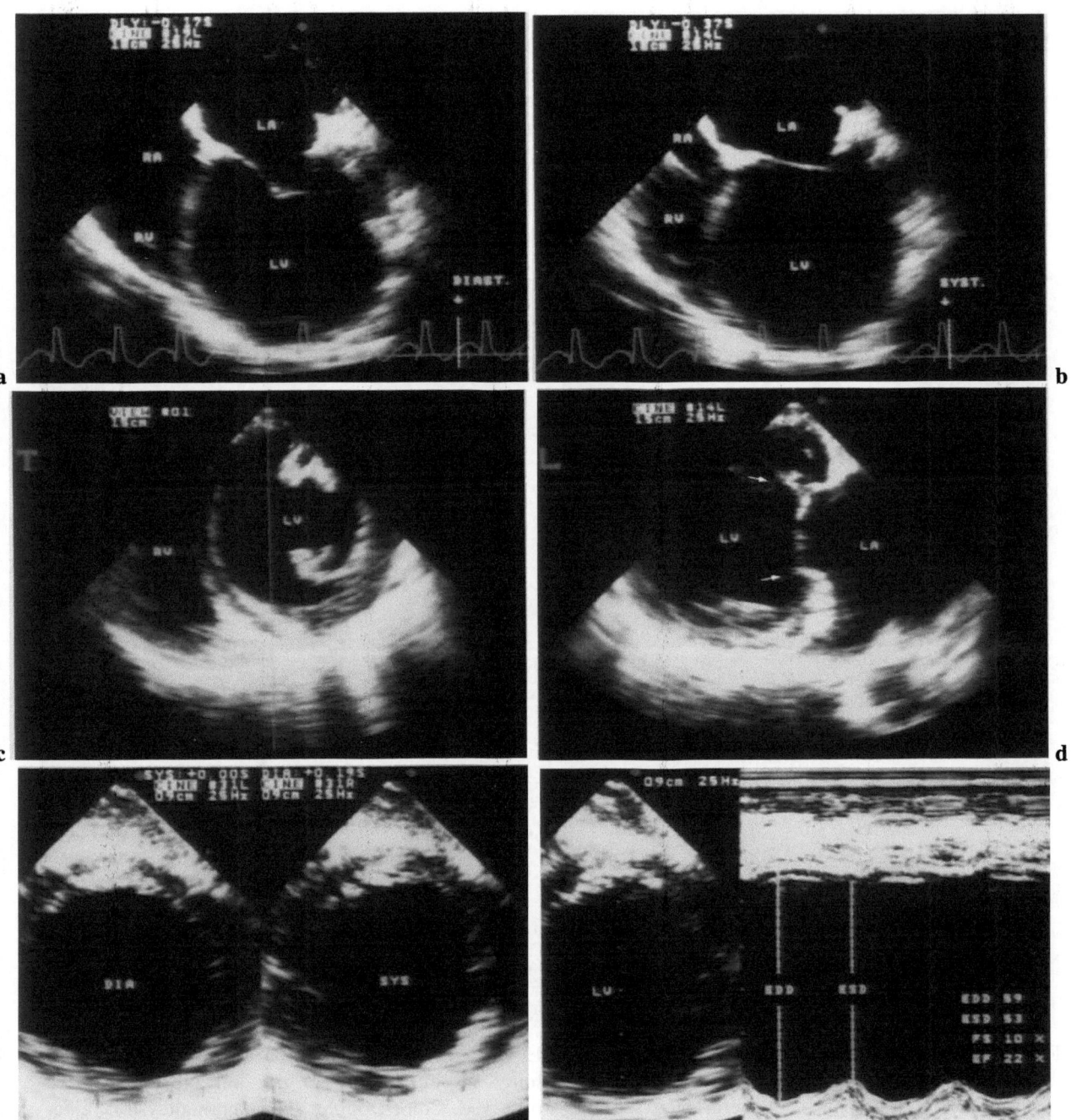

Fig. 2.63a–f. Dilated cardiomyopathy. **a, b** Four-chamber views show massive dilatation of the left ventricle. Left ventricular function is highly impaired (*left*, diastole; *right*, systole). **c, d** Transgastric views of left ventricle. The transverse (**c**) and the corresponding longitudinal (**d**) views show dilatation of the left ventricle. *Arrows*, mitral subvalvular apparatus. **e** Transgastric short-axis view, two-dimension-al echocardiography. The transverse section of the left ventricle shows poor changes in the systodiastol-ic cross-sectional area. **f** Transgastric short-axis view, M-mode echocardiography. Fractional shortening of left ventricular transverse diameter is extremely reduced. *EDD*, End-diastolic diameter; *ESD*, end-systolic diameter; *FS*, fractional shortening; *EF*, ejection fraction.

Hypertrophic Obstructive Cardiomyopathy

Hypertophic obstructive cardiomyopathy is characterized by marked myocardial hypertrophy of unknown cause. The hypertrophy involves especially the upper part of the interventricular septum. This "asymmetrical" septal hypertrophy may cause obstruction to the left ventricular outflow. Hypertrophic cardiomyopathy may occur with or without obstruction.

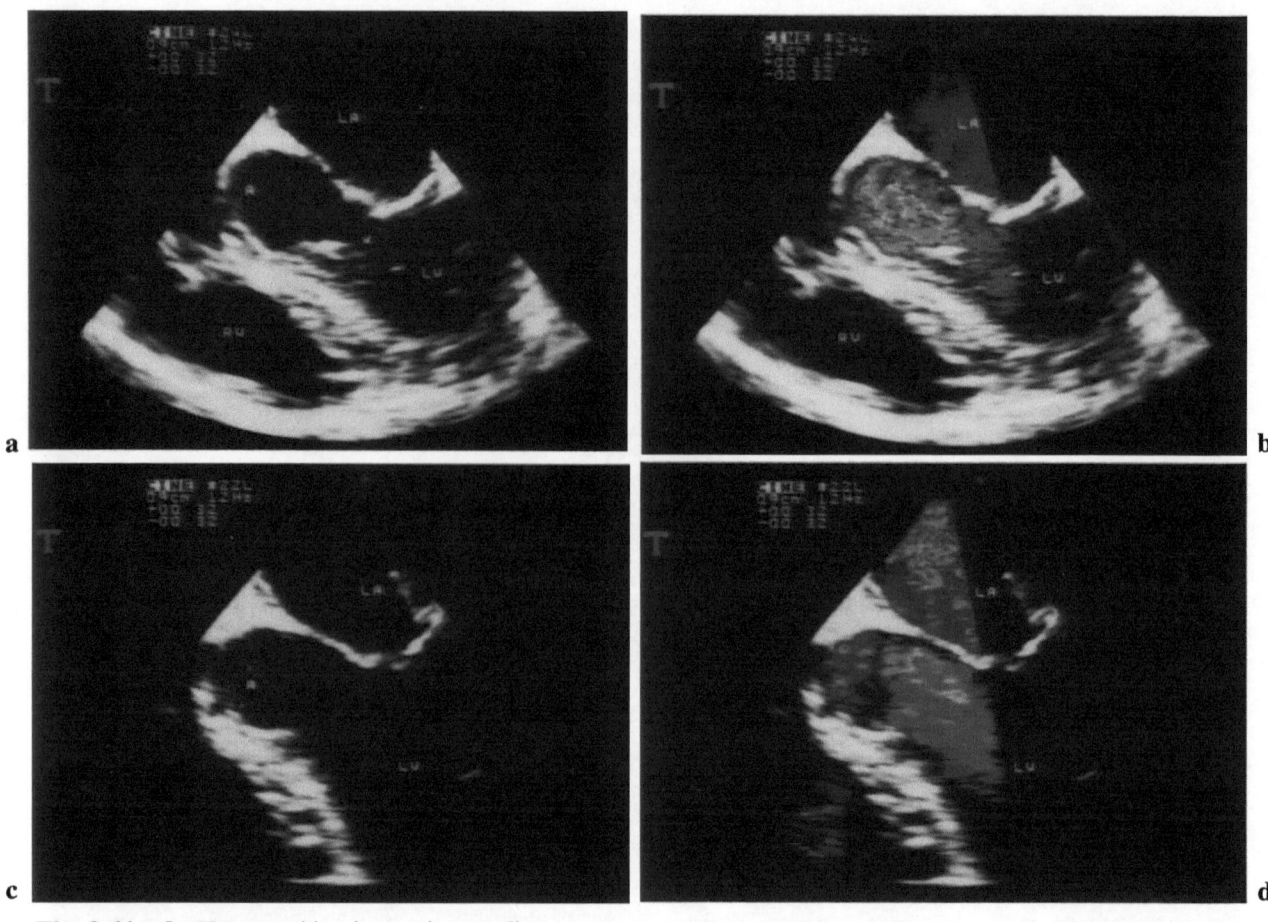

Fig. 2.64a, b. Hypertophic obstructive cardiomyopathy. **a** Two-dimensional TEE, LVOT view. *Arrow*, asymmetrical hypertrophy of the ventricular septum. **b** Color Doppler shows the obstruction to the left ventricular outflow. Turbulent flow (*mosaic*) in the LVOT beyond the obstruction. **c, d** After septal myotomy no obstruction to the left outflow can be observed. Color Doppler shows normal systolic ejection flow (*red*) in the LVOT.

Restrictive Cardiomyopathy

Restrictive cardiomyopathy is characterized by marked myocardial thickening due to interstitial infiltration. The left and the right ventricular cavities are usually small. The hallmark of restrictive cardiomyopathy is diastolic dysfunction. The myocardial thickening makes the heart incapable of receiving an adequate filling volume to maintain sufficient cardiac output.

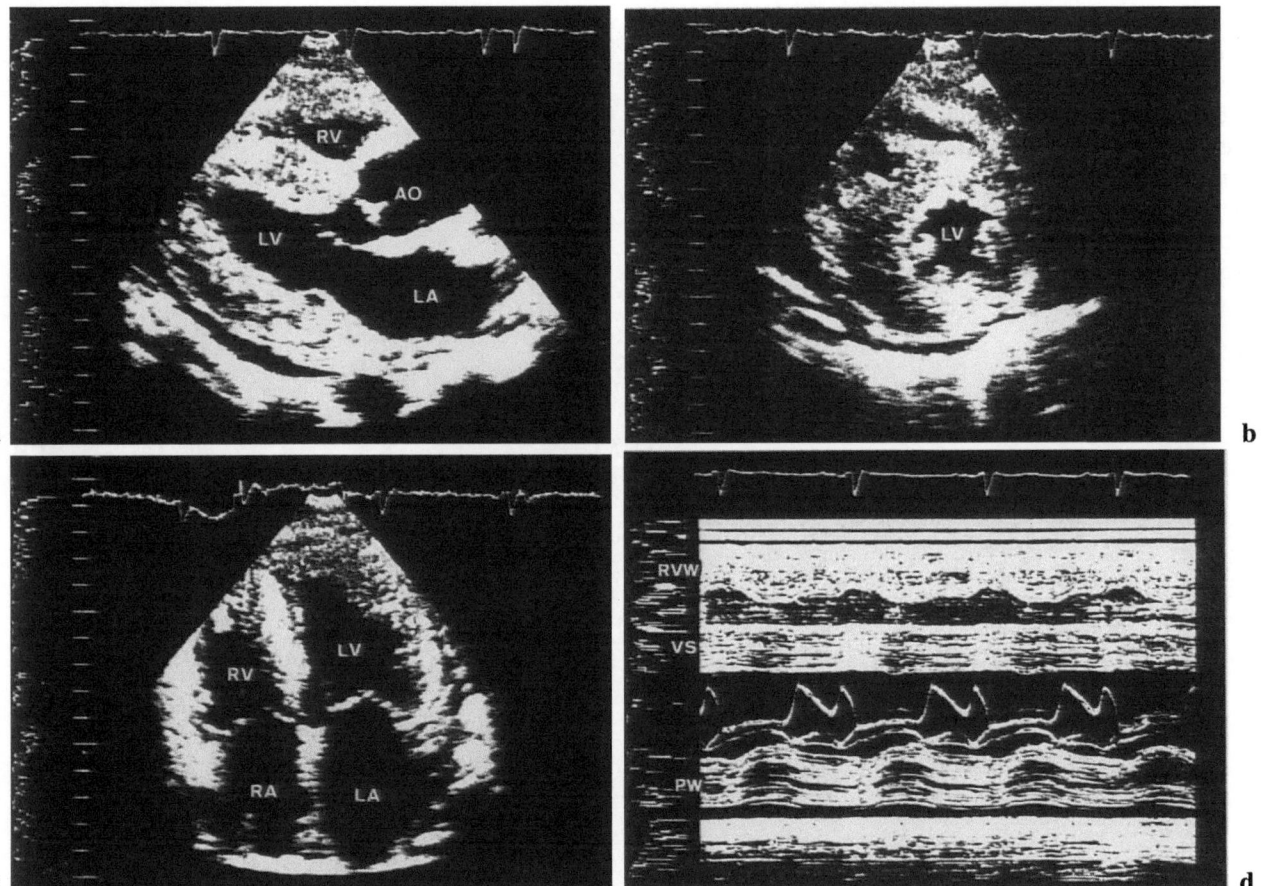

Fig. 2.65 a–d. Restrictive cardiomyopathy in a patient with cardiac amyloidosis. Transthoracic echocardiography. **a** Parasternal long-axis view. **b** Parasternal short-axis view. The myocardial wall is thickened and shows the typical increased refractility known as "granular sparkling." **c** Four-chamber view. The thickening of the right ventricular wall is evident. **d** M-mode shows the global thickening of the myocardial walls, including the posterior wall (*PW*), ventricular septum (*VS*), and right ventricular wall (*RVW*). (From De Simone R et al. (1989) Echocardiographic features of cardiac amyloidosis. Cardiovascular Imaging 1(4):61–64.)

Pericardial Effusion

Pericardial effusion is one of the most frequent complications following cardiac surgery. Echocardiography is very useful for detecting pericardial effusion and the signs of tamponade, such as compression of the right atrium and diastolic collapse of the right ventricle. The following figures show various degrees of pericardial effusion after cardiac surgery. The volume of the pericardial effusion is not predictive of the occurrence of cardiac tamponade.

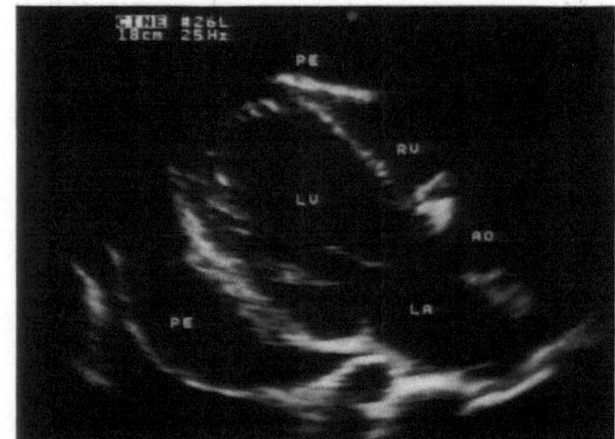

a

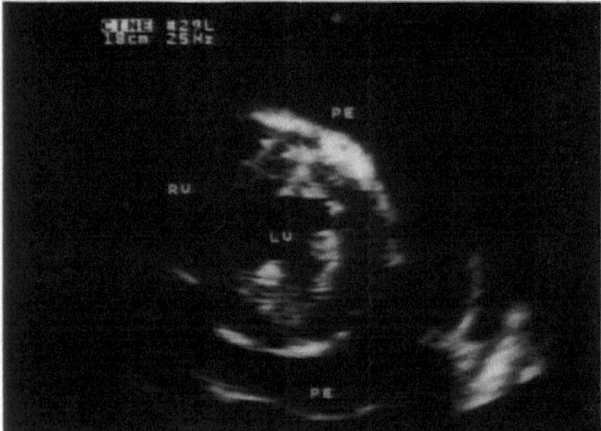

b

Fig. 2.66a, b. Pericardial effusion, transthoracic echocardiography. **a** Parasternal long-axis view. Pericardial effusion (*PE*) surrounding the entire heart. No compression of the right atrium or diastolic collapse of the right ventricle is present. **b** Parasternal short-axis view. Same patient as in **a.**

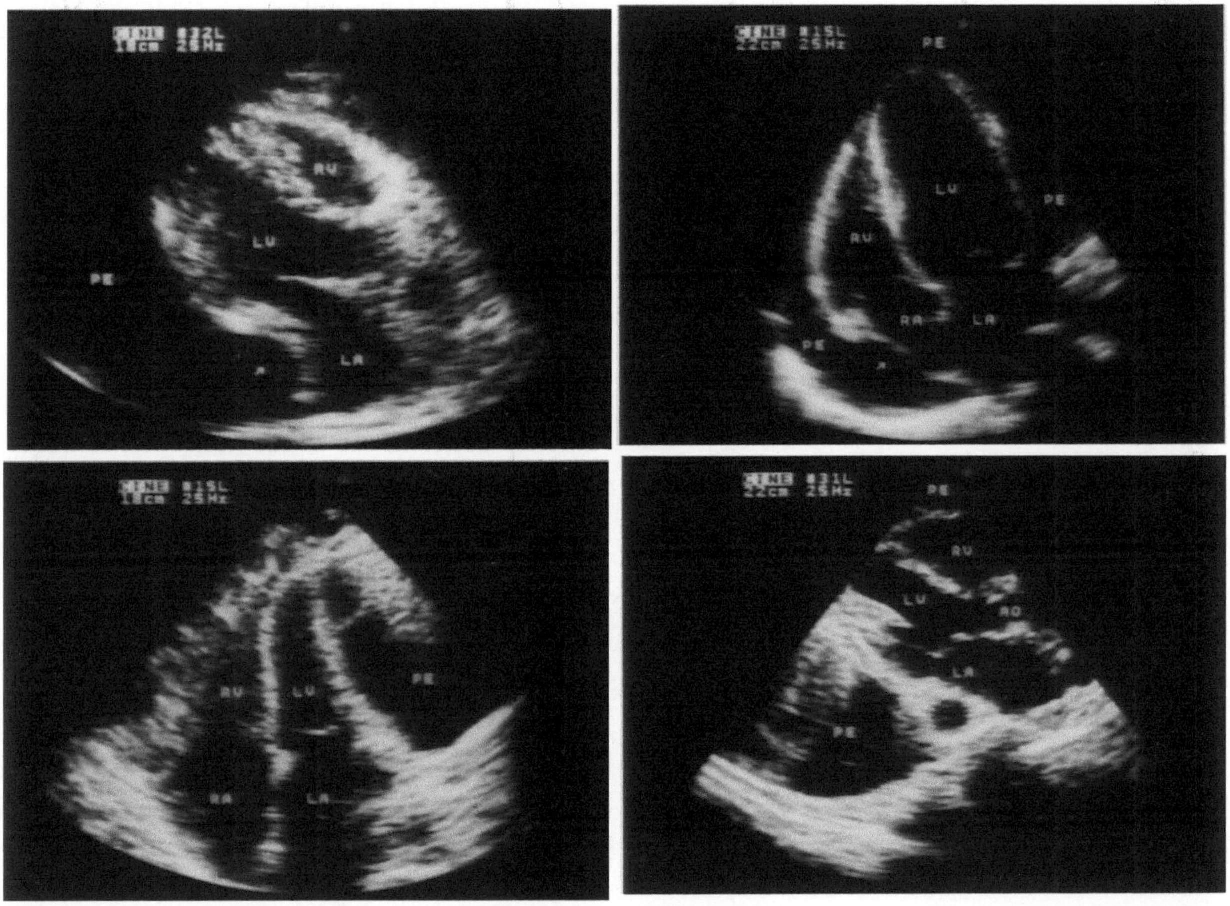

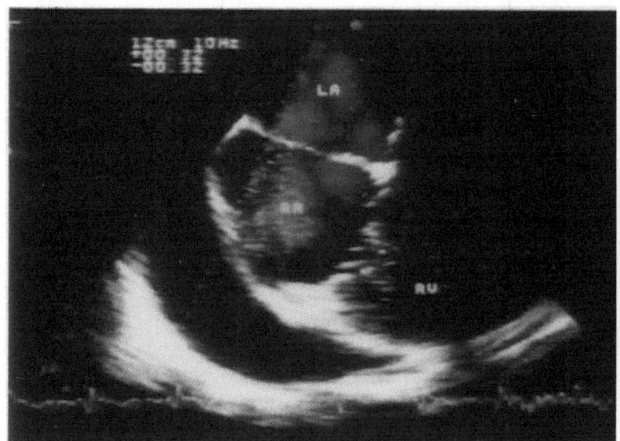

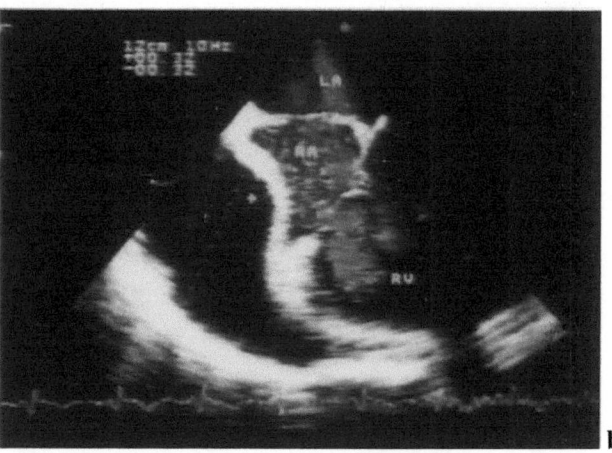

Fig. 2.67 a–d. Cardiac tamponade. Transthoracic echocardiography. **a** Parasternal long-axis view. Pericardial effusion (*PE*) surrounding the heart. The wall of the left atrium shows diastolic compression (*arrow*). **b** Four-chamber view. Pericardial effusion (*PE*) and atrial compression (*arrow*). **c** Four-chamber view shows a large pericardial effusion (*PE*) which compresses the left ventricle. **d** Parasternal long-axis view. Very large pericardial effusion posterior to the heart without signs of cardiac tamponade. Note: the volume of the pericardial effusion is not predictive of the occurrence of cardiac tamponade.

Fig. 2.68 a, b. Cardiac tamponade, TEE. Four-chamber view shows a pericardial effusion (*PE*) posterior to the right atrium. **a** Systole. **b** Diastole. *Arrow* (**b**), diastolic compression of the right atrium, a sign of cardiac tamponade.

Atrial Septal Defects

The diagnosis of atrial septal defect (ASD) can easily be obtained by conventional transthoracic echocardiography. An increasing number of patients with ASD are referred to surgery without angiography.

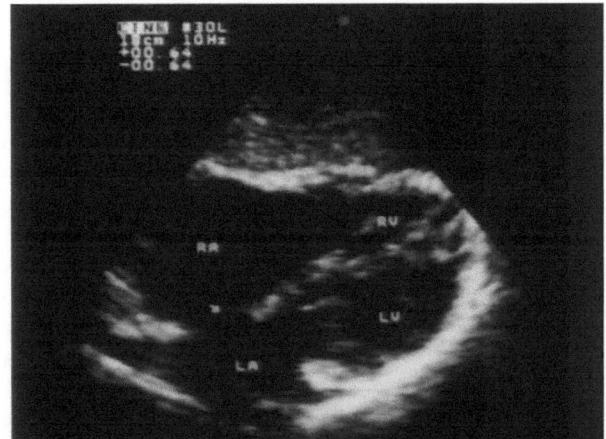

Fig. 3.1a, b. ASD, conventional transthoracic echocardiography, subcostal four-chamber view. **a** A large echo dropout (*arrow*) of the superior portion of the atrial septum. **b** Left-to-right shunt (*red*) across the defect.

3 Congenital Heart Disease

Conventional transthoracic echocardiography is a well-established technique that provides high-quality images for the diagnosis and management of congenital heart disease. Despite the rapid expansion of indications for TEE in adult patients, the use of TEE in pediatric patients is still limited. TEE in children with congenital heart disease has a number of limitations: (a) it cannot be performed without deep sedation; (b) the images produced by pediatric TEE probes are of lesser quality than those for adults since the transducers contain fewer elements; (c) the great arteries of the heart are poorly visualized due to the interposition of the left main bronchus between the esophagus and the heart; and (d) the probes for small children lack biplanar or multiplanar transducers.

Nevertheless, TEE does provide additional information. The structures that can be optimally visualized by TEE are the atrial cavities, atrial septum, atrioventricular valves, and LVOT. The RVOT and ascending aorta can be studied by biplanar TEE.

Patent Foramen Ovale

Patent foramen ovale is due to incomplete fusion of the membrane of the fossa ovalis. The defect can be diagnosed in adult asymptomatic patients.

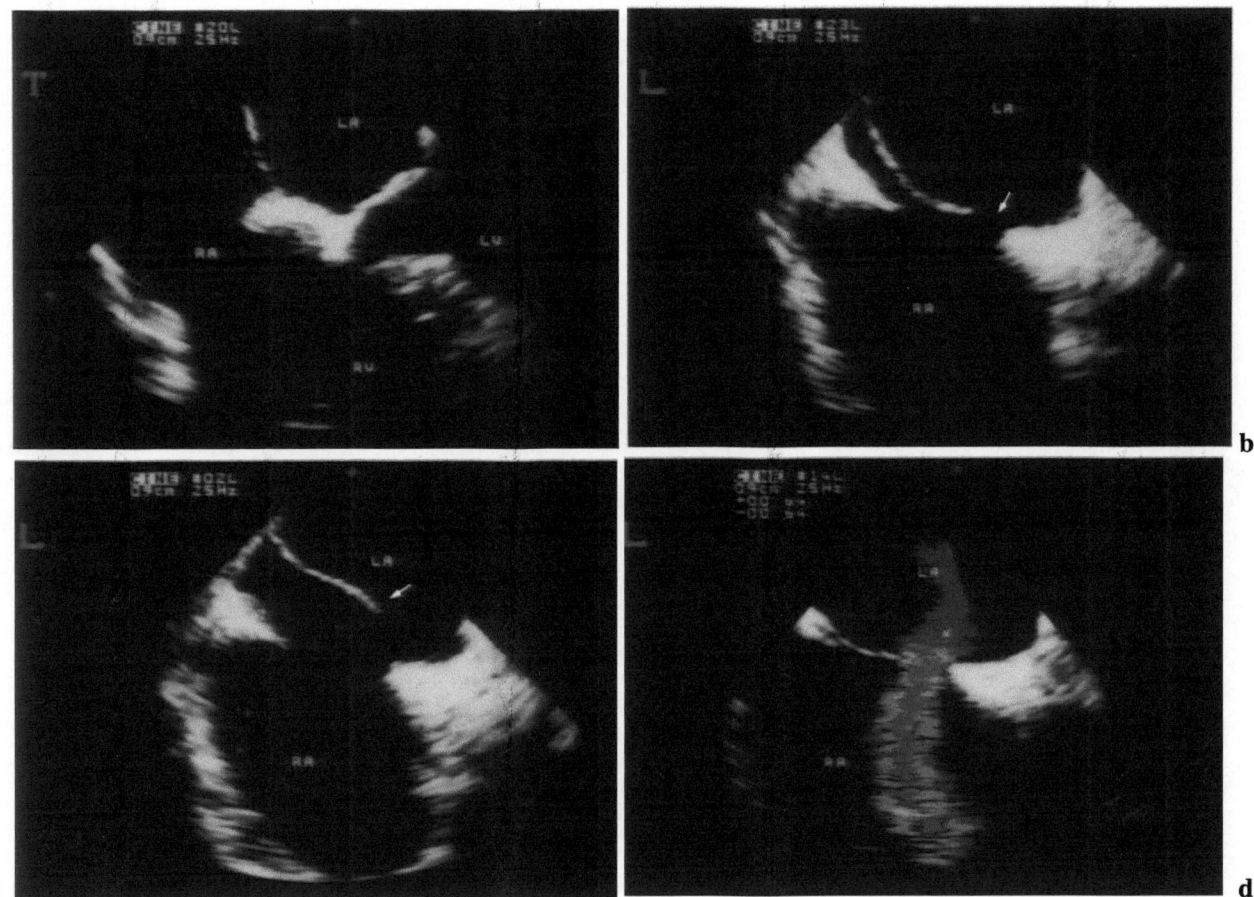

Fig. 3.2a–d. Patent foramen ovale. **a** Two-dimensional TEE, four-chamber view. The ASD cannot be visualized. **b** Caval-atrial septal long-axis view. *Arrow*, ASD. **c** Incomplete closure of the valve of the fossa ovalis. *Arrow*, floating membrane of the fossa ovalis. **d** Color Doppler shows the left-to-right shunt across the defect.

Ostium Secundum ASD

Ostium secundum defect consists of a tissue deficiency of the middle portion of the atrial septum between the orifices of the superior and inferior venae cavae.

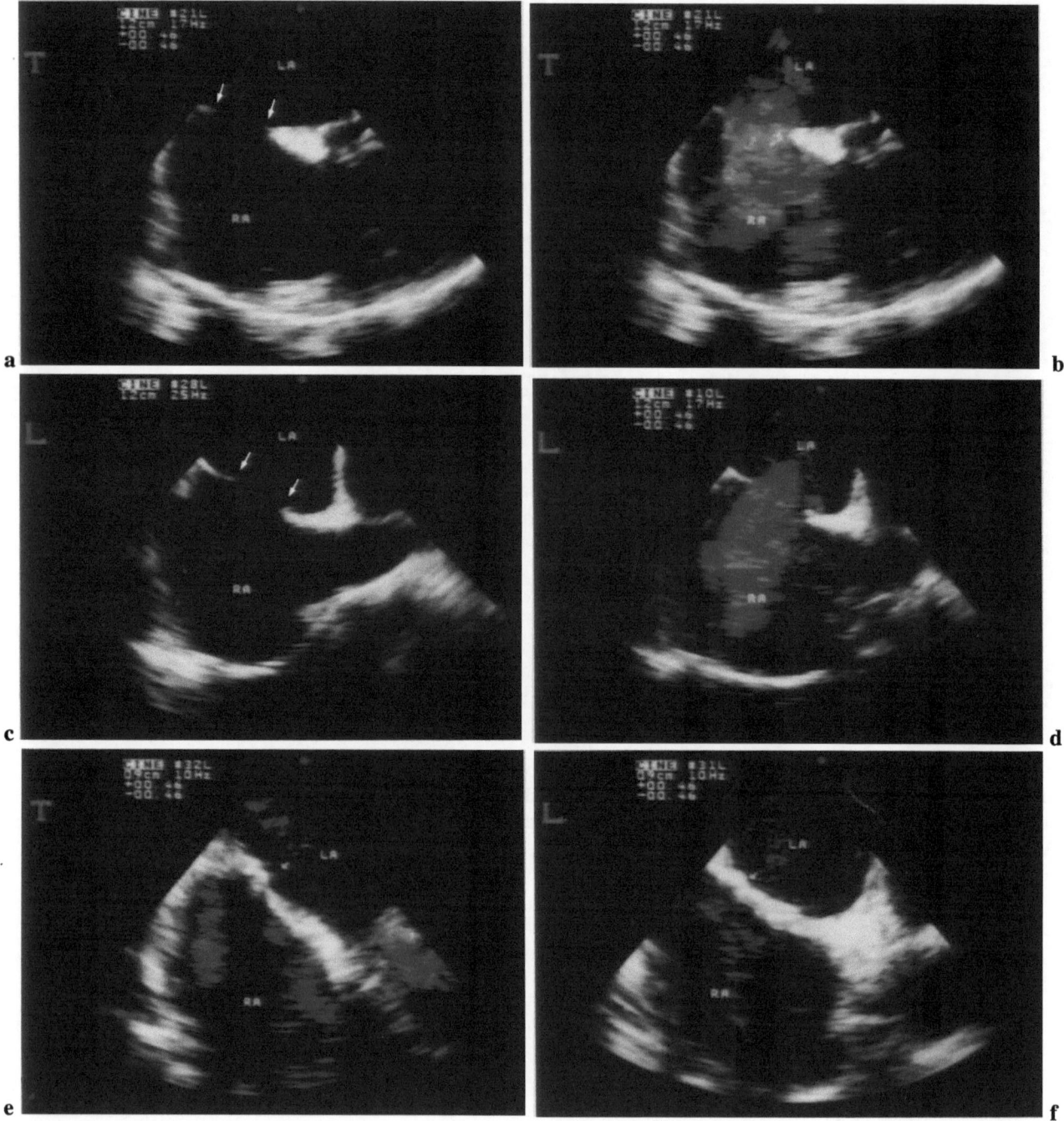

Bidirectional Shunt

In ASD the shunt flow across the defect is directed mainly from the left to the right atrium. Bidirectional shunt or shunt inversion can be observed in patients with pulmonary valve obstruction or high pulmonary vascular resistances.

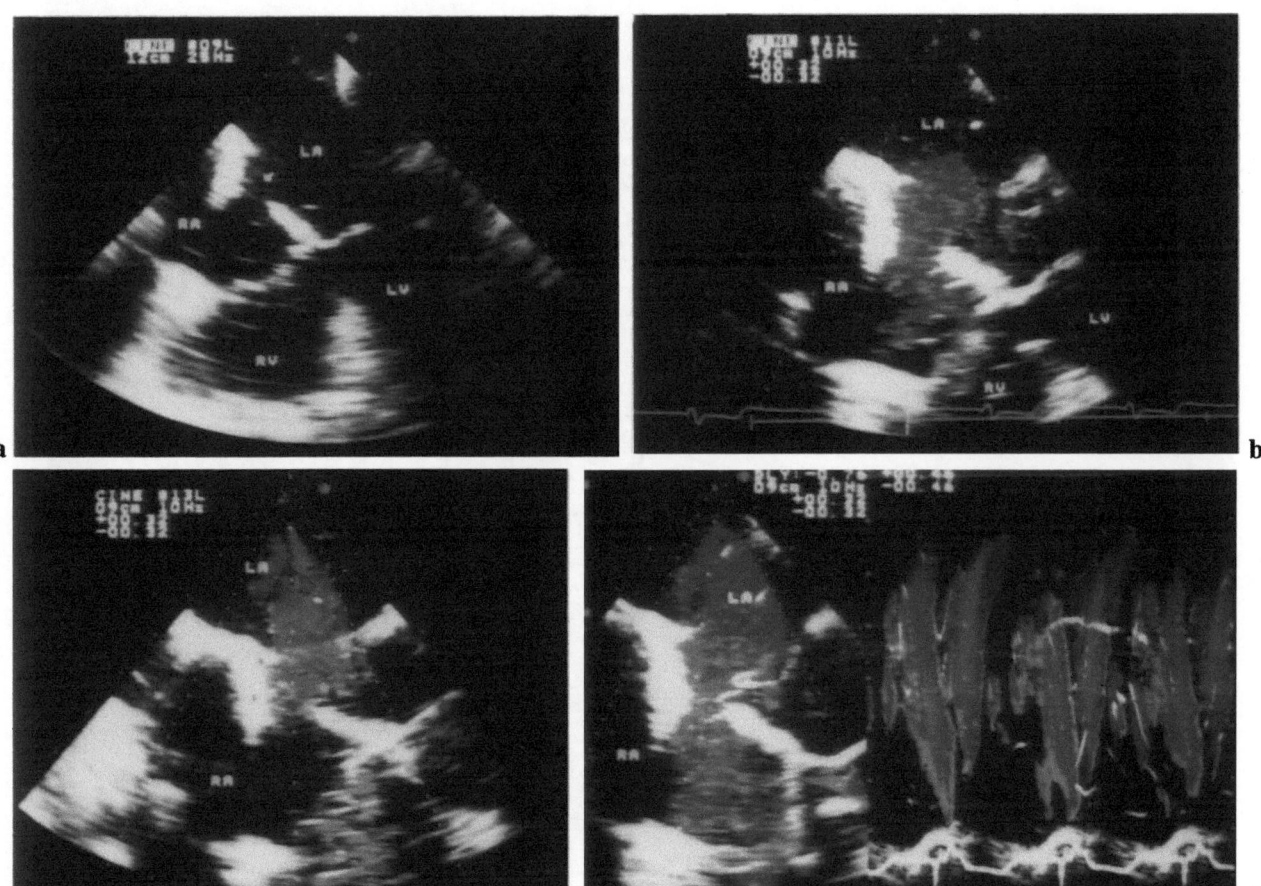

Fig. 3.4a–d. Bidirectional shunt across the ASD in a patient with single ventricle and double outlet right ventricle. **a** Two-dimensional TEE shows the ASD (*arrow*). **b** Left-to-right shunt (*blue*) across the defect. **c** Right-to-left shunt (*red*). **d** M-mode color Doppler. The M-mode line placed across the ASD shows a bidirectional shunt (*blue*, left-to-right shunt; *red*, right-to-left shunt).

Fig. 3.3a–f. Secundum ASD. Two-dimensional TEE shows an echo dropout (*arrows*) of the superior portion of atrial septum (*left*). Color Doppler shows a left-to-right shunt (*blue*) across the defect (*right*). **a,** **b** Transversal four-chamber view. **c, d** Caval-atrial septal long-axis view. **e, f** After repair. *Arrow*, patch. able residual shunt flow. Transversal four-chamber view (**e**) and caval-atrial septal long-axis view (**f**).

Echocontrastography

Venous injection of contrast can improve the value of echocardiography for the diagnosis of ASD. A left-to-right shunt appears as a wash-out of the contrast injected in the right atrium; a right-to-left shunt can be diagnosed by the direct visualization of contrast passage from right to left chambers.

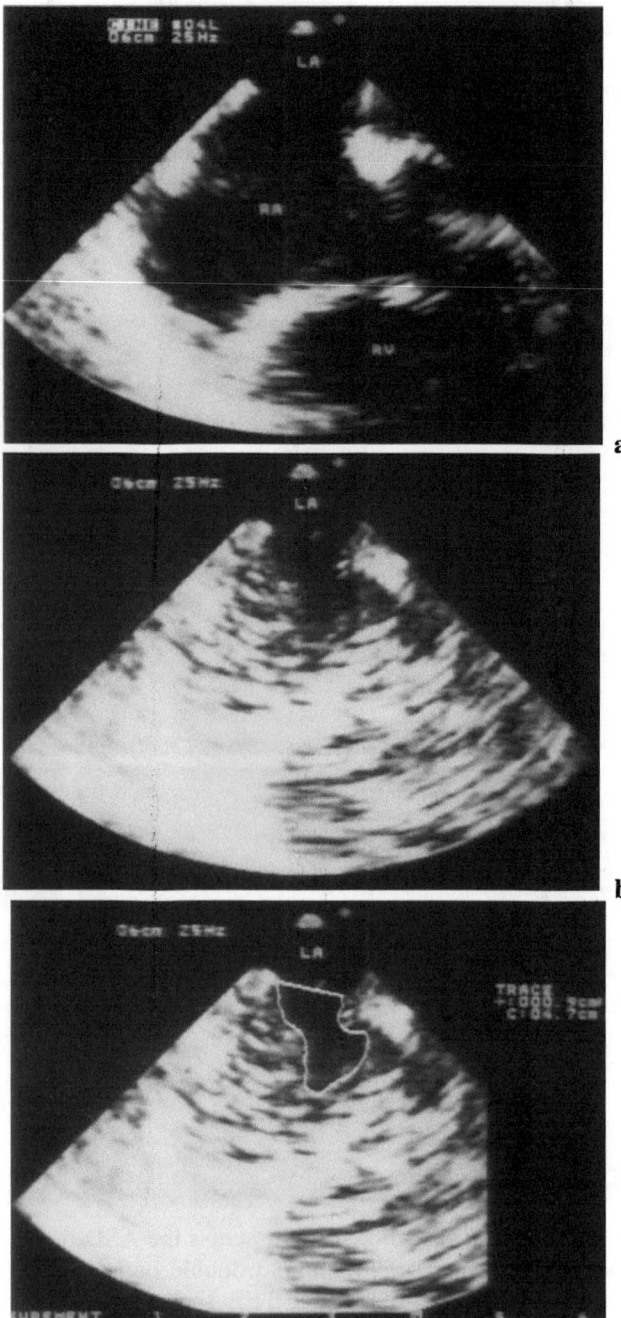

Fig. 3.5 a–c. Contrast echocardiography, secundum ASD. **a** Two-dimensional TEE shows a large ASD. **b** Contrast echocardiography. Agitated human albumin diluted with blood was injected in the right atrium. The left-to-right shunt appears as a negative contrast effect (*outlined* in **c**).

Multiple Defects

Multiple tissue defects of the atrial septum are observed more commonly in patients with primum ASD. The clinical relevance of these defects depends on the magnitude of the shunt flow.

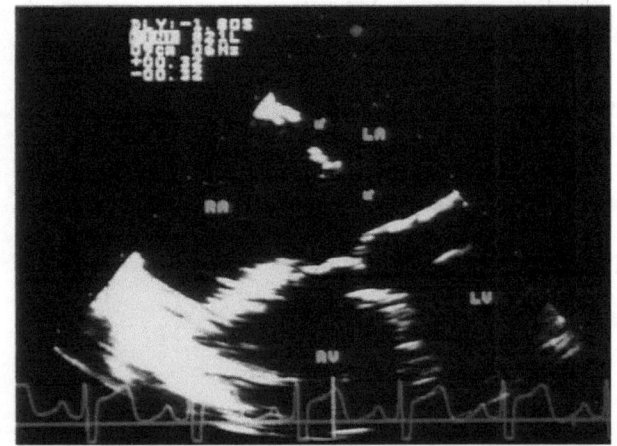

a

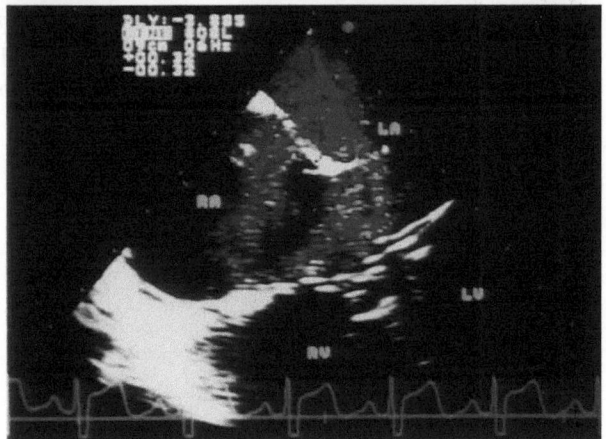

b

Fig. 3.6a, b. Multiple ASD. **a** *Arrows*, two echo dropouts in the atrial septum. **b** Color flow Doppler shows two low-velocity flows shunt across the defects.

Ostium Primum ASD

Ostium primum ASD is characterized by the absence of the lower part of atrial septum. It is often associated with a defect of the anterior mitral leaflet (cleft). Both atrioventricular valves are inserted at the crest of the ventricular septum. The two atrioventricular valves have two distinct annuli.

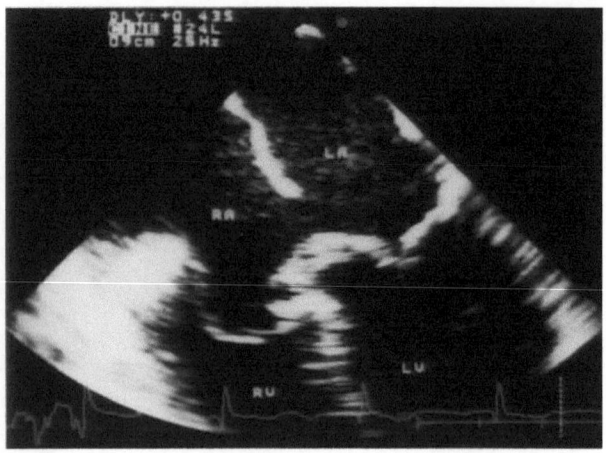

Fig. 3.7. Ostium primum ASD, two-dimensional TEE, four-chamber view. Defect of the lower portion of the atrial septum.

Fig. 3.9a, b. Ostium primum ASD. After surgical repair. **a** Two-dimensional TEE. *Arrow*, atrial patch. The "cleft" of the anterior mitral leaflet was repaired by single sutures. **b** Color Doppler shows the absence of shunt and the competence of the mitral valve in systole.

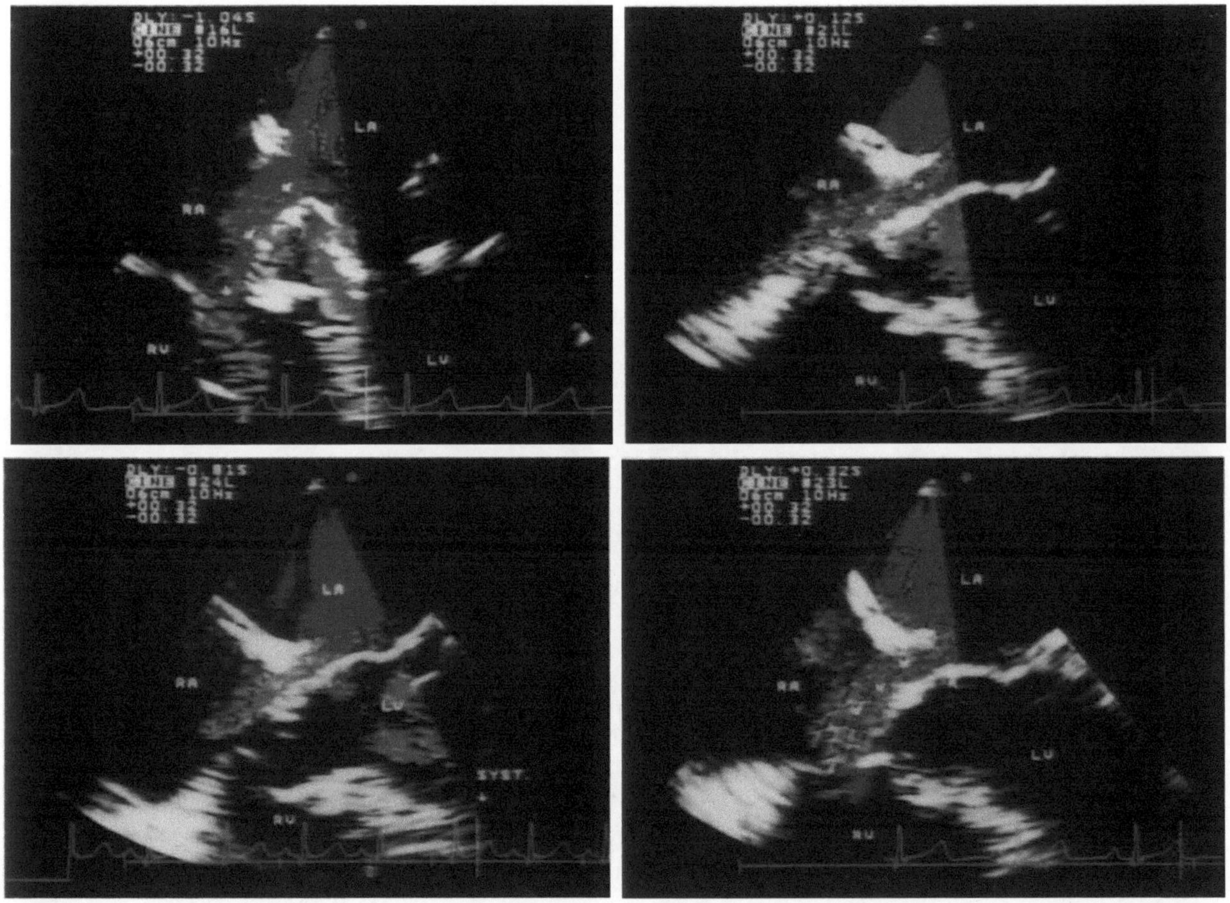

Fig. 3.8a, d. Ostium primum ASD, flow across the defect; same patient as in Fig. 3.7. **a** Color Doppler. Left-to-right shunt across the ASD (*arrows*). Color Doppler shows a diastolic flow (*blue*) directed from the left to the right atrium and to the right ventricle through the tricuspid valve. **b–d** In systole the color Doppler signal of the shunt turns into a turbulent high-velocity jet (*mosaic*). This represents the flow from left ventricle to right atrium through the "cleft" of the anterior mitral leaflet.

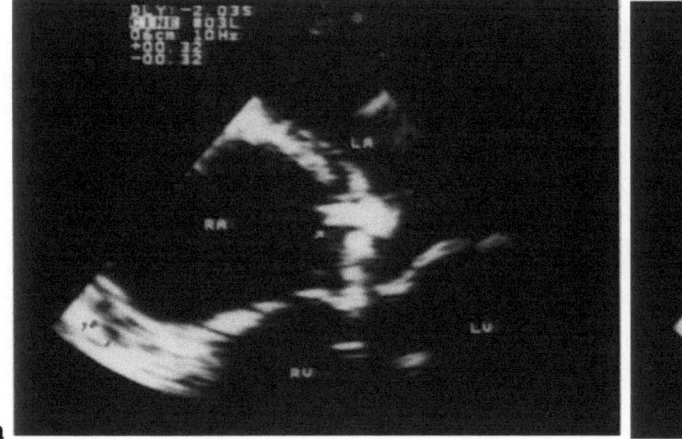

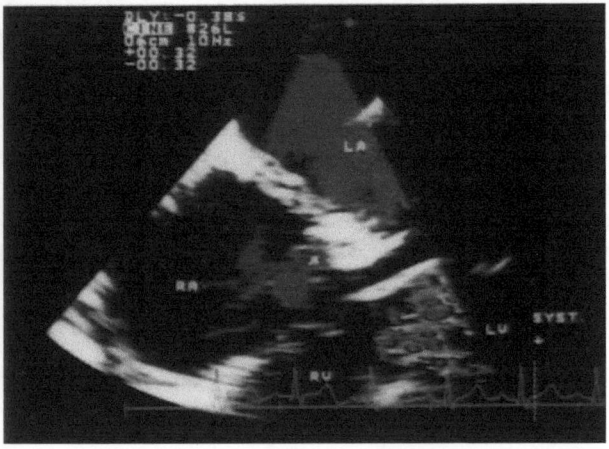

Sinus Venosus ASD

Sinus venosus ASD is a deficiency of the portion of the atrial septum located posterior to the foramen ovalis just beneath the orifice of superior vena cava.

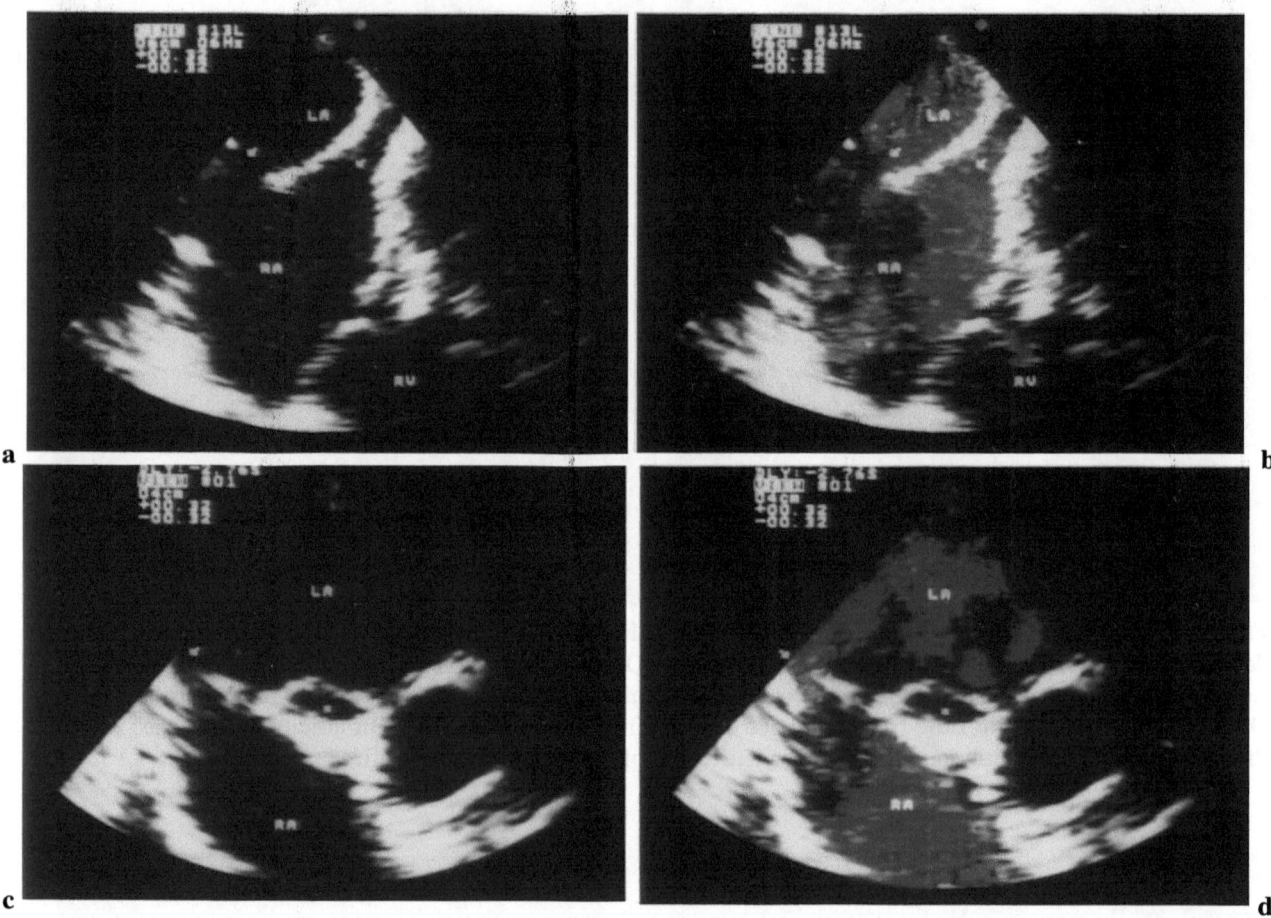

Fig. 3.10a–d. Sinus venosus ASD. **a** Two-dimensional TEE, four-chamber view. Echo dropout of the upper portion of atrial septum close to the entry of the superior vena cava (*upper arrow*). The patient also had an associated anomalous connections of the pulmonary veins. A dilated coronary sinus (lower arrow) drained into the right atrium. **b** Color Doppler flow. Flow across the defect (*upper arrow*) and coronary sinus (*lower arrow*). **c, d** Two-dimensional and color Doppler TEE, basal short-axis view. *Arrows*, sinus venosus ASD. *Asterisks*, cross-sectional view of the dilated coronary sinus.

Atrial Septal Aneurysm

Aneurysm of the atrial septum is an occasional echocardiographic finding in asymptomatic patients. Patent foramen ovale and recurrent systemic embolism are often associated with this anomaly. The clinical relevance of this finding is still controversial.

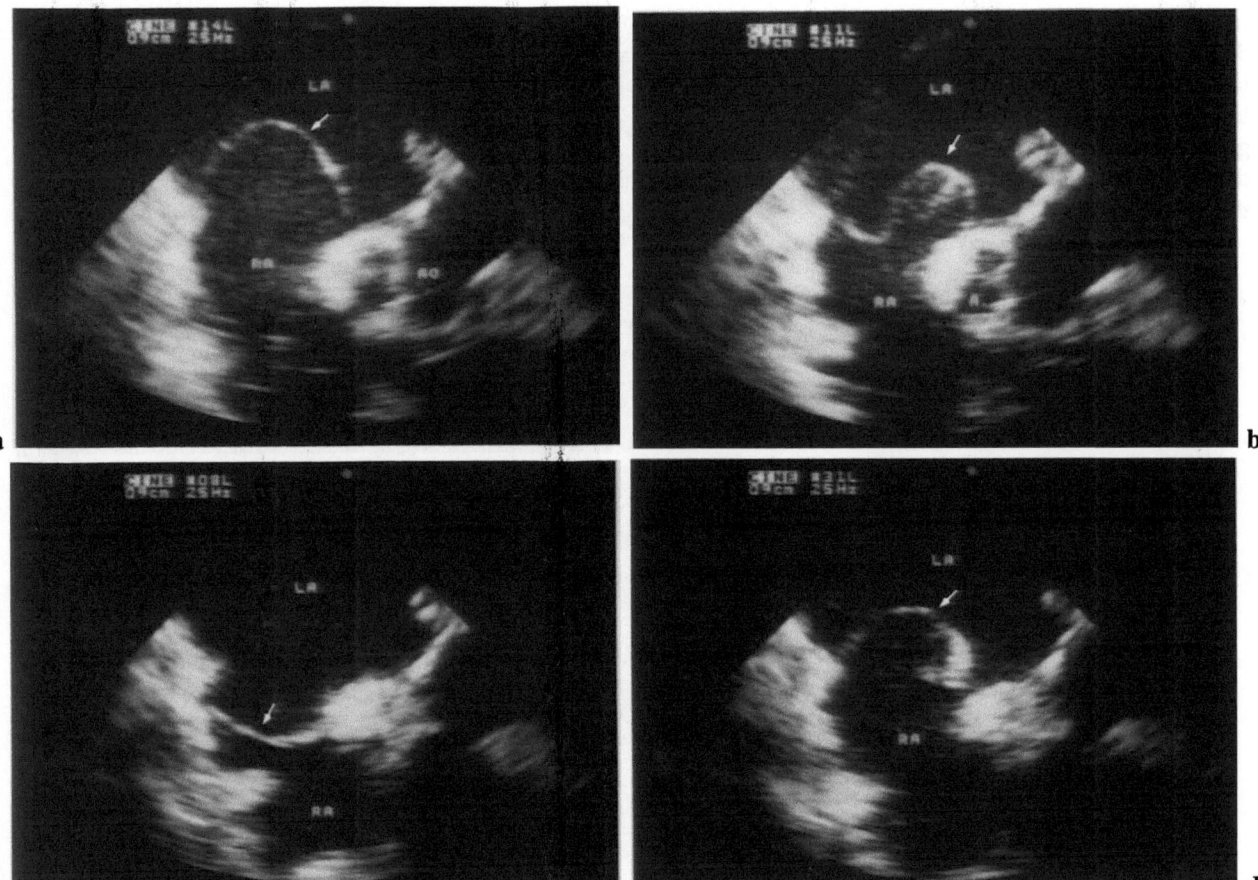

Fig. 3.11a–d. Atrial septal aneurysm, two-dimensional TEE. This sequence shows the bulging of the atrial septum (*arrow*) throughout the cardiac cycle.

Cor Triatriatum

In cor triatriatum an abnormal muscular membrane divides the left atrium into a posterosuperior chamber, which drains the pulmonary veins, and an antero-inferior chamber, leading to the mitral valve. The degree of obstruction to pulmonary venous return varies depending on the size of the orifice from the upper to the lower chamber.

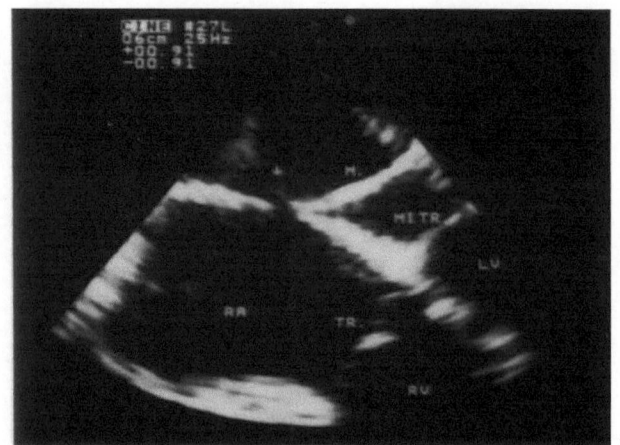

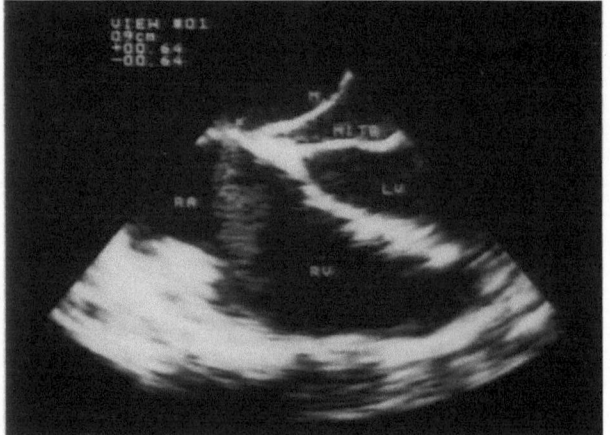

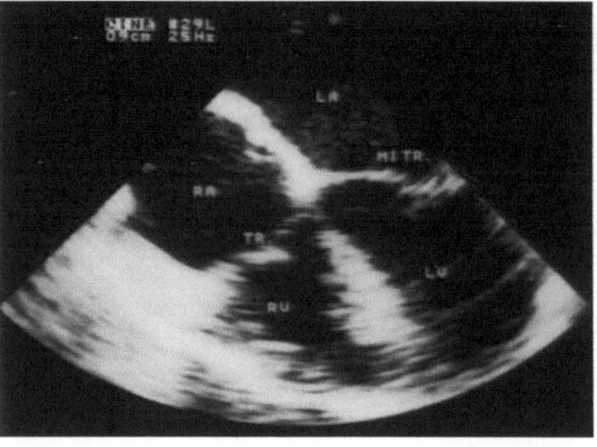

Fig. 3.12a–c. Cor triatriatum. **a** Two-dimensional TEE. *Arrow*, a very small ASD. A membrane (*M*) divides the left atrium into two chambers. **b** Color Doppler shows a high-velocity jet directed from the upper chamber of the left atrium toward the right atrium. **c** After surgical correction. The membrane was resected and the defect closed by single sutures.

Atrioventricular Septal Defects

One of the most profitable applications of intraoperative TEE is evaluating the anatomy and function of the atrioventricular valves during repair of atrioventricular septal defects (AVSD). Surgical correction closes the ASD and ventricular septal defect (VSD) with a patch and reconstructs the atrioventricular valve. Two-dimensional echocardiography allows the study of leaflet motion before and after valve reconstruction. Residual shunts and valve regurgitation can be detected by color Doppler flow imaging. Two forms can be distinguished: partial, or ostium primum ASD, and complete AVSD. Three anatomic types of complete AVSD can be distinguished according to the morphology of the atrioventricular valve: type A, type B, type C.

Partial AVSD

Partial AVSD is characterized by the absence of the lower part of the atrial septum, associated with a defect of the anterior mitral leaflet (cleft). Both atrioventricular valves are inserted at the crest of the ventricular septum. The two atrioventricular valves have two distinct annuli. (See "Ostium Primum ASD").

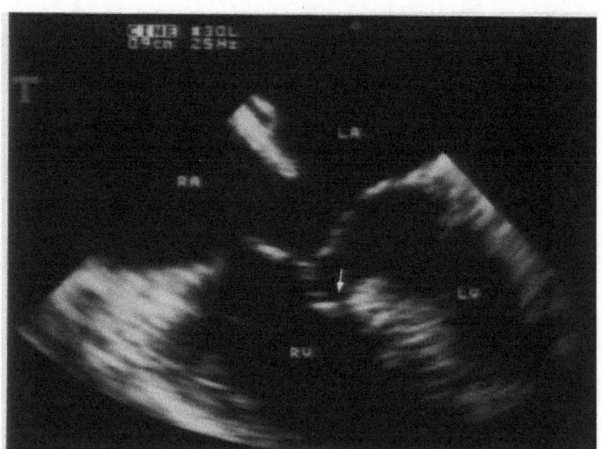

Fig. 3.13. Partial AVSD, two-dimensional TEE, four-chamber view. Defect of the lower portion of the atrial septum. The insertion of both right and left atrioventricular valves is to the crest of the ventricular septum (*arrow*). There is no VSD.

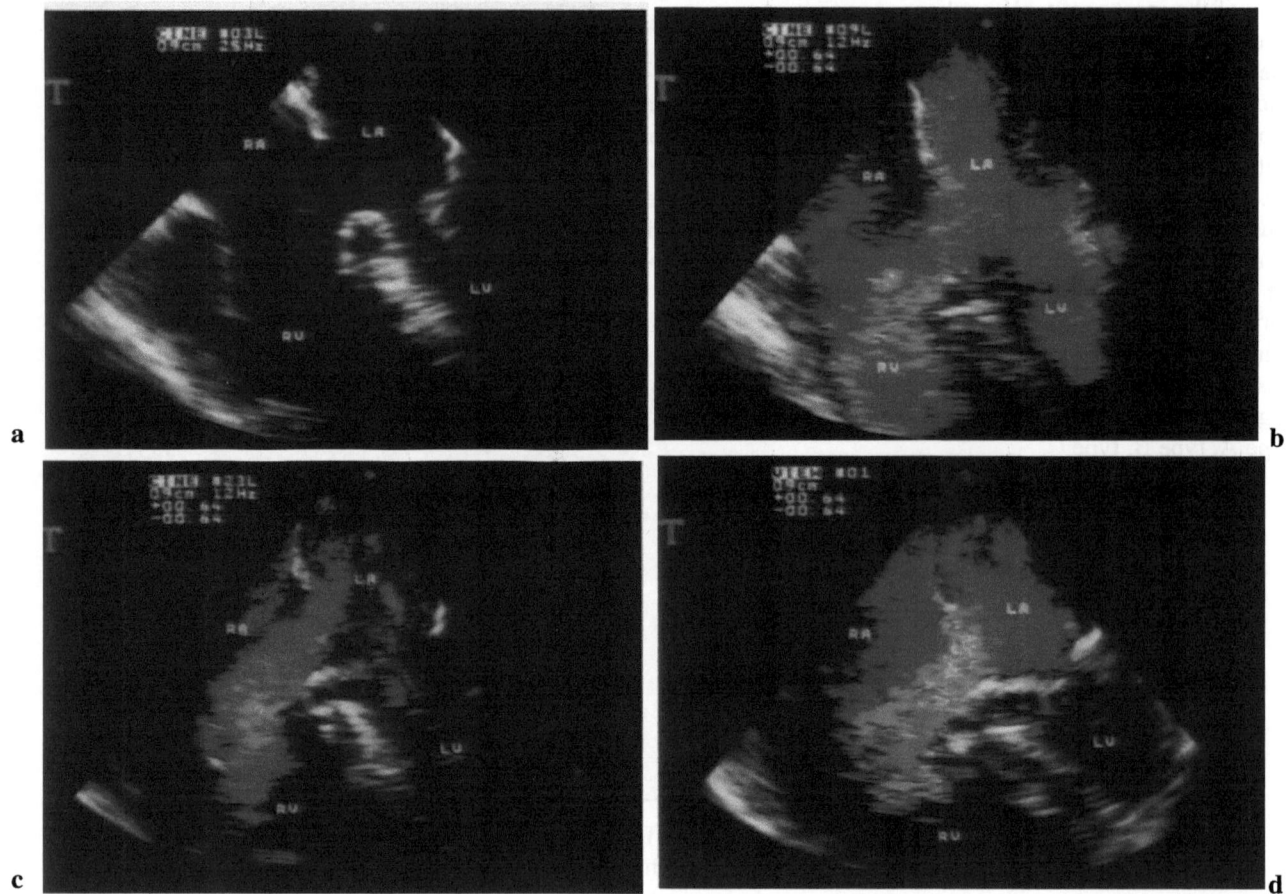

Fig. 3.14a–d. Partial AVSD. **a** Two-dimensional TEE, four-chamber view, shows a dilated right ventricle. **b** Color Doppler shows the diastolic flow across the mitral and tricuspid valves, and the left-to-right shunt across the ASD. **c** Color Doppler shows the flow (*blue*) directed from left to right atrium and to the right ventricle through the tricuspid valve in diastole. **d** In systole the color Doppler signal of the shunt turns into turbulent high-velocity jet (*mosaic*). This represents the flow from left ventricle to right atrium through the "cleft" of the anterior mitral leaflet.

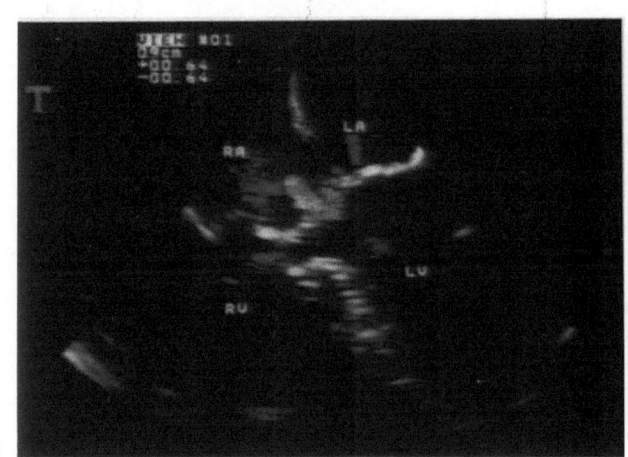
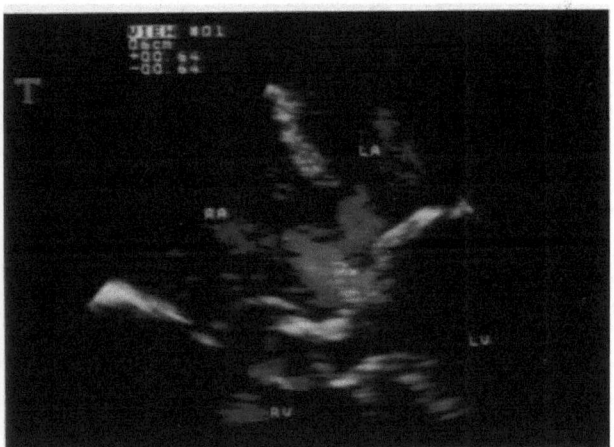

Fig. 3.15a, b. Partial AVSD. "Cleft" of the mitral valve. Color Doppler shows a regurgitant jet (*red*) originating from the cleft of the anterior mitral leaflet.

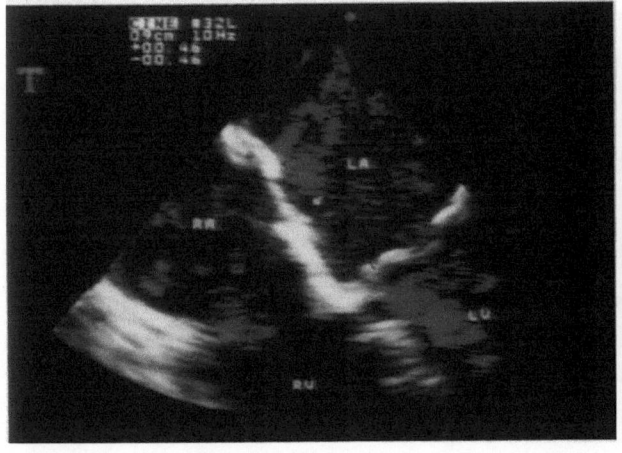
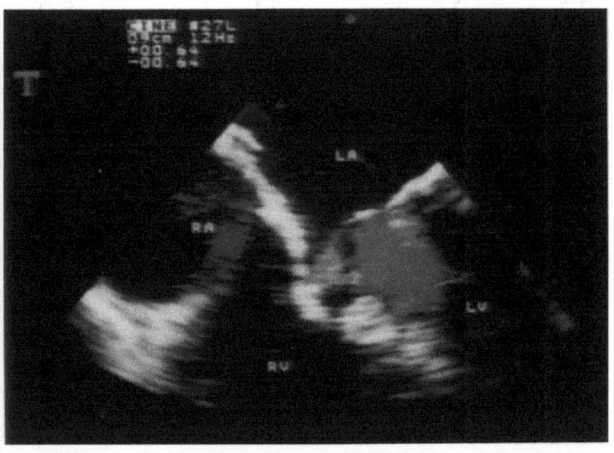

Fig. 3.16a, b. Partial AVSD. After surgical repair; same patient as in Fig. 3.15. **a** *Arrow*, atrial patch. Color Doppler shows the absence of atrial shunt. **b** The cleft of the anterior mitral leaflet was closed by single sutures. Color Doppler shows the competence of the mitral valve in systole.

Complete AVSD

Complete AVSD is characterized by absence of the lower portion of the atrial septum and upper portion of the ventricular septum. Between the atria and the ventricles there is a common atrioventricular valve. Rastelli´s classification is based on the configuration of the anterior leaflet and on the location of right-sided chordal insertions for the anterior leaflet. In type A the anterior bridging leaflet is divided into mitral and tricuspid portions and is attached by short cords to the crest of the interventricular septum. In type B the anterior leaflet is attached to an anomalous anterior papillary muscle adjacent to the septum in the right ventricle. In type C the anterior leaflet is attached to the anterior papillary muscle, at the right ventricular free wall. The membranous septum is present in type A and is absent in types B and C.

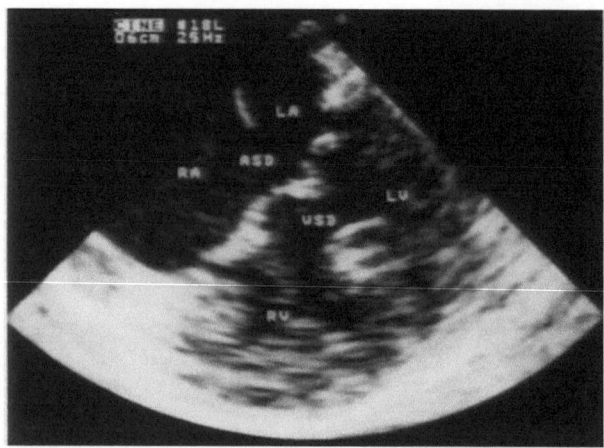

Fig. 3.17. Complete AVSD, two-dimensional TEE, four-chamber view. Defects of the lower portion of the atrial septum (*ASD*) and of the upper portion of the ventricular septum (*VSD*). A common atrioventricular valve divides the atria from the ventricles.

Type A

In AVSD type A the anterior bridging leaflet is divided into mitral and tricuspid portions and is attached by short cords to the crest of the interventricular septum.

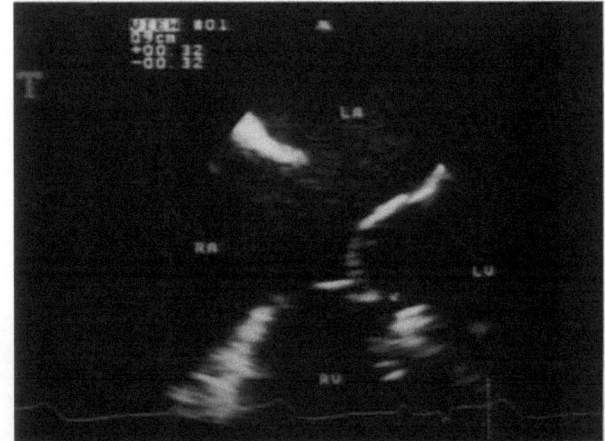

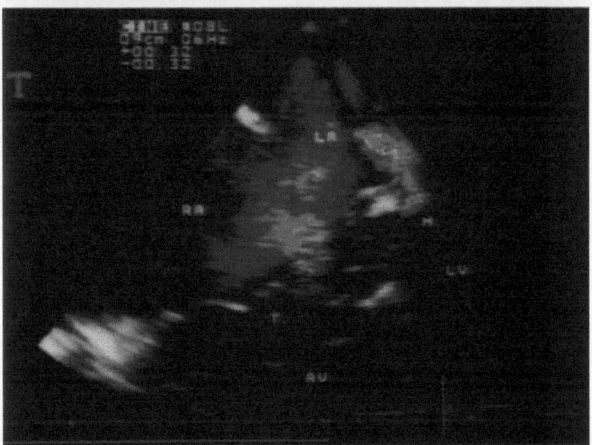

Fig. 3.18a–c. Complete AVSD, type A. **a** Two-dimensional TEE, four-chamber view. Large defect of the lower portion of the atrial septum. *Arrow*, a small defect of the upper portion of the interventricular septum. Short chordae from the anterior leaflet are attached to the crest of the interventricular septum. **b** Color Doppler shows two small regurgitant jets arising from the mitral portion (*M*) of the common atrioventricular valve and from the commissure adjacent to the tricuspid portion of the valve (*T*). The color Doppler signal (*blue*) represents the left-to-right shunt across the ASD. **c** The arrow shows the left-to-right shunt across the small VSD.

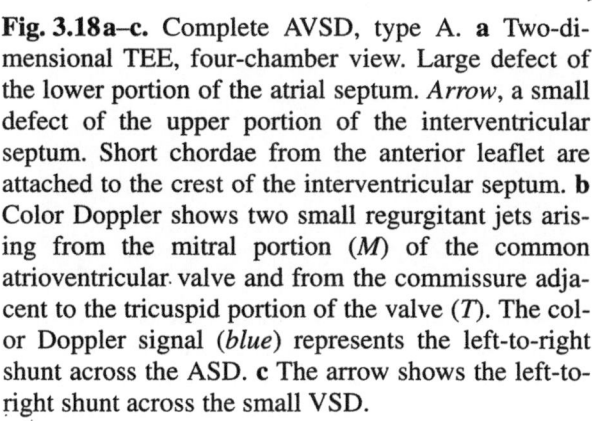

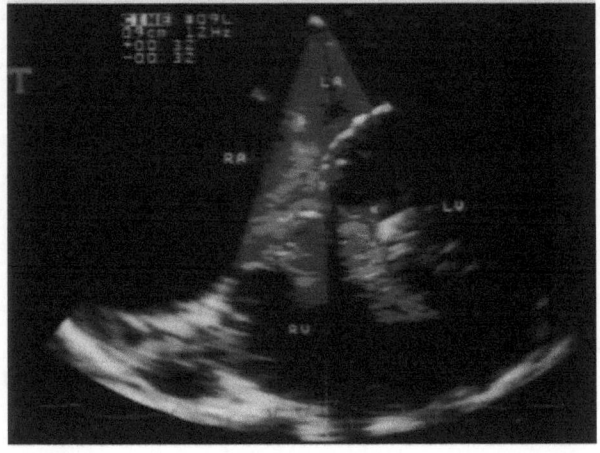

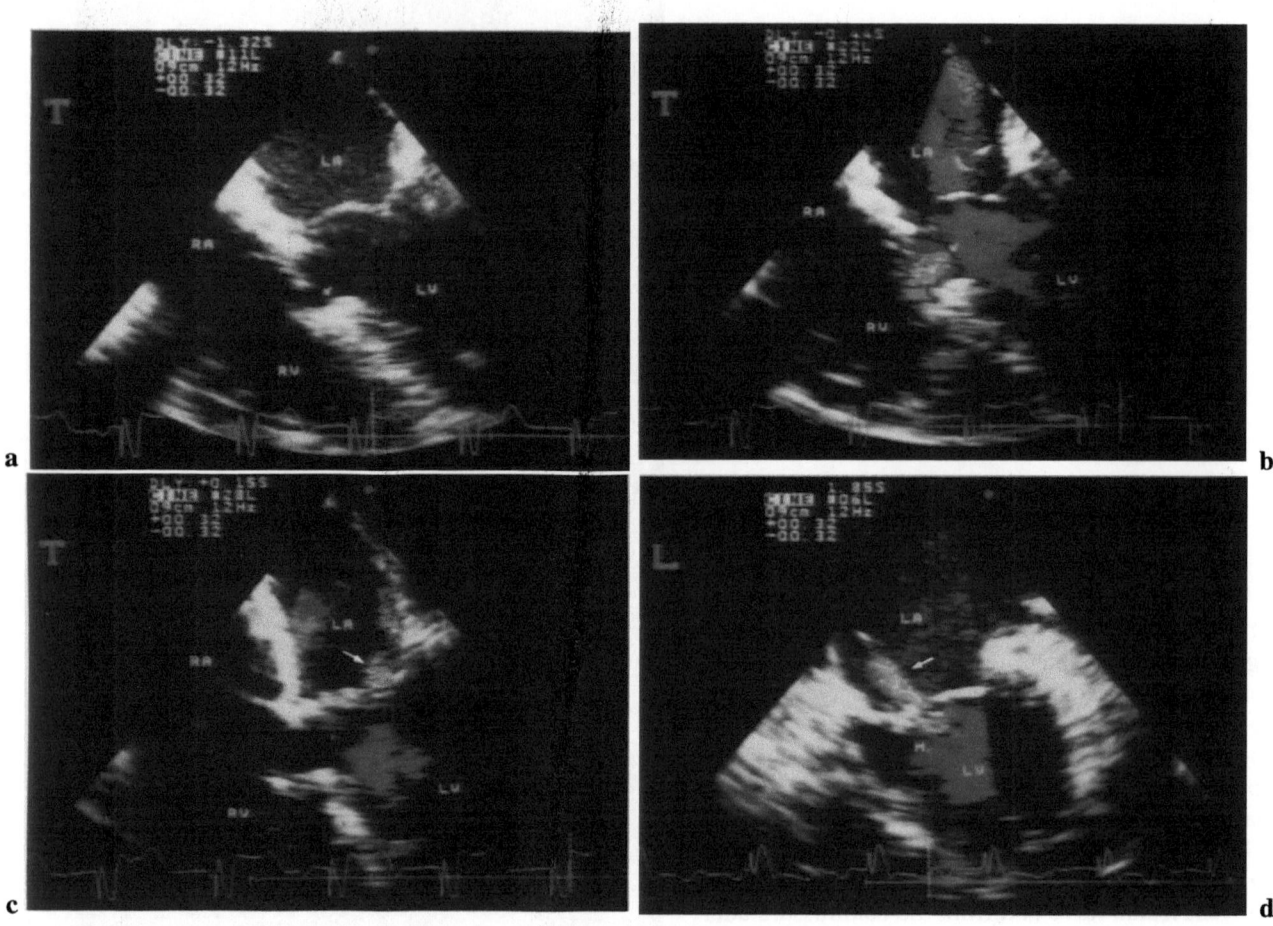

Fig. 3.19a–d. Complete AVSD, after repair; same patient as in Fig. 3.18. **a** Two-dimensional TEE shows repair of the ASD and VSD. *Arrow*, small echo dropout in the ventricular septum. **b** Color Doppler shows a small residual flow across the VSD. **c, d** Color Doppler shows the competence of the two atrioventricular valves. A small jet directed posteriorly can be observed in the left atrium. **c** Transversal view. **d** Longitudinal view.

Type B

In AVSD type B the anterior leaflet is attached to an anomalous anterior papillary muscle adjacent to the septum in the right ventricle. The membranous septum is absent.

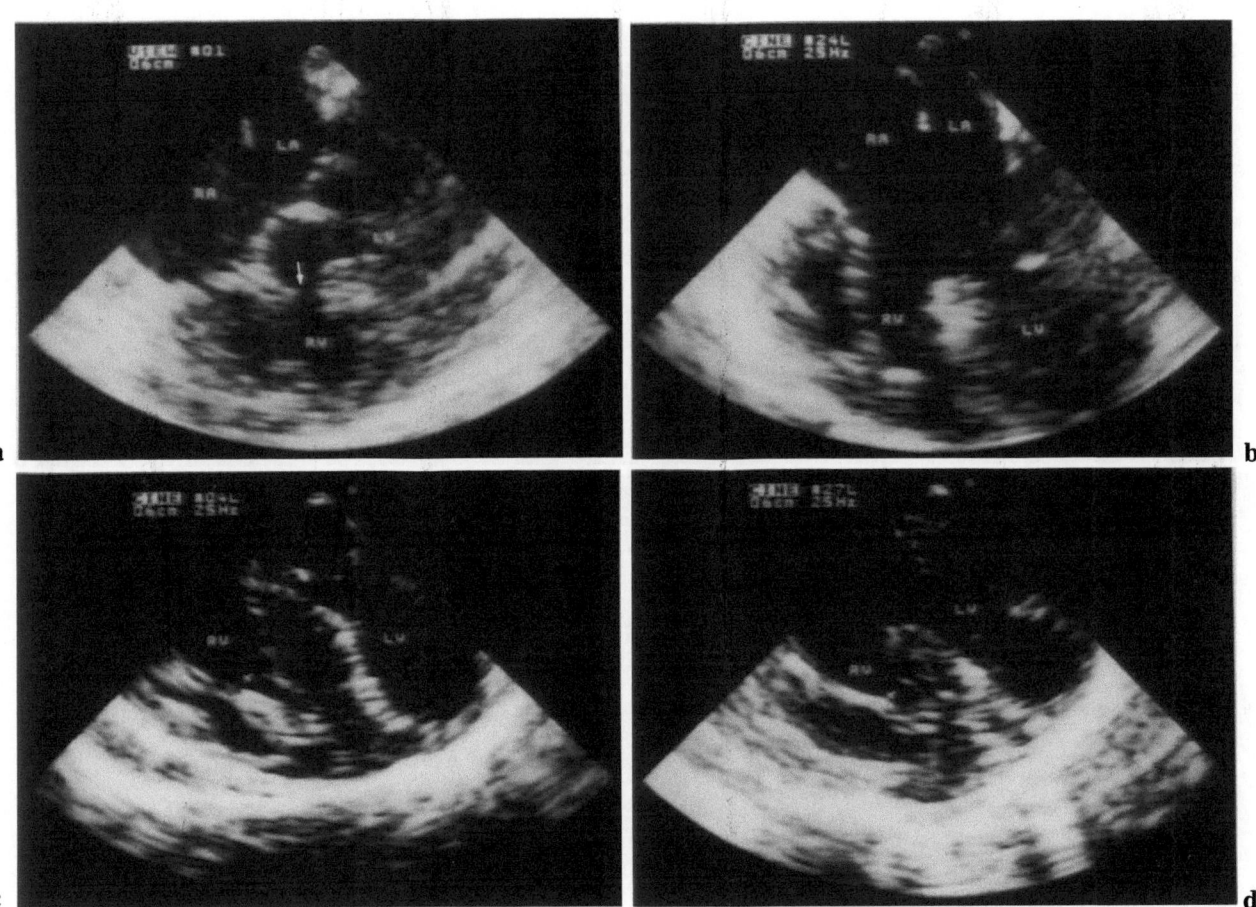

Fig. 3.20a–d. Complete AVSD, type B. **a, b** Two-dimensional TEE, four-chamber view. Large ASD and VSD. The chordae of the anterior bridging leaflet (*arrow*) are attached onto the right side of the ventricular septum. **a** Systole. **b** Diastole. **c, d** Detail showing the attachment of the chordae to the septum.

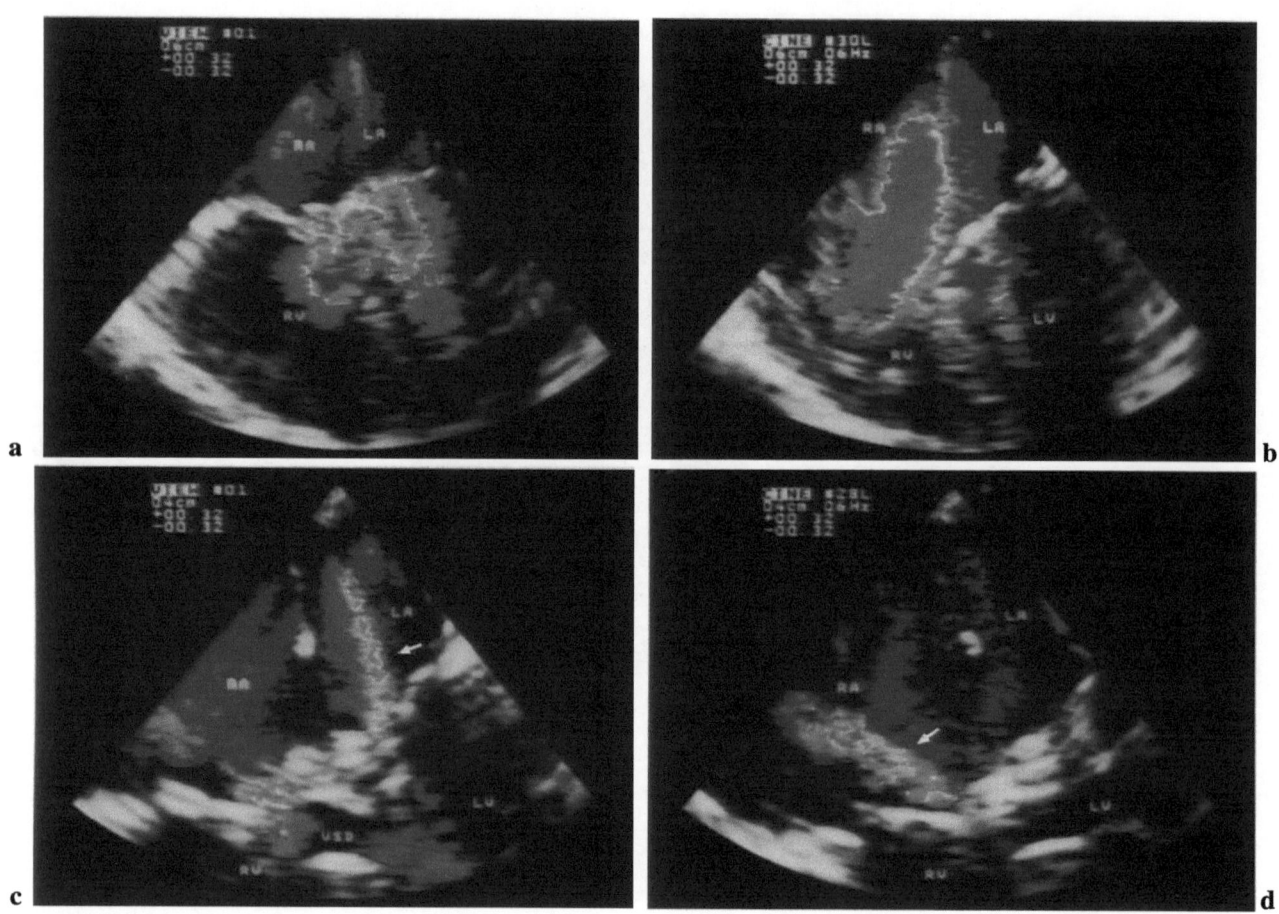

Fig. 3.21a–d. Complete AVSD, type B. **a** Color Doppler shows the shunt across the VSD. **b** Increased diastolic flow across the tricuspid orifice can be observed due to the confluence of the left-to-right shunt through the ASD and the systemic venous return. **c, d** Color Doppler shows the incompetence of the atrioventricular valve. Two regurgitant jets originate from the mitral (**c**) and tricuspidal (**d**) portions of the valve, respectively.

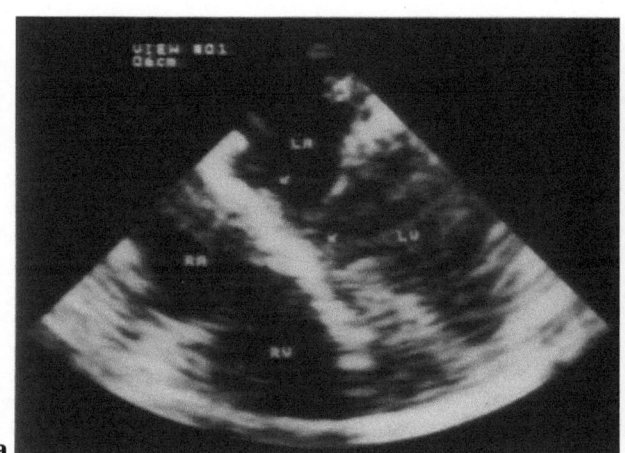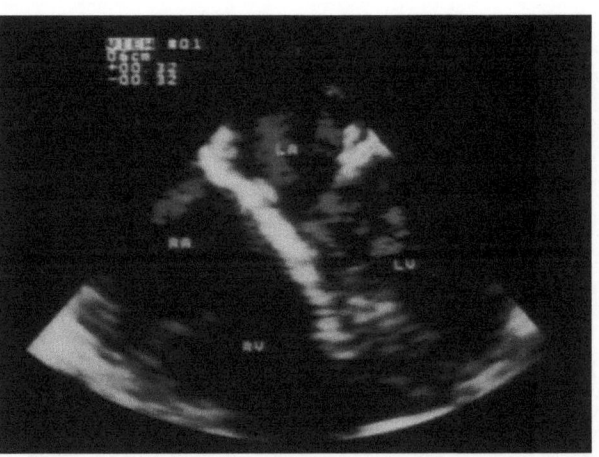

a

b

Fig. 3.22a,b. Complete AVSD, after repair; same patient as in Fig. 3.21. **a** Two-dimensional TEE shows repair of the ASD and VSD. *Arrows*, position of the atrial and ventricular patches. **b** Color Doppler shows the absence of valve insufficiency and of a residual shunt.

Type C

In this of AVSD the anterior leaflet is attached to the anterior papillary muscle, at the right ventricular free wall. The membranous septum is absent.

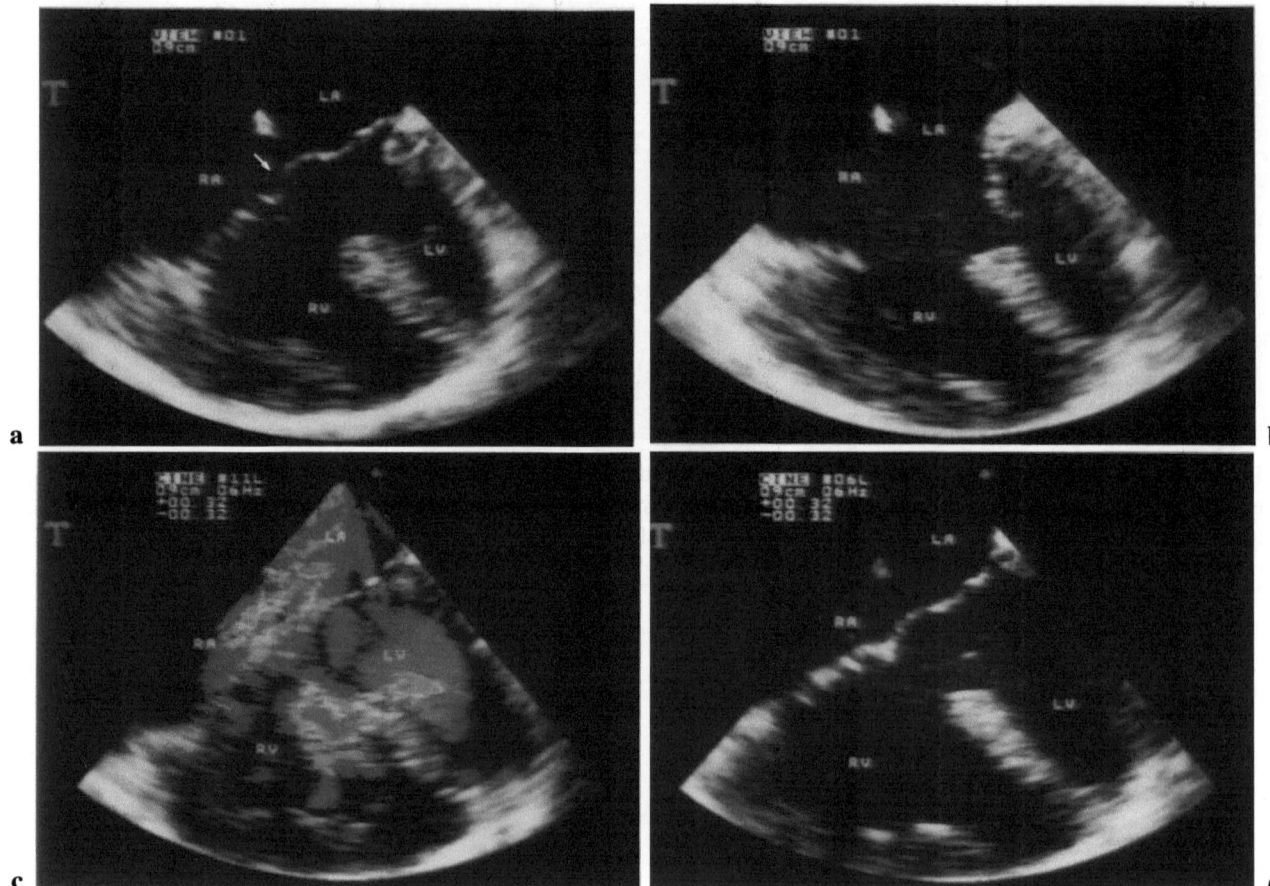

Fig. 3.23a–d. Complete AVSD, type C. **a, b** Two-dimensional TEE, four-chamber view. Large ASD and VSD. The anterior bridging leaflet of the atrioventricular valve (*arrow*) straddles the large VSD and has a free-floating appearance. The chordae of the bridging leaflet are attached to an anomalous papillary muscle in the right ventricle. The right ventricle is dilated and hypertrophied. An obstruction to the RVOT secondary to the infundibular hypertrophy is present (see Fig. 3.49). **a** Systole. **b** Diastole. **c** Color Doppler shows two shunts across the ASD and VSD. The common atrioventricular valve shows no regurgitation. **d** The same frame as in **c**, without the color Doppler signal.

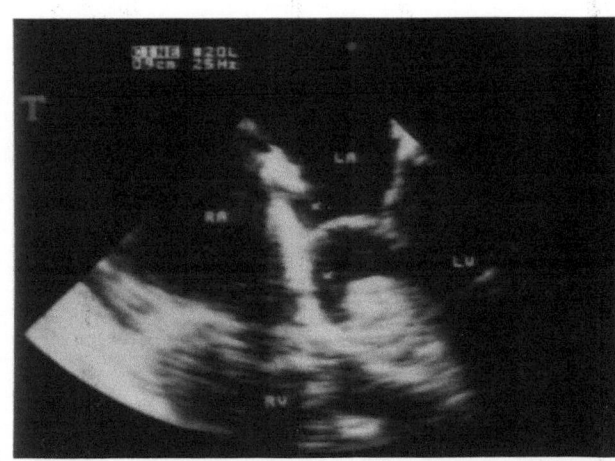
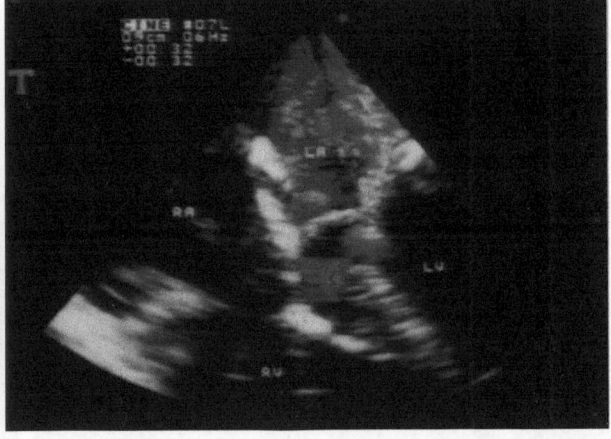

a

b

Fig. 3.24a, b. Complete AVSD, after repair. Same patient as in Fig. 3.23. **a** Two-dimensional TEE, four-chamber view. *Arrows*, position of the patches. The ventricular patch has been attached to the right side of the ventricular septum. **b** Color Doppler shows the absence of left-to-right shunts. A small regurgitant jet originating from the mitral portion of the valve is directed posteriorly into the left atrium.

Ventricular Septal Defects

Two-dimensional echocardiography allows assessment of the dimension and location of VSD. Color Doppler flow imaging permits detection of the shunt and assessment of the flow direction.

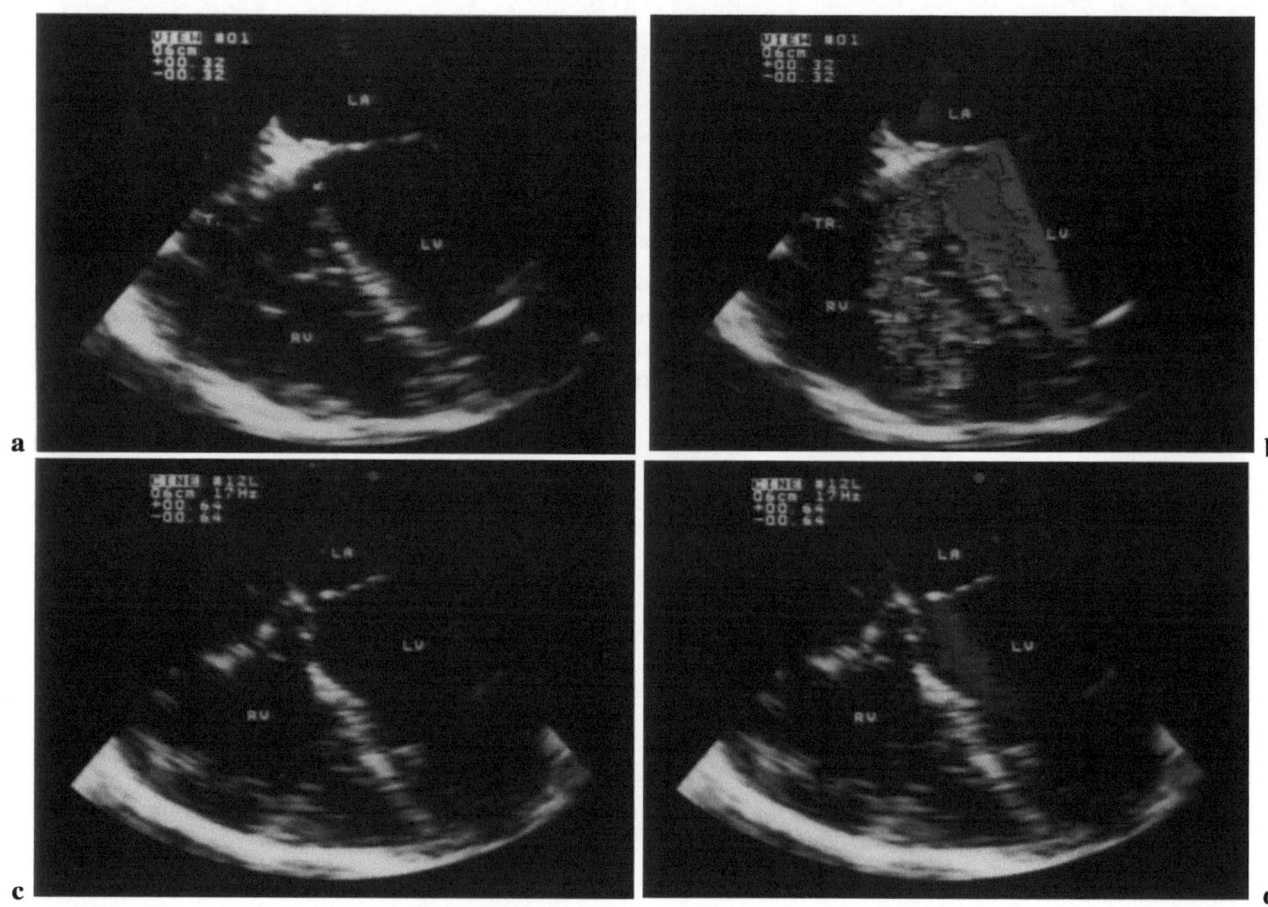

Fig. 3.25a–d. Perimembranous VSD. **a** Two-dimensional TEE. *Arrow*, defect of the membranous portion of the ventricular septum. **b** Color flow Doppler shows a large left-to-right shunt. Turbulent flow (*mosaic*) in the right ventricle originating from the defect. Normal (*aliased*) systolic ejection flow is displayed in the left outflow tract (*red + blue*). **c, d** Two-dimensional and color Doppler echocardiography after the closure of the defect with a patch. No residual shunt was present after the repair. (*T, TR,* Tricuspid valve).

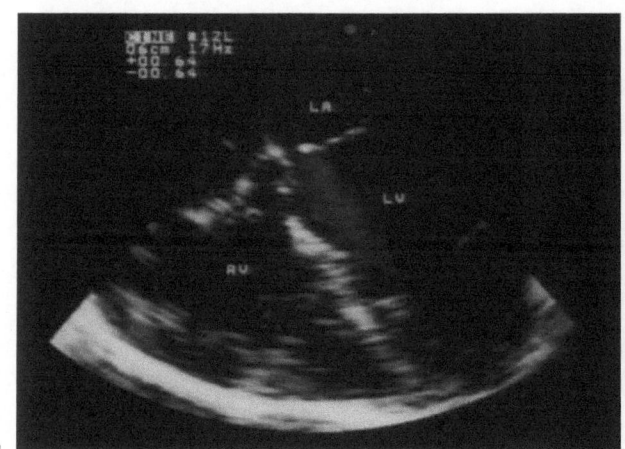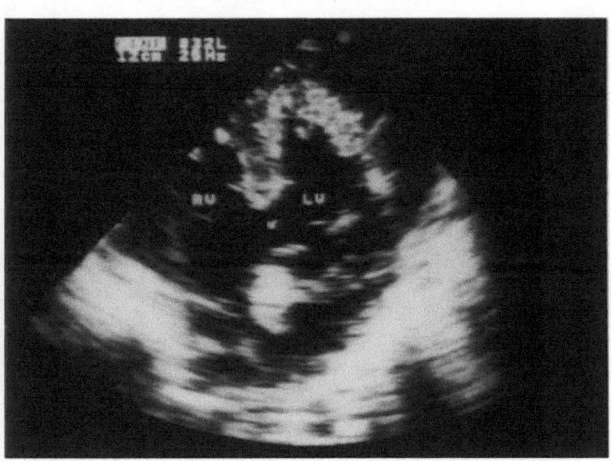

Fig. 3.26a, b. VSD and double outlet right ventricle, preoperative transthoracic echocardiography. Large VSD including the membranous and a large portion of the muscular ventricular septum. **a** Parasternal long-axis view. *Arrow*, large defect of the upper portion of the ventricular septum. **b** Parasternal short-axis view of the same patient. *Arrow*, VSD.

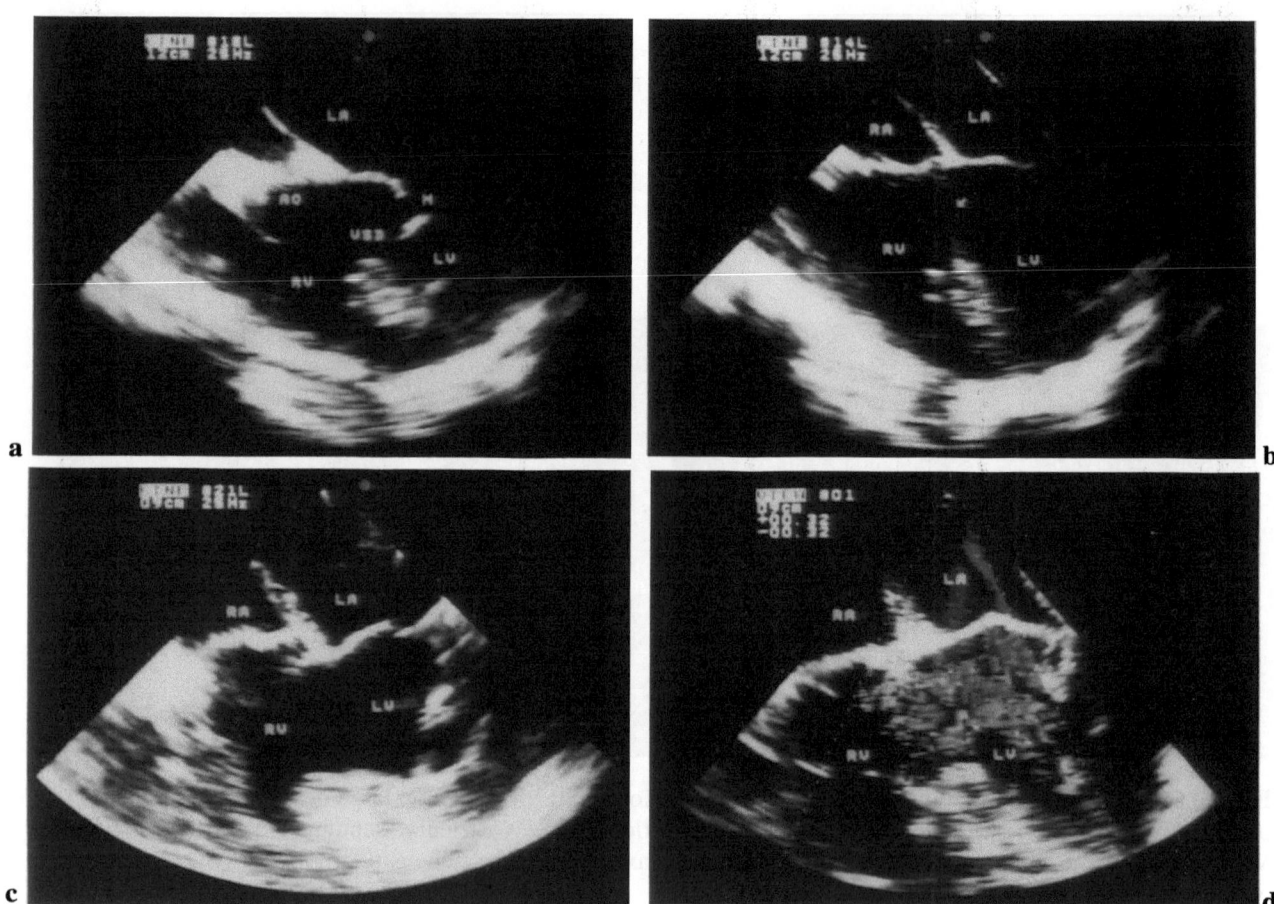

Fig. 3.27 a–d. VSD; same patient as in Fig. 3.26. Intraoperative TEE shows a very large VSD, acting functionally as a single ventricle. Closure of the defect was not possible. A modified Fontan operation was performed. **a** Basal short-axis view shows a VSD immediately beneath the aortic valve. **b** Four-chamber view shows the absence of the membranous portion of the interventricular septum **c** Advancing the transducer more deeply into the esophagus, a much larger defect including a large portion of the muscular septum can be visualized. **d** Color Doppler shows a bidirectional shunt with low velocity flow signal across the large defect.

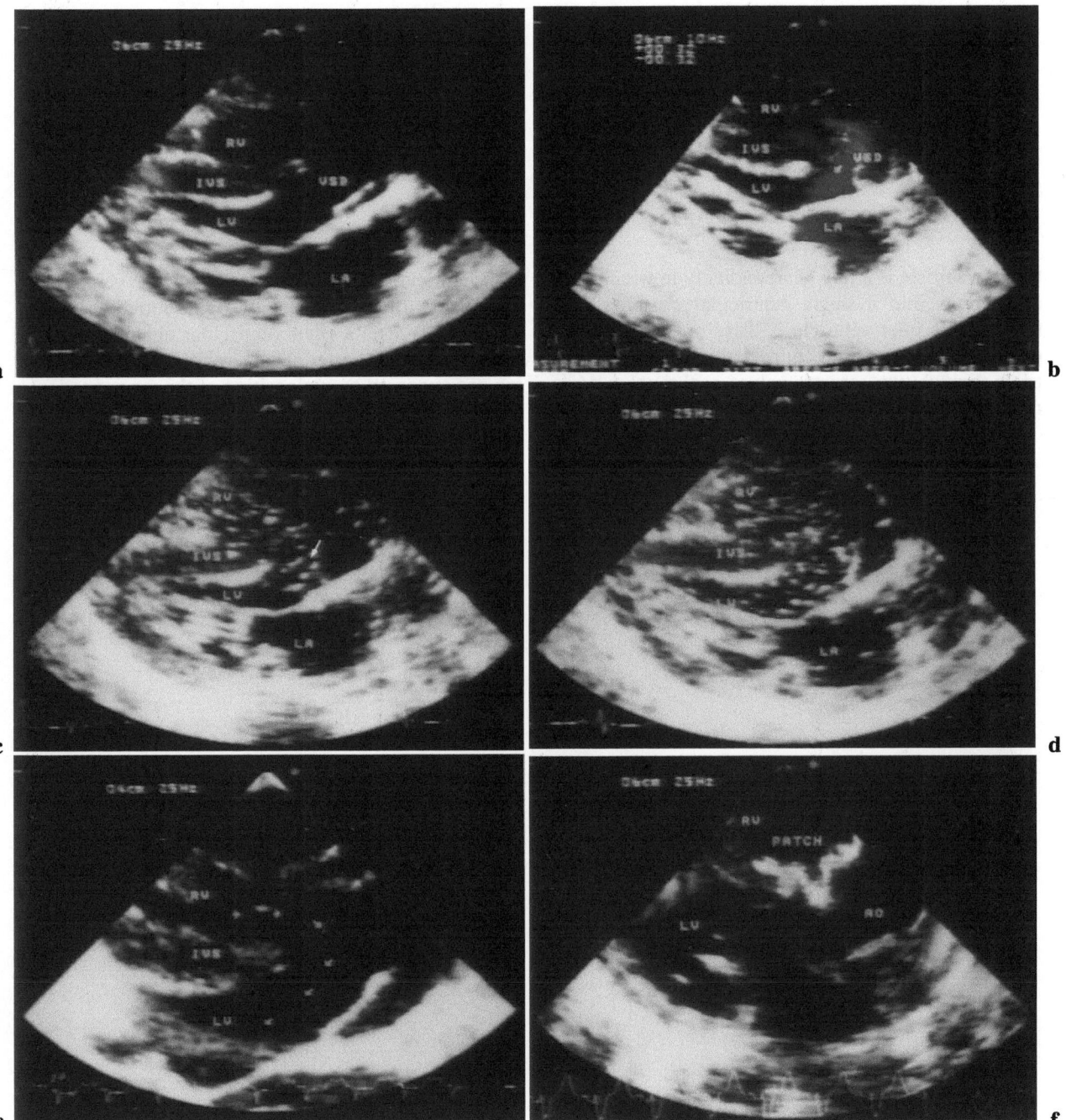

Fig. 3.28a–f. VSD, shunt direction. A patient with VSD, double outlet left ventricle, and infundibular pulmonary stenosis. Epicardial echocardiography, parasternal long-axis equivalent view. **a** Large subaortic VSD. **b** The flow of the right-to-left shunt through the defect is visualized as low velocity signal (*blue*).

c, d Contrast echocardiography. Human albumin diluted with blood was injected into the right atrium. The sequence shows that the contrast appears first in the right ventricle and is then directed into the left ventricle. **e** *Arrows*, flow direction of the contrast. **f** Ventricular patch after surgical closure of the defect.

Single Ventricle

Single ventricle is a rare heart anomaly in which both atria empty into a single ventricular chamber. The term double inlet ventricle is therefore more appropriate. The two atria are connected to the single ventricle through two separate valves or through a common atrioventricular valve. Most commonly the single ventricle is morphologically a left ventricular chamber with a rudimentary right outlet chamber. More rarely it is a right ventricular chamber with a rudimentary left outlet chamber. This anomaly is often accompanied by malposition of the great arteries.

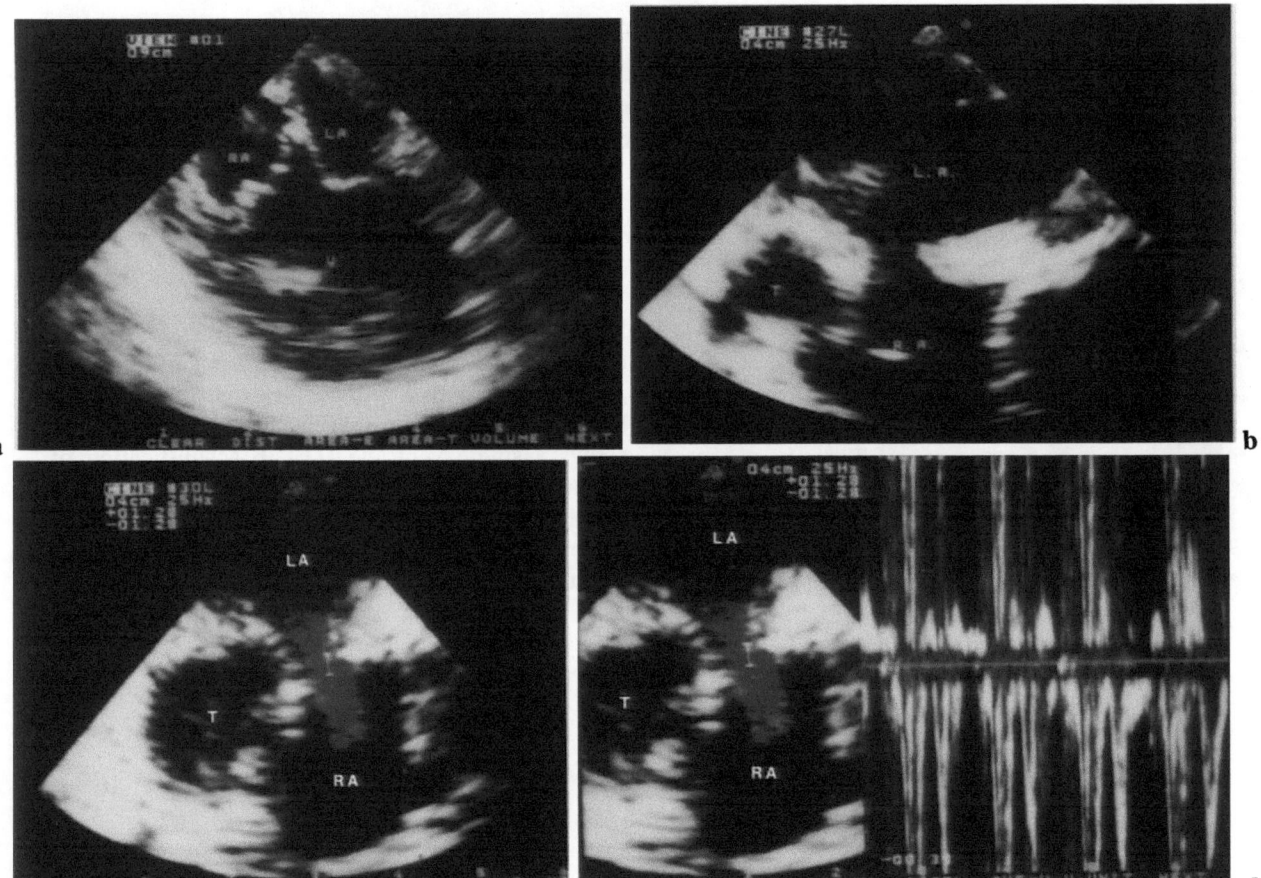

Fig. 3.29 a–d. Single ventricle with left transposition of the great arteries. **a** "Four"-chamber view shows a single ventricle (*V*) with two atria and two atrioventricular valves. **b** After surgery. A total cavopulmonary connection was performed. An intra-atrial tunnel (*T*) connected both superior and inferior venae cavae to the main pulmonary artery. An ASD was enlarged surgically. **c, d** Color flow and pulsed Doppler indicate that the flow through the ASD is directed from the left to the right atrium.

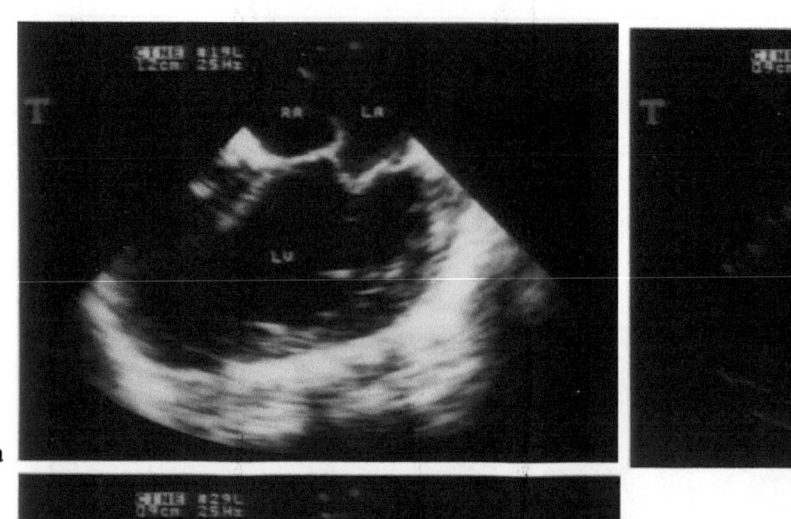

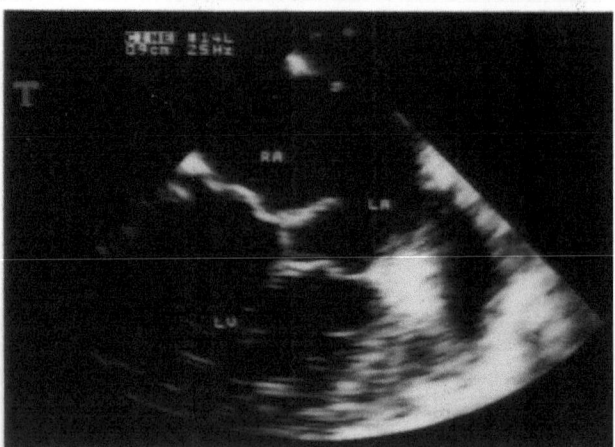

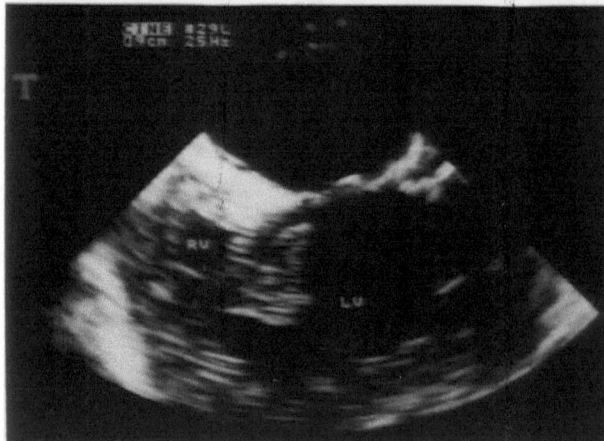

Fig. 3.30a–c. Double inlet left ventricle. Dextrocardia with situs solitus, right transposition of the great arteries with a rudimentary right outlet chamber. **a** Two-dimensional TEE. "Four"-chamber view shows a single ventricle (*LV*). **b** Magnification of the atrioventricular valves. The tricuspid valve is dysplastic. **c** Detail of the rudimentary right ventricle (*RV*), in communication with the left chamber through a restrictive foramen bulboventricularis.

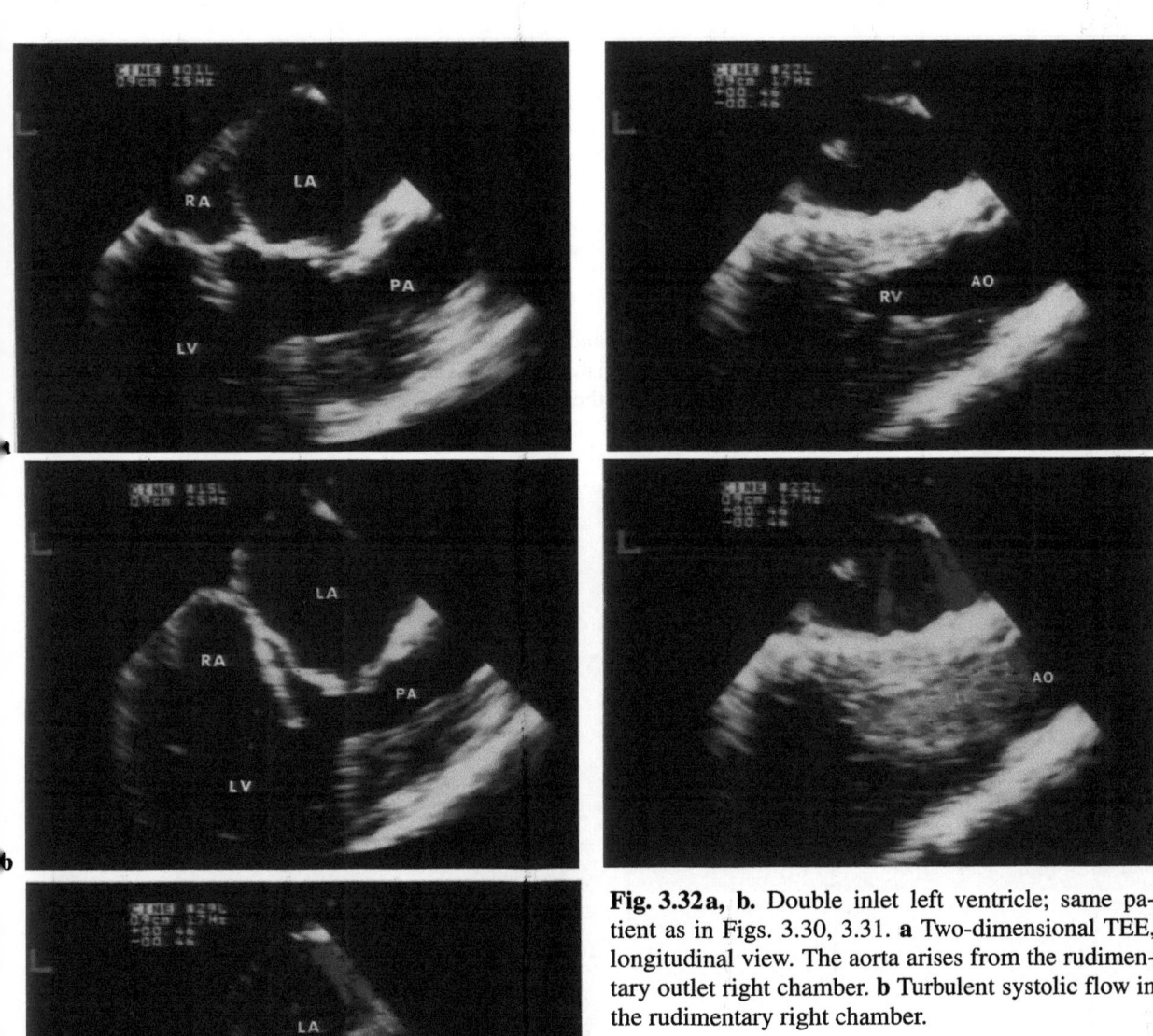

Fig. 3.32a, b. Double inlet left ventricle; same patient as in Figs. 3.30, 3.31. **a** Two-dimensional TEE, longitudinal view. The aorta arises from the rudimentary outlet right chamber. **b** Turbulent systolic flow in the rudimentary right chamber.

Fig. 3.31a–c. Double inlet left ventricle; same patient as in Fig. 3.30. **a, b** Two-dimensional TEE, longitudinal view (intermediate view between RVOT long-axis and ascending aorta-atrial septum long-axis view), showing the single chamber and the atrioventricular valves in systole (**a**) and in diastole (**b**). The tricuspid valve is dysplastic. The pulmonary artery (*PA*) arises from the left ventricle. **c** Regurgitant jet across the tricuspid valve. Note: the standard TEE views cannot be used in complex anomalies of the heart.

Tetralogy of Fallot

The four characteristics of Fallot's tetralogy are: VSD, aortic root overriding the ventricular septum, obstruction to the right ventricular outflow, and right ventricular hypertrophy. Pulmonary valve stenosis and hypoplasia of the pulmonary arteries may coexist. Biplanar TEE provides unique visualization of the VSD and the RVOT.

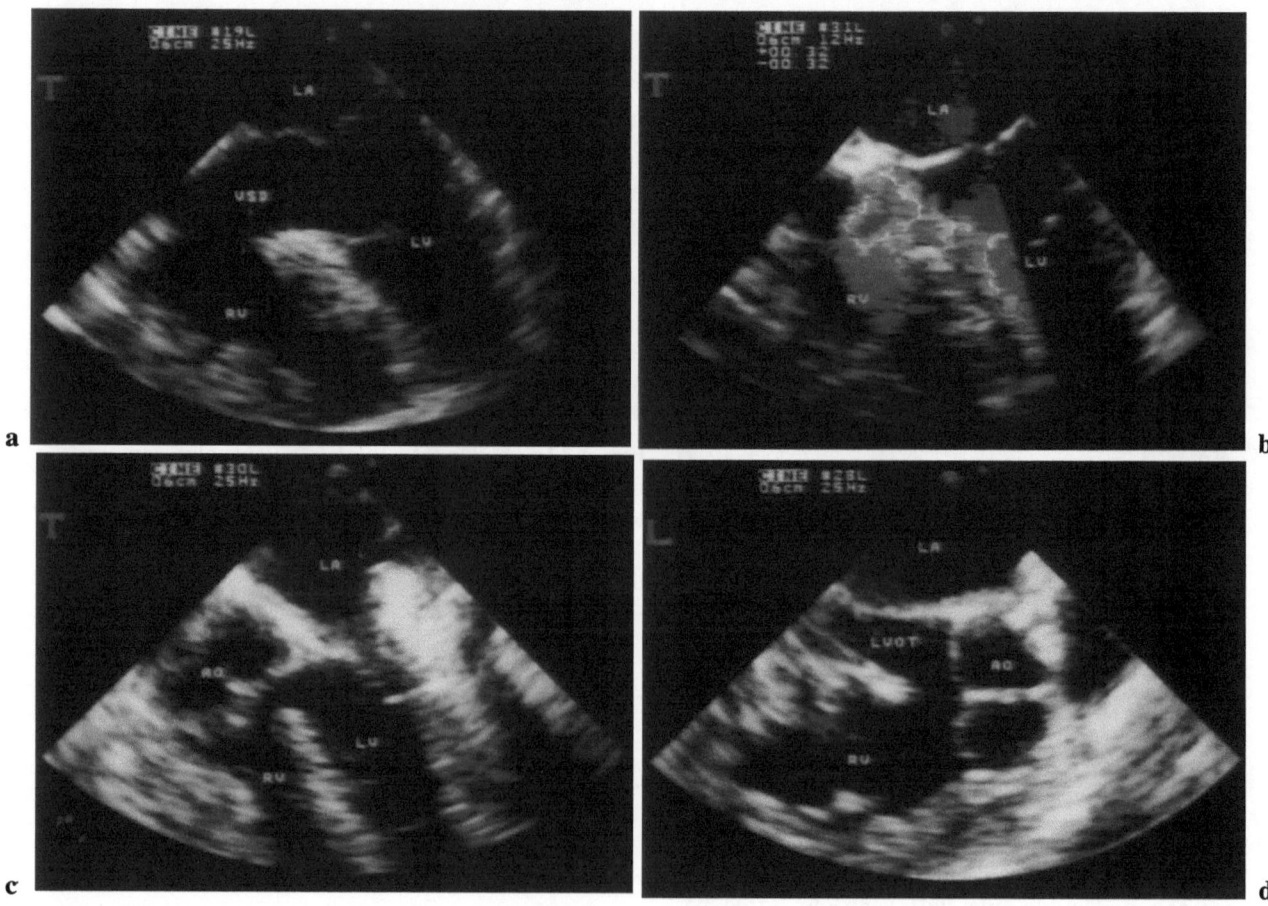

Fig. 3.33a–d. Tetralogy of Fallot. **a** Two-dimensional TEE, transversal four-chamber view, shows the VSD. **b** Color Doppler flow signal through the defect. **c** LVOT view shows the aortic root overriding the ventricular septum. **d** Biplanar TEE, long-axis view of the LVOT. The aortic valve overrides the ventricular septum.

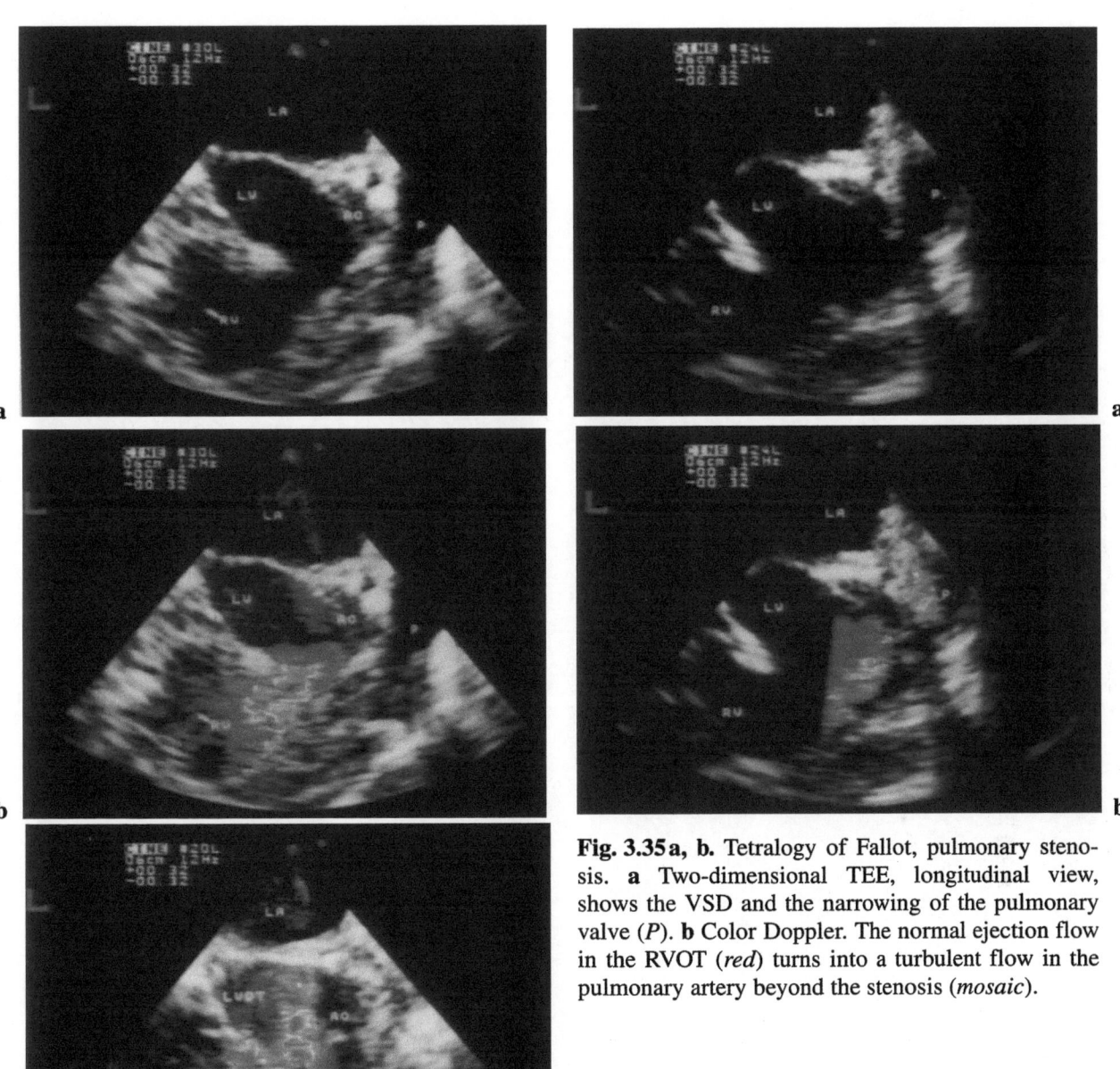

Fig. 3.35 a, b. Tetralogy of Fallot, pulmonary stenosis. **a** Two-dimensional TEE, longitudinal view, shows the VSD and the narrowing of the pulmonary valve (*P*). **b** Color Doppler. The normal ejection flow in the RVOT (*red*) turns into a turbulent flow in the pulmonary artery beyond the stenosis (*mosaic*).

Fig. 3.34 a–c. Tetralogy of Fallot, bidirectional shunt through the VSD; same patient as in Fig. 3.33. **a** Two-dimensional TEE, longitudinal view, shows the VSD just beneath the aortic root. **b** Right-to-left shunt through the defect (*red*). *Blue*, aliasing. **c** Left-to-right shunt through the defect (*blue*). *Red*, aliasing.

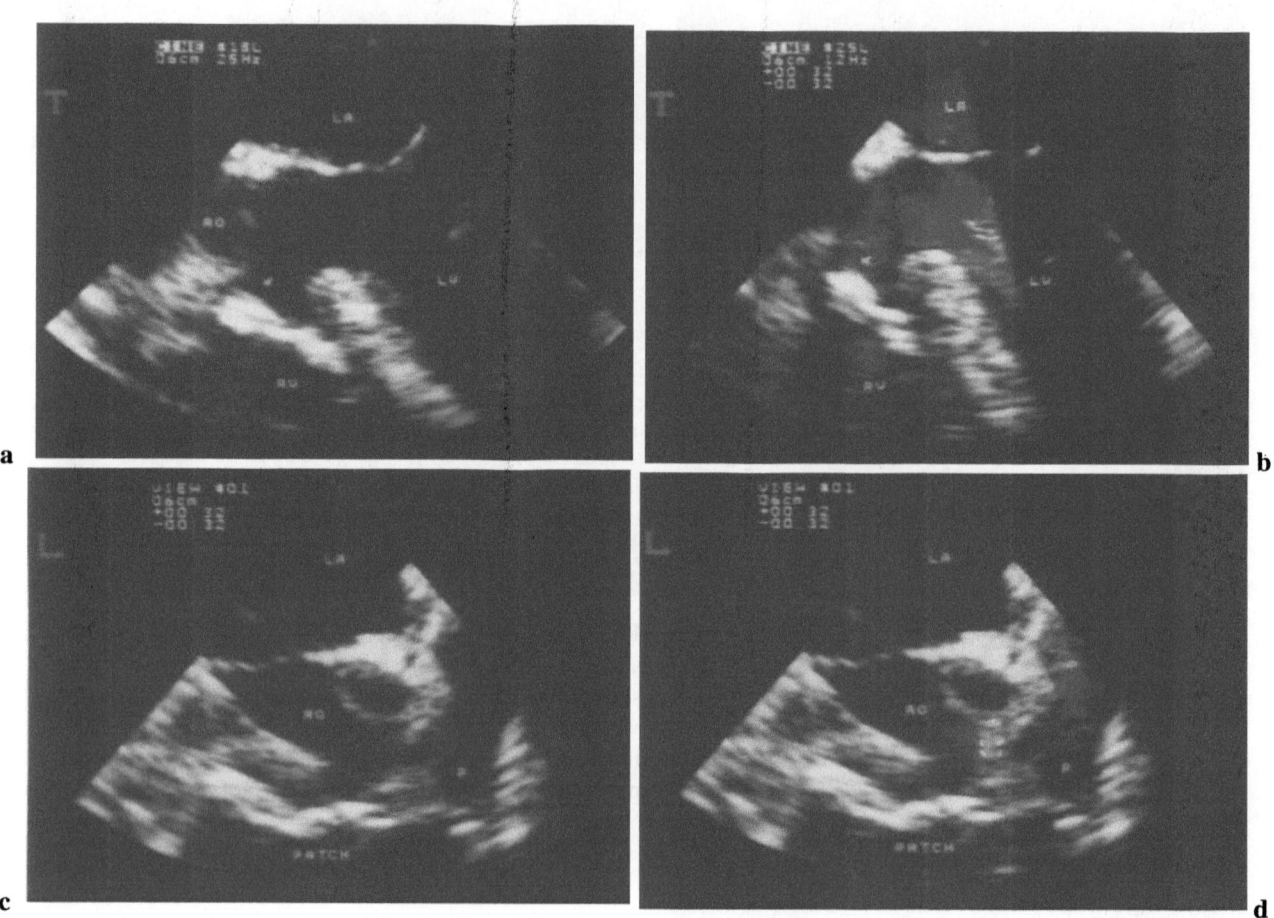

Fig. 3.36a–d. Tetralogy of Fallot, after surgical correction. **a** Two-dimensional TEE. *Arrow*, the patch that separates the two ventricles and deviates the left ventricular ejection flow into the overriding aorta. **b** Color Doppler shows no residual shunt. **c** Two-dimensional TEE. *Arrow*, patch. **d** Color Doppler shows normal flow in the pulmonary artery after commissurotomy of the pulmonary valve.

Double Outlet Right Ventricle

The anomaly of double outlet right ventricle is characterized by a subaortic or subpulmonary VSD from which the two great arteries arise. More than 50% of both great arteries arise from the right ventricle, whereas the main outlet from the left ventricle is the VSD. Pulmonary valve or infundibular stenosis is common, and the hemodynamics and symptoms are therefore similar to those in the tetralogy of Fallot.

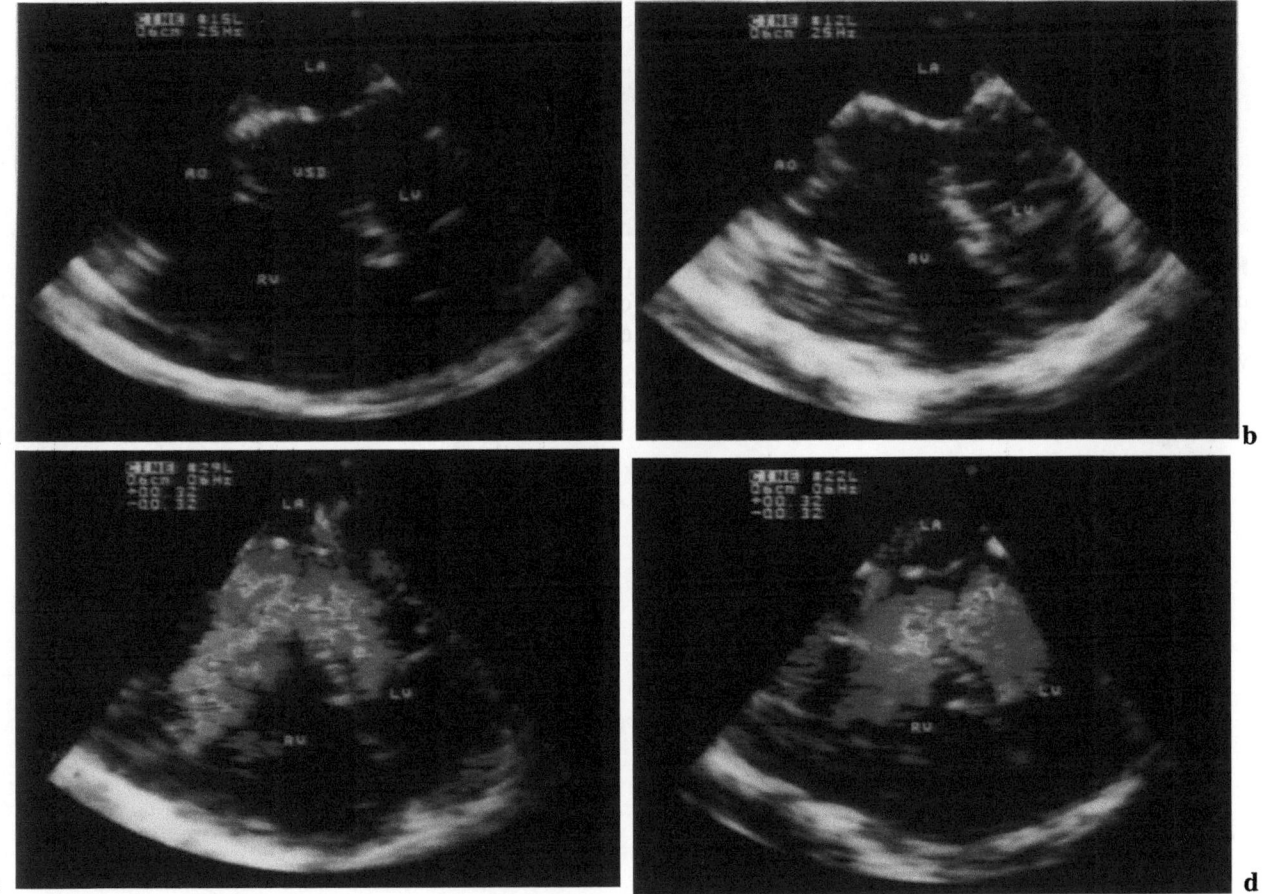

Fig. 3.37a–d. Double outlet right ventricle. **a** Two-dimensional TEE, transversal four-chamber view, shows the VSD. **b** LVOT view shows the aorta overriding the right ventricle. More than 50% of the aortic root arises from the right ventricle. **c, d** Bidirectional shunt through the VSD. **c** left-to-right shunt (*mosaic*). **d** Right-to-left shunt (*red*).

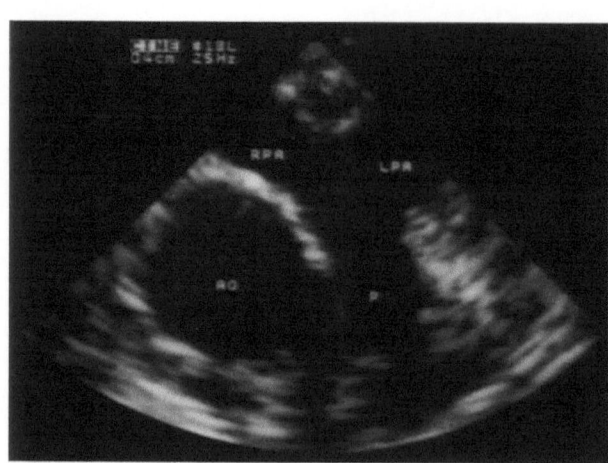 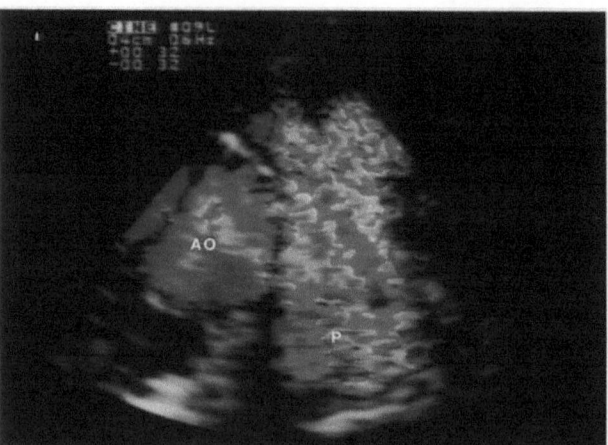

a

b

Fig. 3.38a, b. Double outlet right ventricle. Obstruction to right ventricular outflow. Same patient as in Fig. 3.37. **a** Two-dimensional TEE, basal short-axis view shows the relationship between aorta and pulmonary artery. The diameter of the aorta is twice that of the pulmonary artery. **b** Turbulent pulmonary ejection flow due to the stenosis.

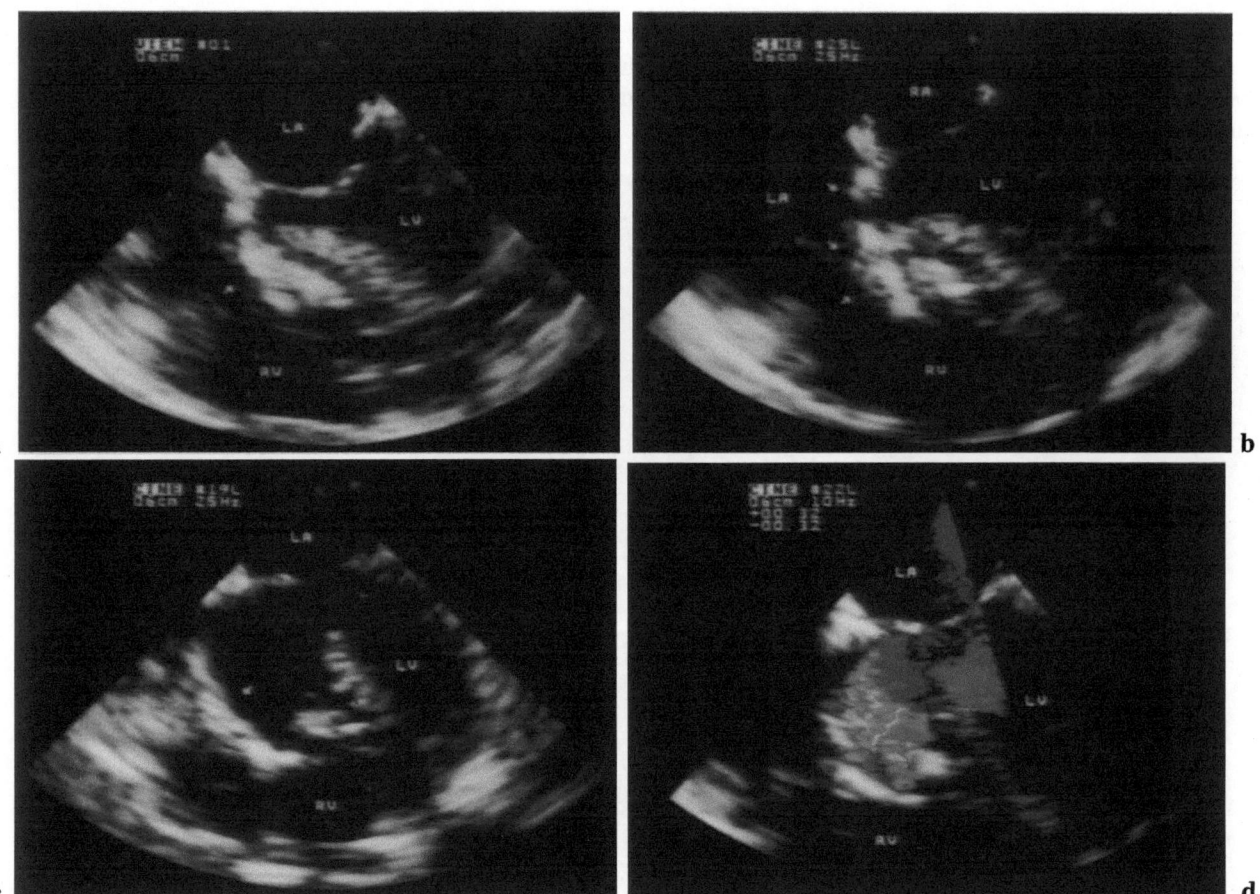

Fig. 3.39a–d. Double outlet right ventricle, after surgical repair. **a–c** Two-dimensional TEE, transversal four-chamber view, shows the position of the ventricular patch (*arrows*) that deviates the left ventricular outflow into the aorta. **d** Color Doppler shows the flow in the LVOT and the absence of residual shunt.

Dextrocardia

Dextrocardia is characterized by malposition of the heart and cardiac apex. The cardiac apex is located in the right side of thorax. Two types of dextrocardia can be distinguished: that with situs solitus and that with situs inversus. In dextrocardia with situs solitus the morphological left atrium is to the patient's left; in situs inversus it is to the right.

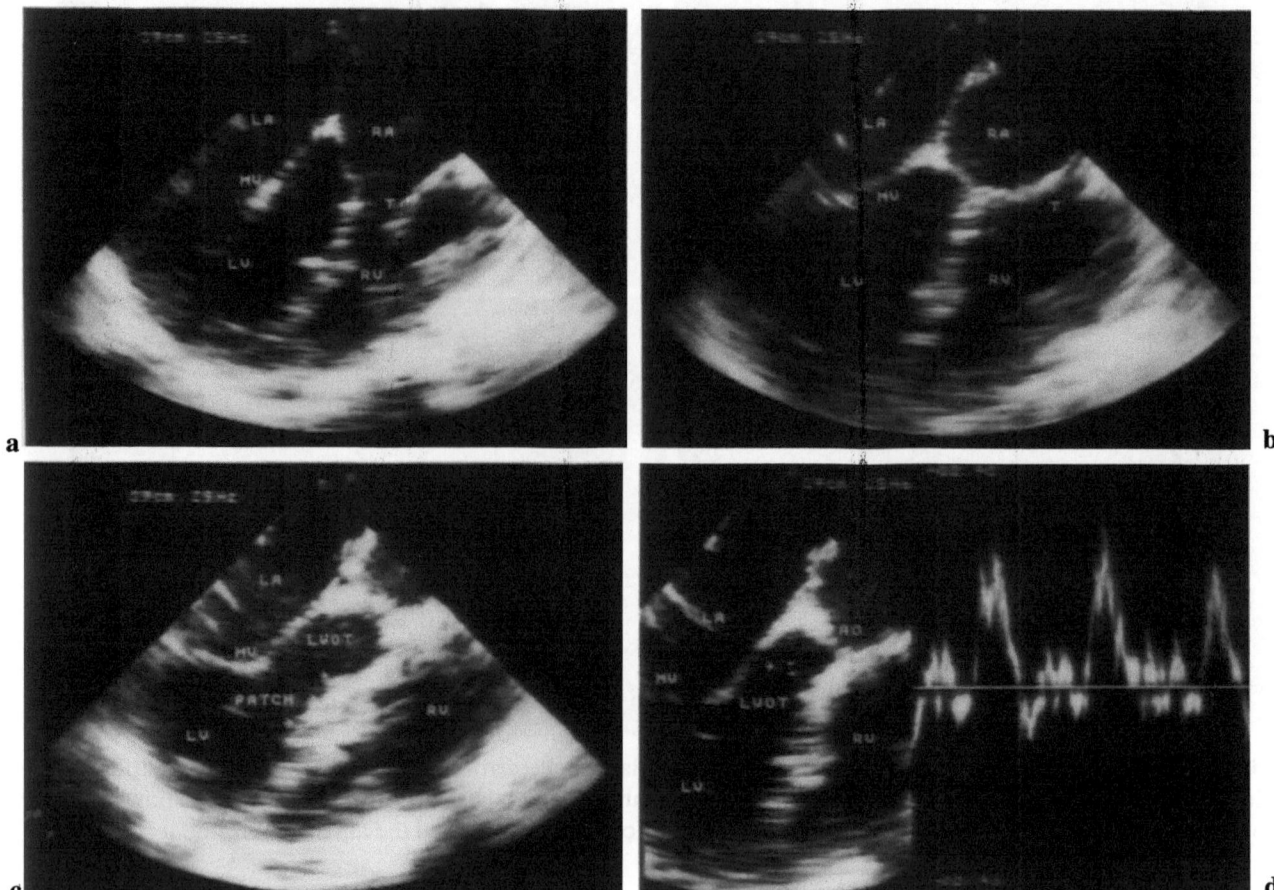

Fig. 3.40a–d. Dextrocardia with situs inversus, post-operative two-dimensional TEE. The patient underwent cardiac surgery for closure of a VSD. **a, b** Four-chamber view shows the position of cardiac chambers in diastole (**a**) and systole (**b**). The morphological left atrium and morphological left ventricle are to the patient´s right (*left in the figure*). The morphological right atrium and morphological right ventricle are to the patient´s left (*right in the figure*). **c** LVOT view. *Arrow*, the patch that closes the defect. **d** Pulsed-wave Doppler. *Arrow*, the sample volume placed in the LVOT. *Right*, Doppler curve shows laminar flow, demonstrating no obstruction to the left ventricular ejection. Note: dextrocardia with situs solitus and levocardia with situs inversus are associated with a characteristic curvature of the atrial septum, while dextrocardia with situs inversus does not show the characteristic curvature.

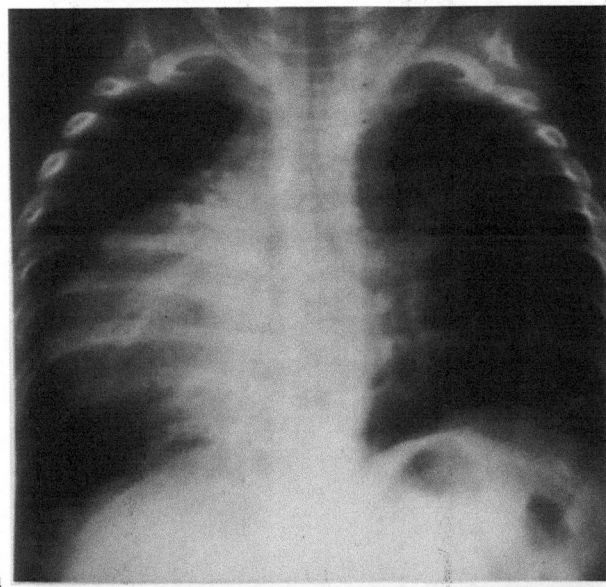

Fig. 3.41a–c. Dextrocardia with situs solitus. The patient underwent cardiac surgery for closure of an ASD. **a** Chest roentgenogram shows the heart malposition. The heart apex is located in the right side of thorax. **b, c** Two-dimensional TEE, four-chamber view, shows the position of cardiac chambers in diastole (**b**) and in systole (**c**). The morphological left atrium and morphological left ventricle are to the patient´s left (*right in the figure*). The morphological right atrium and morphological right ventricle are to the patient´s right (*left in the figure*). The cardiac apex (*arrow*) looks toward the right side (*left in the figure*).

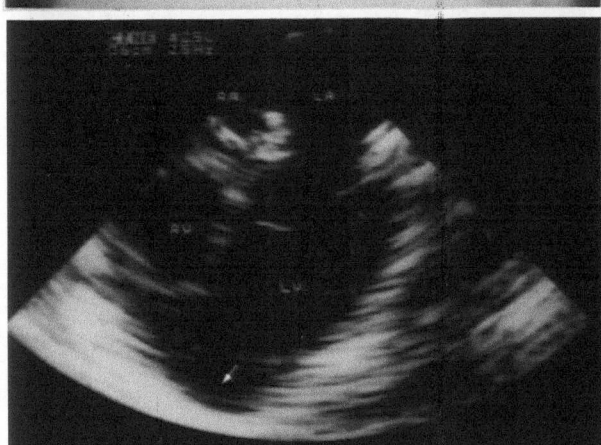

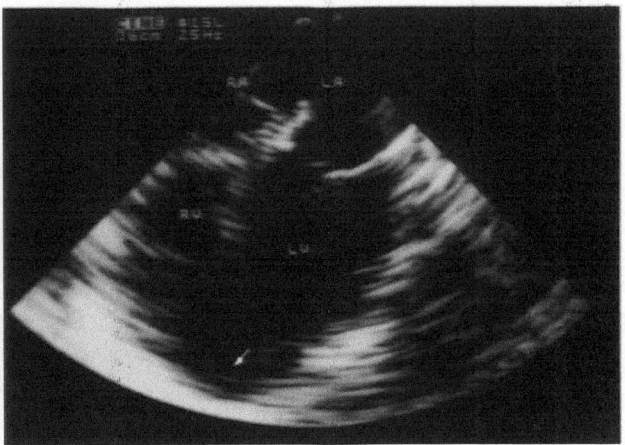

Transposition of the Great Arteries

In transposition of the great arteries (TGA) the aorta arises from the morphological right ventricle and the pulmonary artery from the morphological left ventricle, in the setting of a concordant atrioventricular connection.

Noncorrected TGA

Noncorrected TGA is not compatible with life if no other associated septal defect is present. If untreated, about one-third of patients die within the first week of life. Generally TEE provides poor visualization of the great arteries of the heart. However, the great arteries can be imaged and their reciprocal relationship determined by withdrawing the transducer systematically from the level of the four-chamber view toward the basis of the heart.

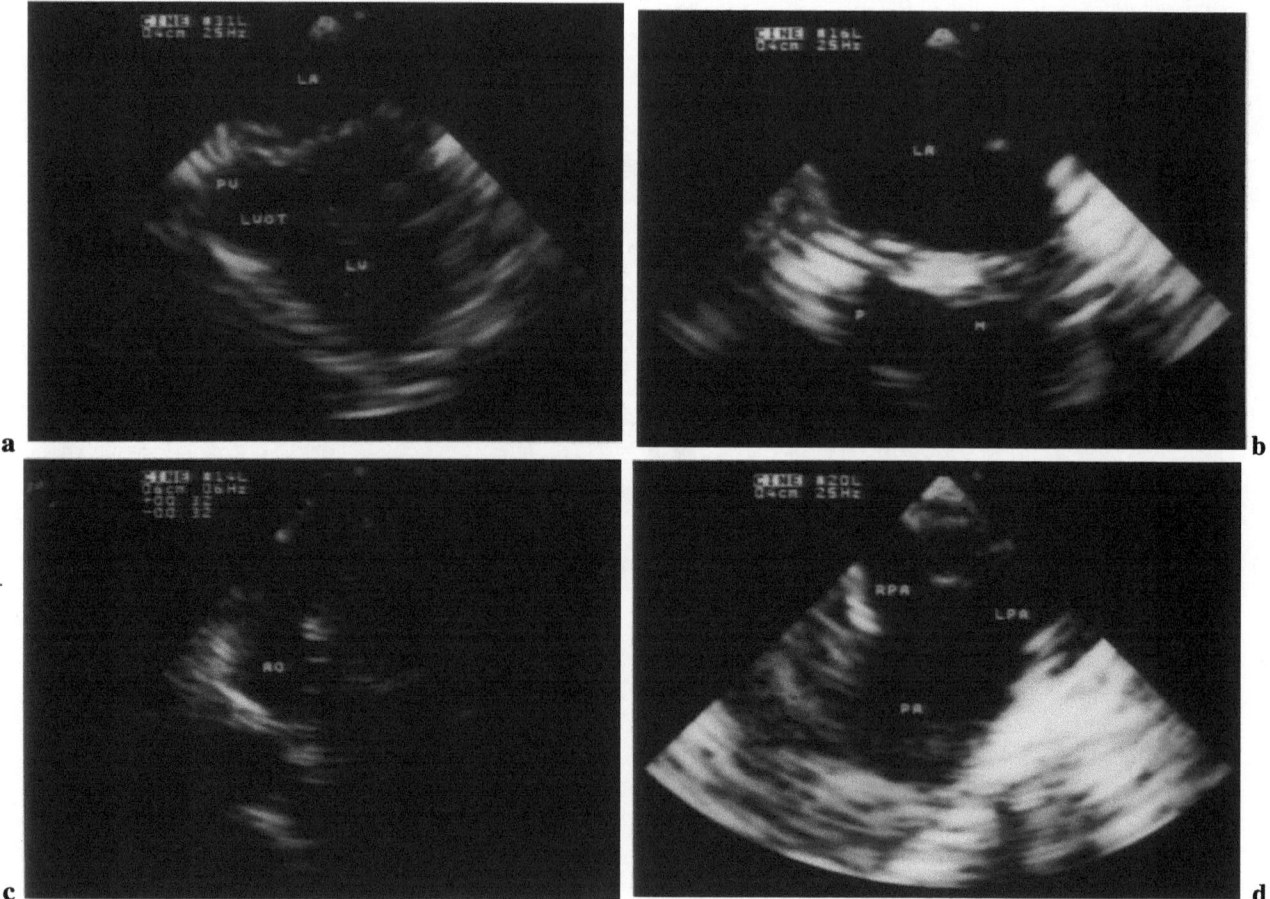

a

b

c

d

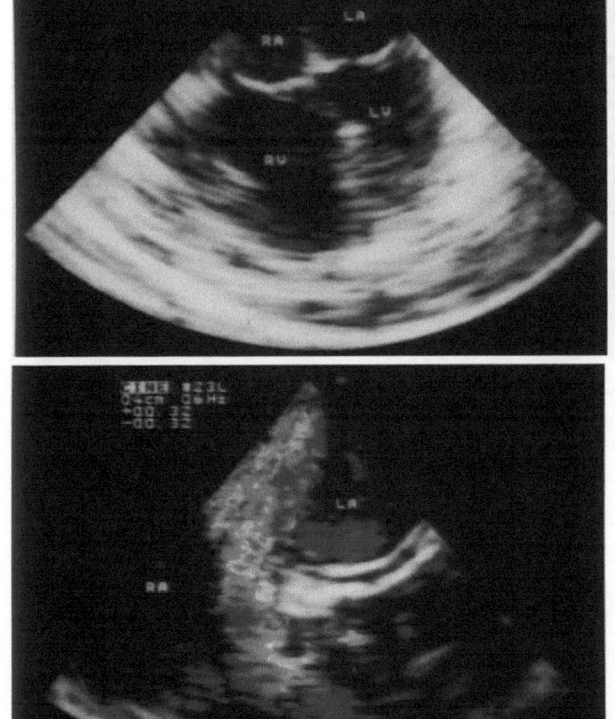

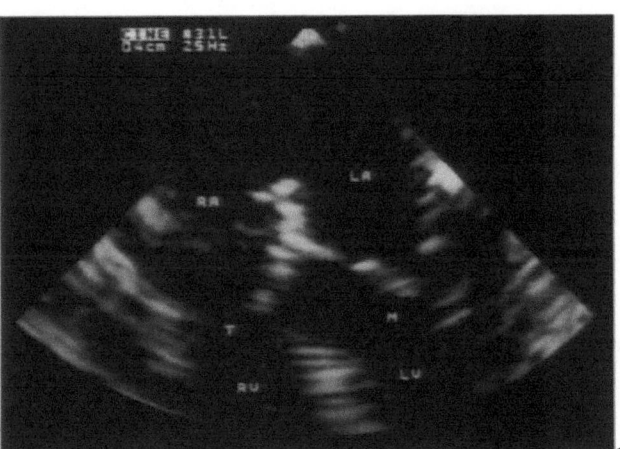

Fig. 3.43 a–c. TGA; same patient as in Fig. 3.42. Intraoperative TEE in a 3-day-old newborn. **a, b** Four-chamber view showing the normal position of the four chambers and the atrioventricular valves. *Arrow*, a large ASD achieved by rupturing the valve of the foramen ovale with a balloon catheter (Rashkind´s procedure). **c** Color Doppler flow signal of the shunt through the defect.

Fig. 3.42 a–d. TGA. **a, b** LVOT view shows that the pulmonary artery arises from the morphological left ventricle through the LVOT. **c, d** Basal short-axis view of the aorta and main pulmonary artery and the bifurcation. The aorta is markedly smaller than the pulmonary artery. *RPA*, Right pulmonary artery; *LPA*, left pulmonary artery. Note: the basal short-axis views are taken at different levels since the aorta and pulmonary artery could not be visualized in the same view.

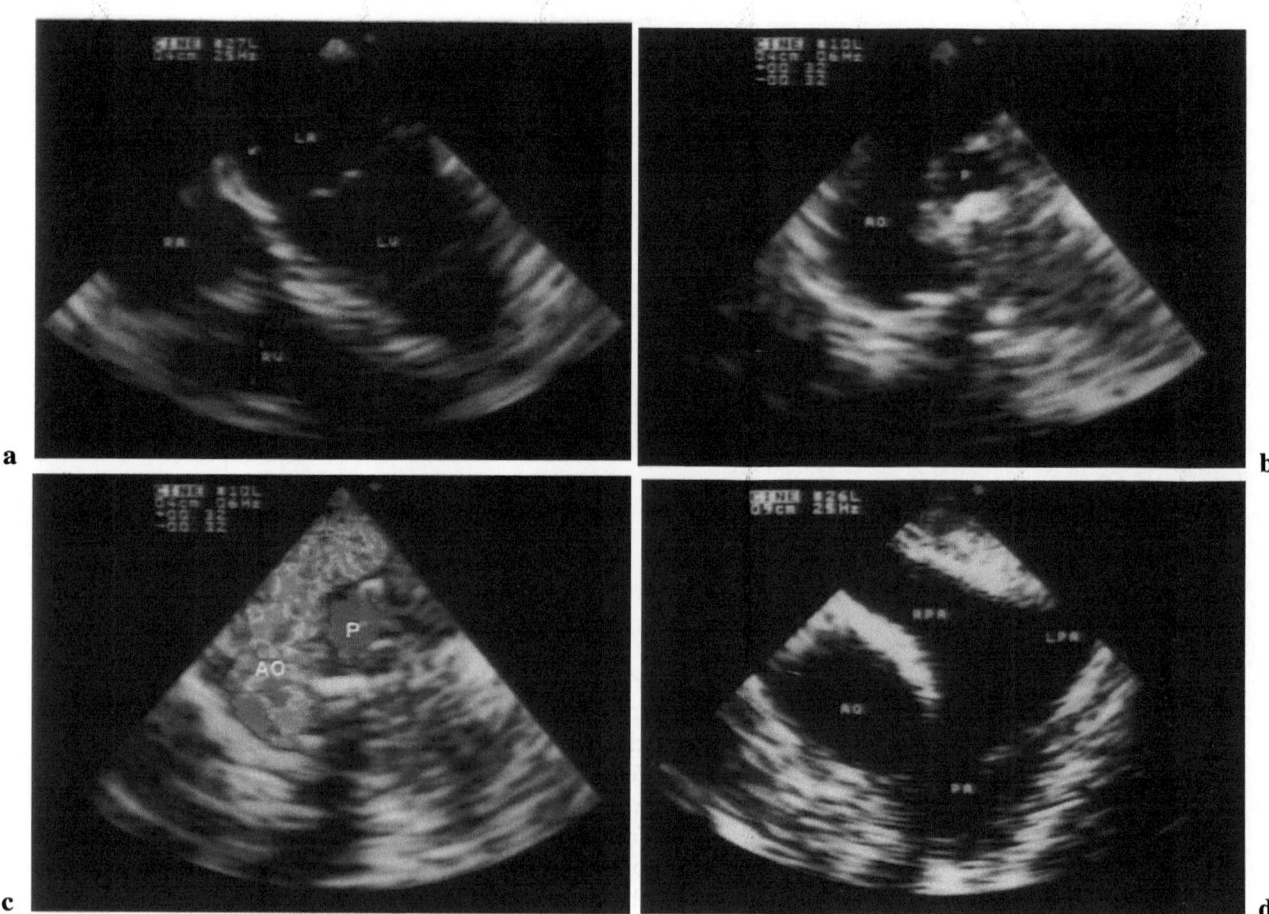

Fig. 3.44a–d. TGA, after arterial switch procedure; same patient as in Fig. 3.43. **a** Four-chamber view. *Arrow*, patch closure of the ASD caused by the Rashkind´s procedure. **b** Basal short-axis view shows the relative position of the great arteries after the switch procedure. **c** Color Doppler flow imaging shows turbulent flow in the aorta. **d** Normal position of the great arteries, basal short-axis view. The aorta is visualized to the patient´s right (*left in the figure*) in its transversal section. The pulmonary artery and its bifurcation are visualized to the patient´s left. Note: the turbulent flow in the aorta was not associated with a significant pressure gradient.

Congenitally Corrected TGA

In congenitally corrected TGA the aorta arises from the morphological right ventricle and the pulmonary artery from the morphological left ventricle, in the setting of a discordant atrioventricular connection. The anatomical left ventricle lies to the patient's right and connects the right atrium to a posterior and right-sided pulmonary artery. The anatomical right ventricle lies to the patient's left and connects the left atrium to an anterior and left-sided aorta.

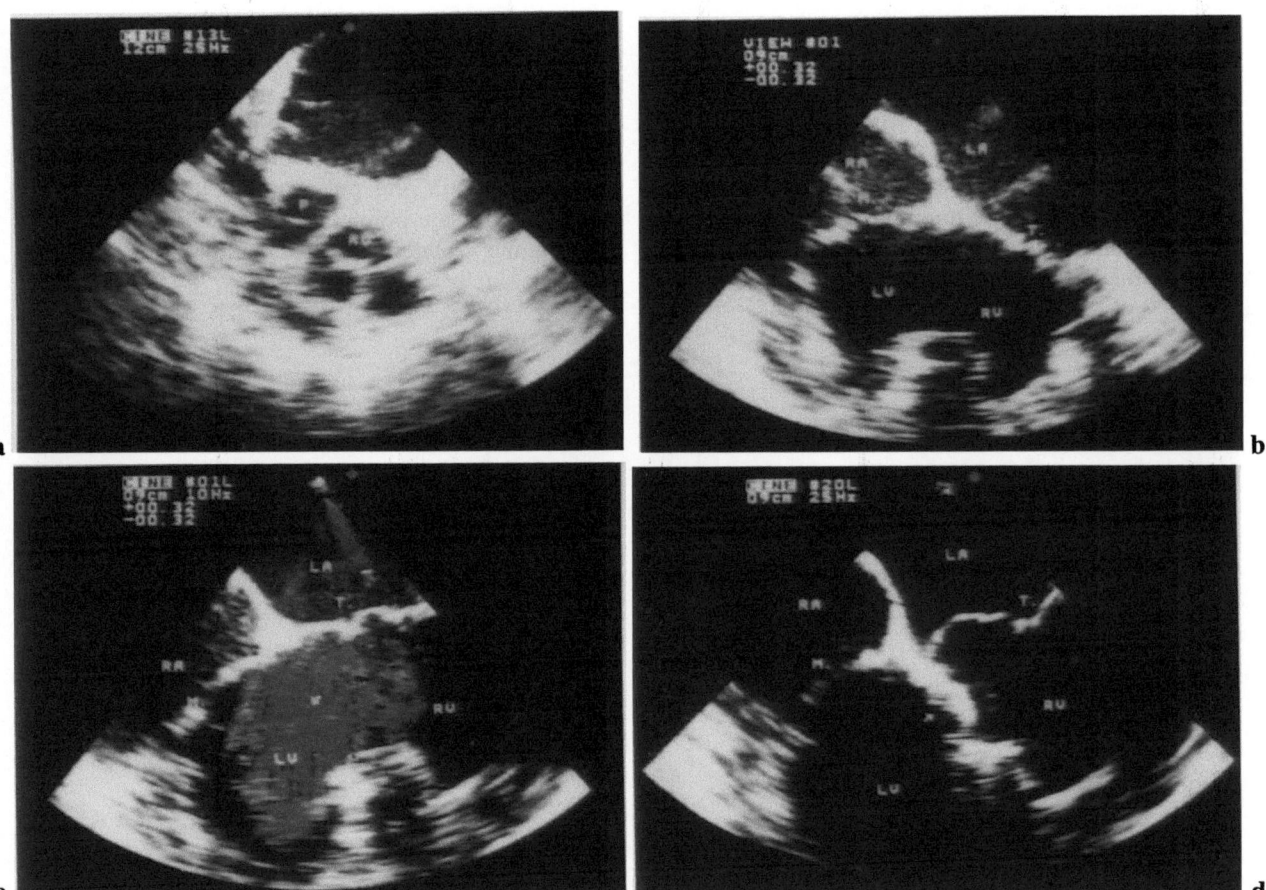

Fig. 3.45a–d. Congenitally corrected TGA. **a** Basal short-axis view of the great arteries. The aortic valve is anterior and to the patient's left (*right in the figure*), the pulmonary artery is posterior and to the patient's right (*left in the figure*). **b** Four-chamber view shows the atrioventricular discordance: the morphological left ventricle and mitral valve are to the patient's right. The morphological right ventricle and tricuspid valve are to the patient's left. An associated large VSD is present. **c** Color Doppler flow imaging of the bidirectional shunt through the defect. Note the low velocity signal of the ventricular shunt due to the absence of gradient between the two ventricles. **d** After surgical closure of the VSD. *Arrow*, the patch.

Truncus Arteriosus

Persistent truncus arteriosus is an anomaly in which a single vessel (truncus) arises from both ventricles through a VSD. Systemic, pulmonary and coronary circulation originate from the truncus, which is provided with a common valve. Four types of truncus arteriosus may be distinguished according to the degree of blood flow to the lung. In type I, the common type, a rudimentary separate pulmonary trunk gives origin to the left and right pulmonary arteries. In type II a separate pulmonary trunk is absent; the left and the right pulmonary arteries originate from the left side of the common trunk. In type III the left and right pulmonary arteries originate from the left and right side of the common trunk, respectively. In the so-called type IV the pulmonary arteries are completely absent; the pulmonary circulation is supplied by systemic collateral arteries arising from the descending aorta.

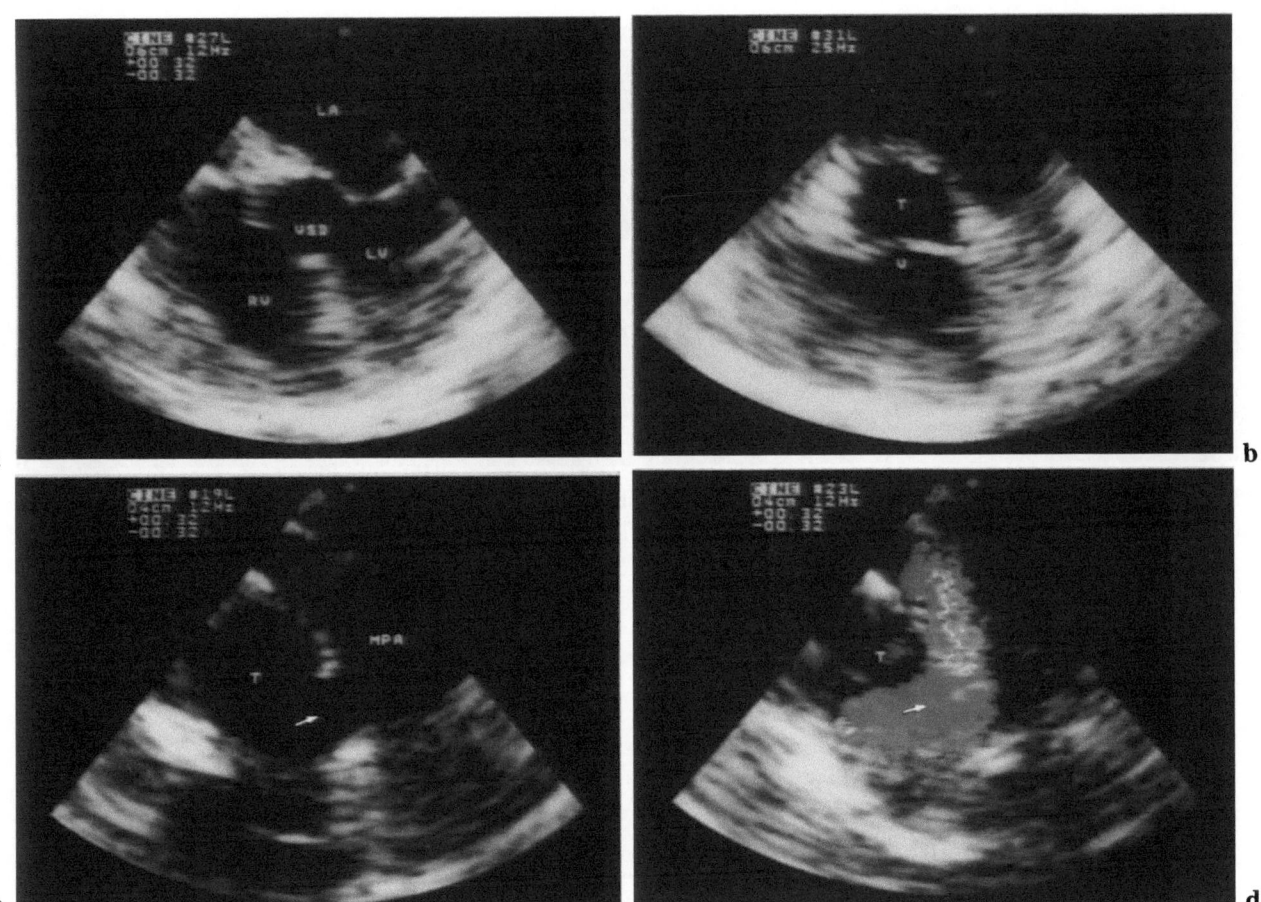

Fig. 3.46a–d. Persistent truncus arteriosus, type I. The truncus arteriosus gives origin to the main pulmonary artery. **a** Four-chamber view shows the VSD. **b** By withdrawing the esophagoscope from the four-chamber view toward the basis of the heart, the truncus root (*T*) and the valve (*V*) can be visualized. **c** Basal short-axis view. *Arrow*, communication between the truncus and pulmonary artery. **d** Color Doppler shows the shunt flow from the truncus (*T*) to the pulmonary artery across the communication.

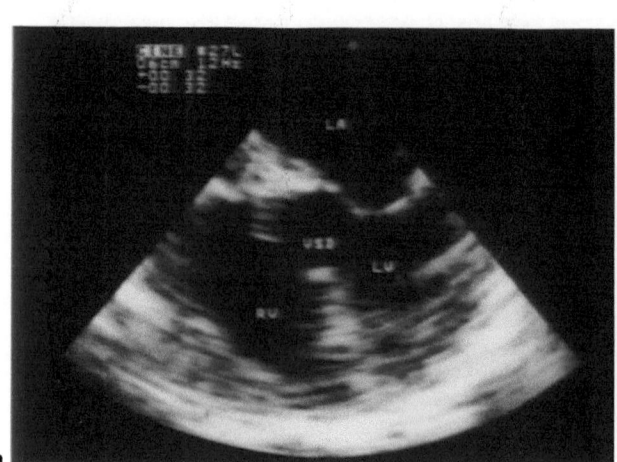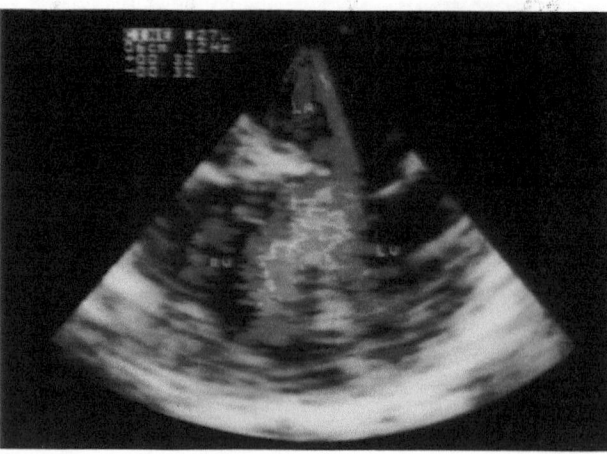

Fig. 3.47a, b. Persistent truncus arteriosus, type I; same patient as in Fig. 3.46. **a** Four-chamber view shows the VSD. **b** Color Doppler shows the shunt flow across the VSD.

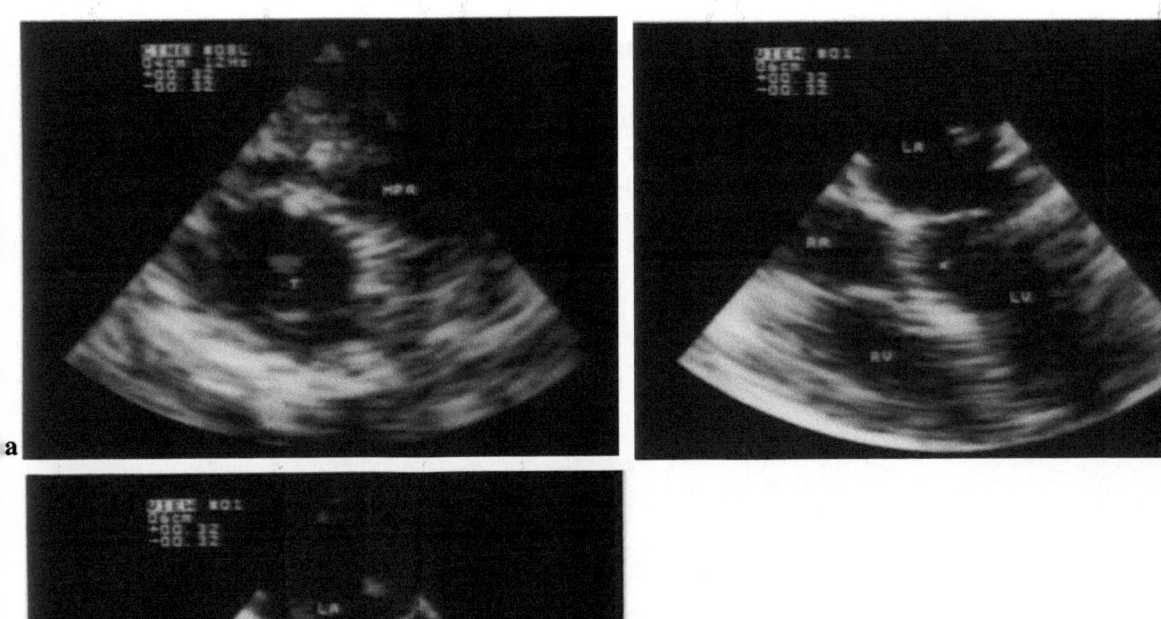

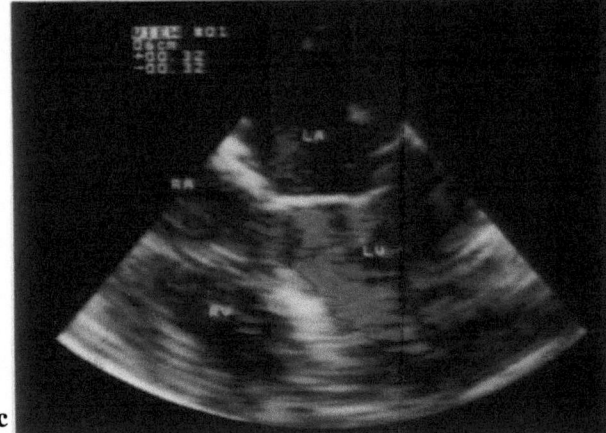

Fig. 3.48a–c. Persistent truncus arteriosus, after surgical repair. **a** Basal short-axis view. The truncus has been separated into systemic and pulmonary vessels. **b** Four-chamber view shows the position of the patch closing the VSD. **c** Color Doppler shows the absence of residual shunt flow across the ventricular septum.

Congenital Pulmonary Stenosis

Obstructions to pulmonary arterial flow may be localized at the RVOT, the pulmonary valve, or the pulmonary artery and its peripheral branches. Pulmonary stenosis is frequently associated with other cardiac malformations. Valvular stenosis cannot always be visualized directly by monoplanar transverse TEE, but color Doppler can show the characteristics of poststenotic turbulent flow. Pulmonary valve and right ventricular infundibular obstructions can be clearly visualized by longitudinal views of biplanar TEE. Peripheral stenoses of pulmonary artery cannot be visualized by TEE.

Infundibular Stenosis

Narrowing of the infundibulum of the right ventricle is often associated with other heart malformations that cause right ventricular hypertrophy.

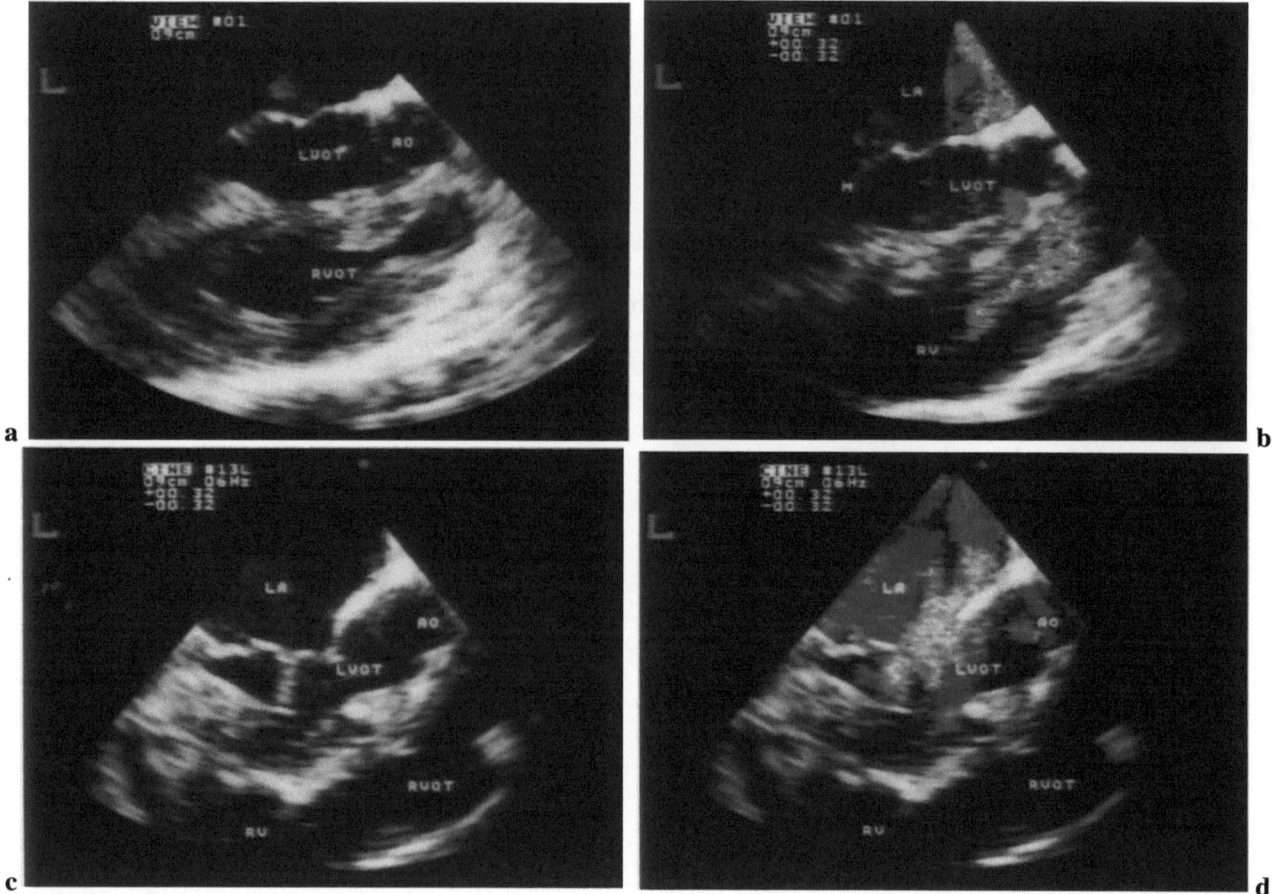

Pulmonary Valve Stenosis

Congenital stenosis of the pulmonary valve results from fusion of the valve commissures. Hypertrophy of the right ventricle and associated secondary obstruction of the right ventricular infundibulum is often observed in these patients.

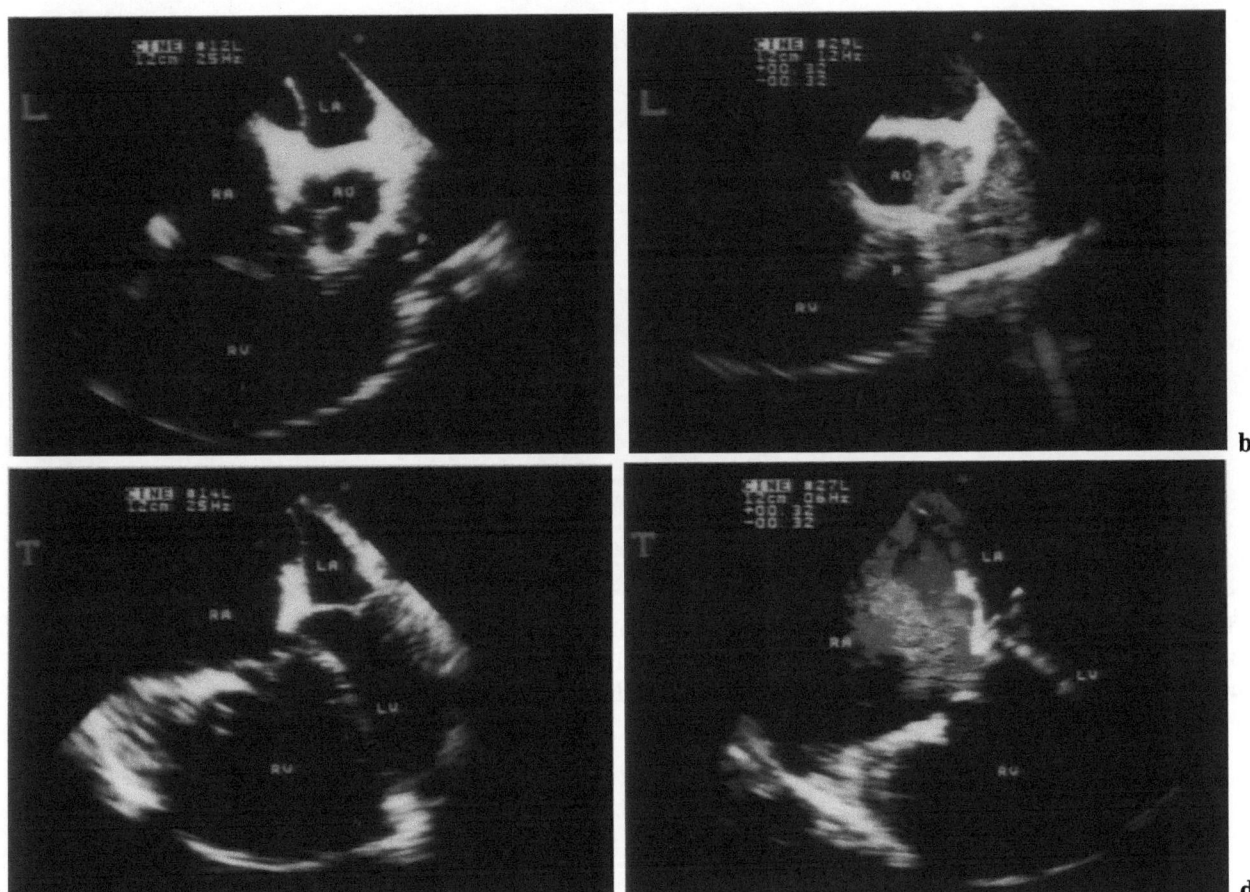

Fig. 3.50 a–d. Pulmonary valve stenosis. **a** Two-dimensional TEE, RVOT long-axis view, shows narrowing of the pulmonary valve (*P*). **b** Color Doppler shows turbulent poststenotic flow (*mosaic*) in the main pulmonary artery. **c** Two-dimensional TEE, four-chamber view, shows hypertrophy and dilatation of the right ventricle. **d** Color Doppler shows relative insufficiency of the tricuspid valve due to right ventricular dilatation.

Fig. 3.49 a–d. Infundibular stenosis, AVSD and obstruction to the RVOT due to right ventricular hypertrophy, same patient as in Fig. 3.23. **a** Longitudinal RVOT view shows hypertrophy of the right ventricle and narrowing of the infundibular tract. **b** Color Doppler shows turbulent systolic flow in the RVOT. **c, d** After surgical repair. Longitudinal RVOT view shows enlargement of the RVOT after the infundibulectomy. No turbulent systolic flow is present in the RVOT.

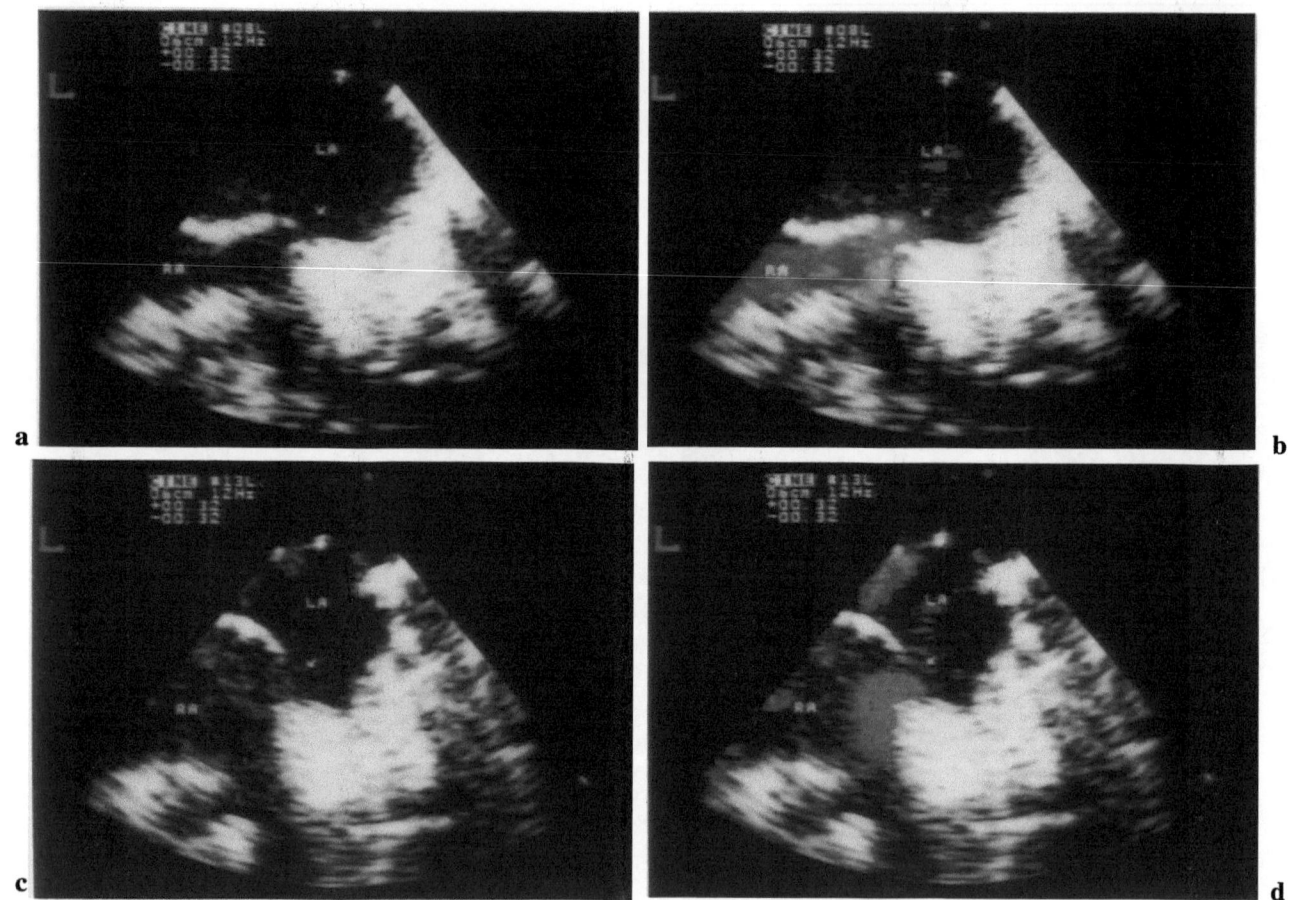

Fig. 3.51a–d. Pulmonary valve stenosis, patent foramen ovale; same patient as in Fig. 3.50. **a, c** Two-dimensional TEE, RVOT long-axis view shows incomplete closure of the fossa ovalis. Color Doppler shows a bidirectional shunt. **b** Left-to-right shunt (*blue*). **d** Right-to-left shunt (*red*).

Banding of the Pulmonary Artery

Banding of the pulmonary artery is aimed at preventing the occurrence of pulmonary vascular obstructive disease in patients with left-to-right shunts. It represents one of the most frequent obstructions to right outflow. Early correction of cyanotic heart diseases represents a new tendency in modern heart surgery.

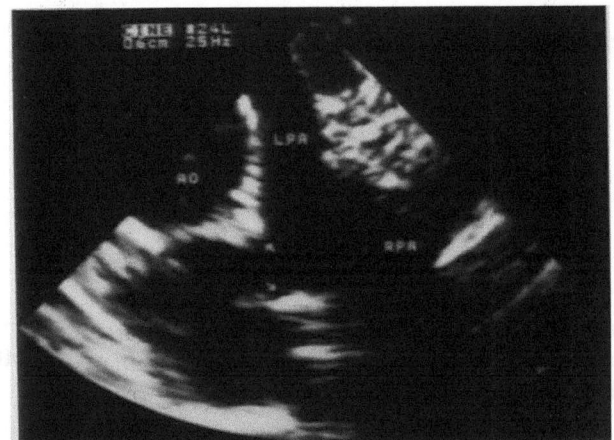

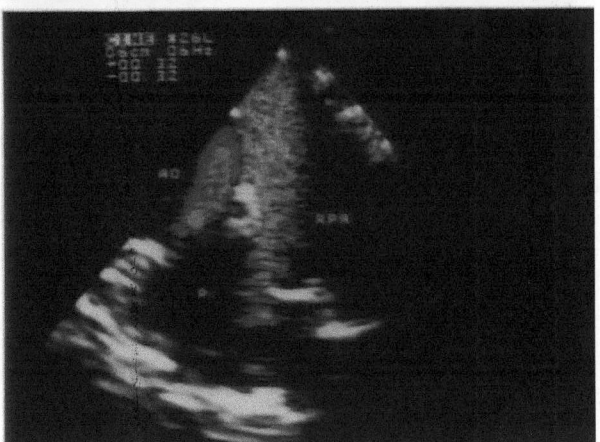

Fig. 3.52a, b. Banding of the pulmonary artery, patient with AVSD. **a** Two-dimensional TEE, basal short-axis view. *Arrows*, narrowing of the main pulmonary artery due to banding. **b** Color Doppler shows turbulent systolic flow in the pulmonary bifurcation beyond the banding. The patient underwent correction of the AVSD, enlargement of the RVOT and debanding of the pulmonary artery. *LPA*, Left pulmonary artery; *RPA*, right pulmonary artery.

Congenital Aortic Stenosis

Congenital aortic stenosis includes subvalvular obstruction to left ventricular outflow, valvular stenosis, and narrowing of the supravalvular ascending aorta.

Subvalvular Stenosis

Subvalvular aortic stenoses are generally due to a membranous fibromuscular diaphragm obstructing the LVOT just beneath the aortic valve.

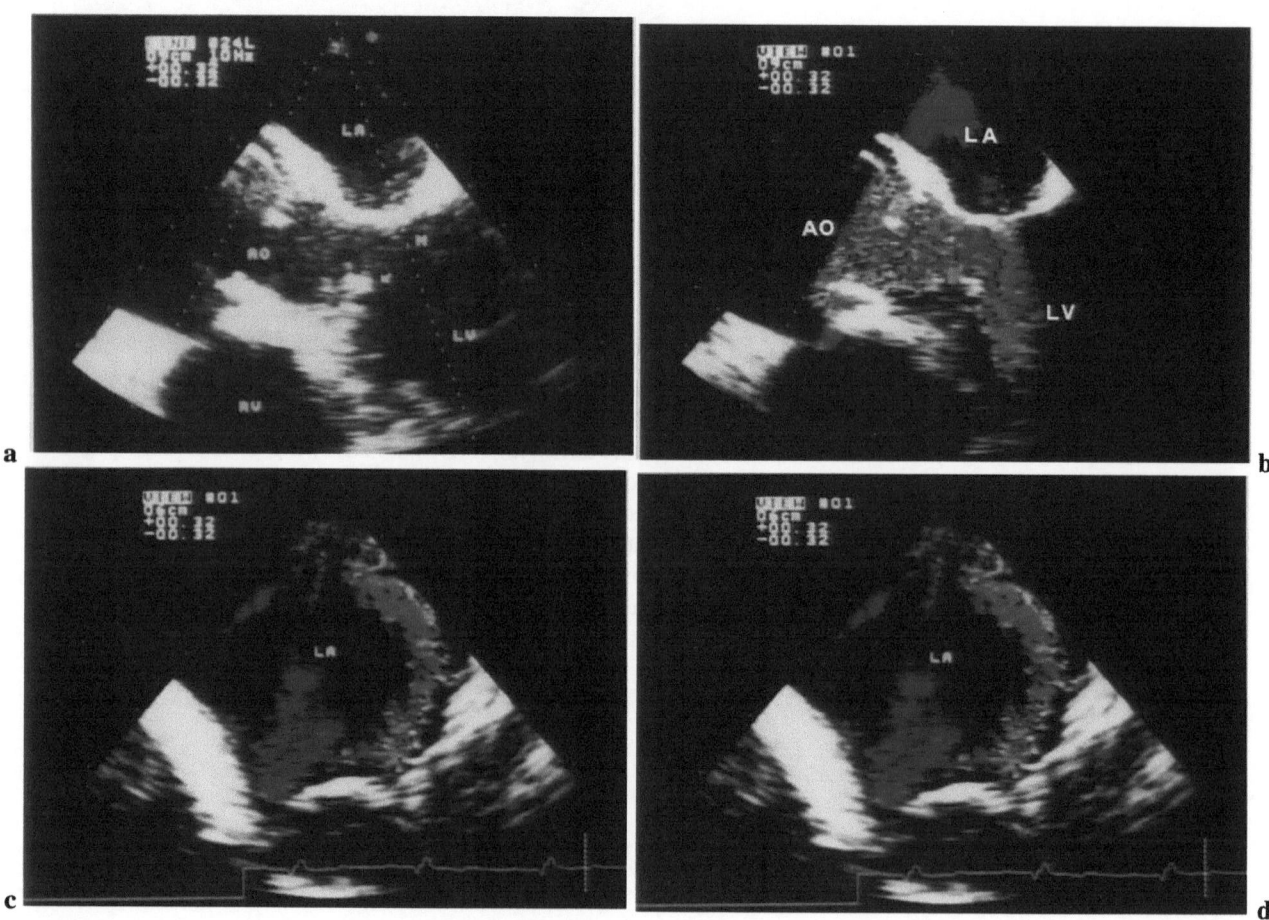

Fig. 3.53a–d. Subvalvular aortic stenosis. **a** LVOT view. *Arrow*, fibromuscular membrane just beneath the aortic valve, obstructing left ventricular outflow. **b** Color Doppler. Left ventricular ejection flow (*red*) turns into turbulent high-velocity flow (*mosaic*) beyond the obstruction. **c** LVOT view. Systolic anterior movement of the anterior mitral leaflet (*arrow*) increases the degree of obstruction to left ventricular outflow. **d** Color Doppler shows a small mitral regurgitant jet directed posteriorly, due to the systolic anterior movement of the anterior mitral leaflet.

Aortic Valve Stenosis

Various degrees of fusion of the aortic commissures
can be observed in congenital stenosis of the aortic
valve. These include the tricuspid, bicuspid, and unicuspid aortic valves.

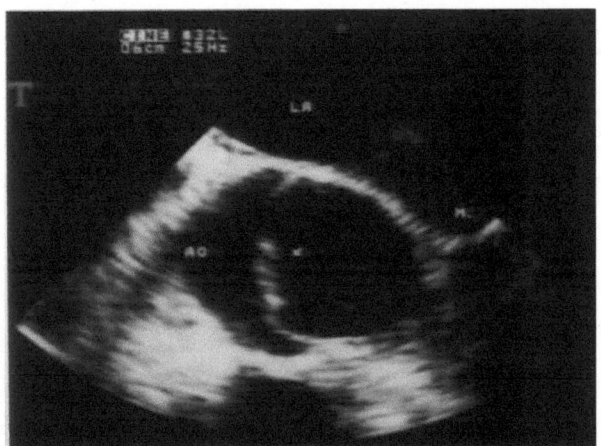

a

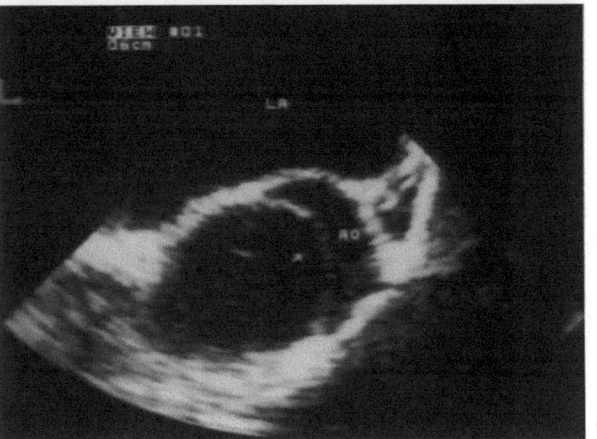

b

Fig. 3.55a, b. Aortic valve stenosis, congenitally bicuspid aortic valve. Two-dimensional TEE, transversal (*T*) and longitudinal (*L*) basal views The "doming" of the aortic cusps in systole (*arrow*) is a typical
landmark of aortic valve stenosis.

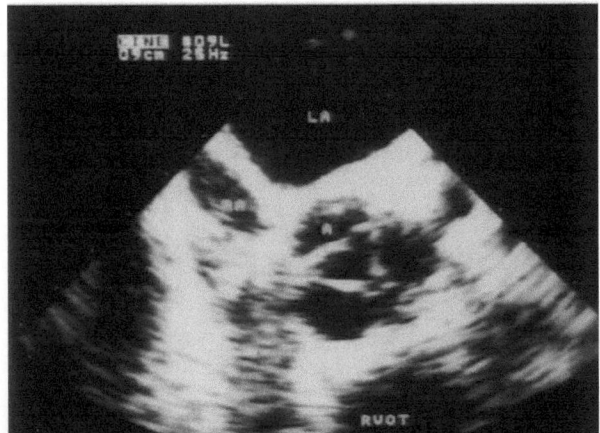

a

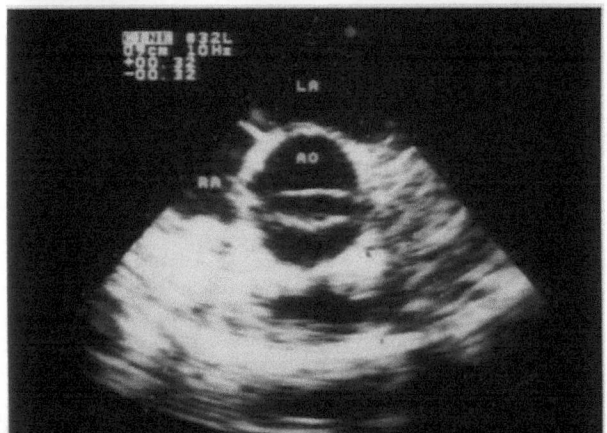

b

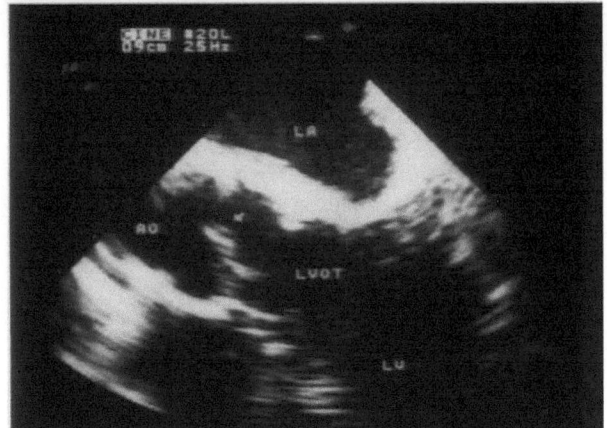

c

Fig. 3.54a–c. Aortic valve stenosis. **a** Basal short-
axis view, tricuspid aortic valve. Impaired systolic separation of the three aortic cusps. **b** Bicuspid aortic
valve, impaired systolic separation of the two aortic
leaflets. **c** LVOT view, unicuspid aortic valve. *Arrow*,
a single aortic leaflet.

Supravalvular Stenosis

Three types of obstructions to the ascending aorta have been described: the hourglass, membranous, and tubular types.

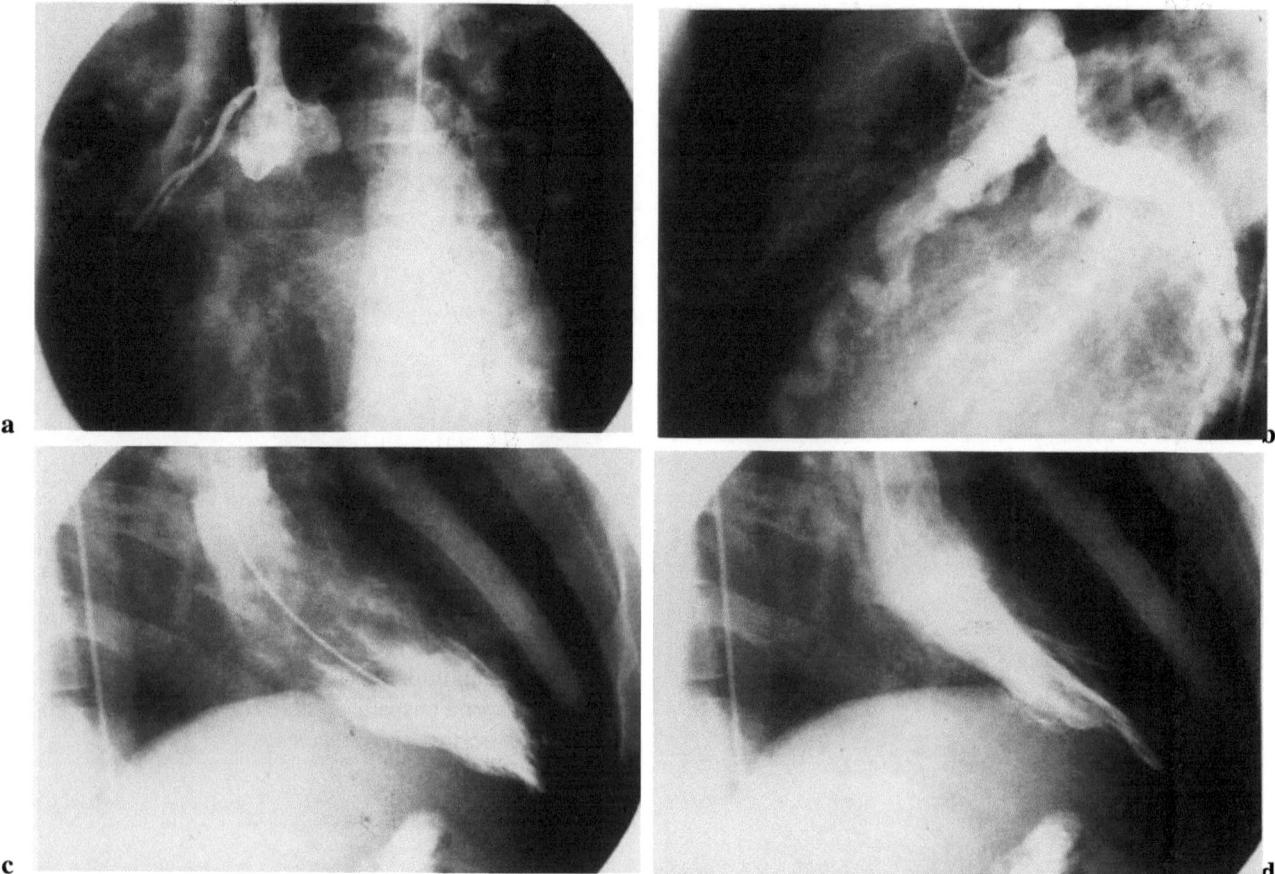

Fig. 3.56a–d. Supravalvular aortic stenosis. **a** Angiography of the aorta showing a tubular narrowing of the ascending aorta beginning just above the aortic sinuses, extending up to the transverse aortic arch. The internal diameter of the ascending aorta is narrowed to only 5–6 mm. A small right coronary artery arises from the narrowed portion and shows 70% ostial stenosis. **b** The left coronary system, arising proximal to the narrowing, is enormously dilated and tortuous. The diameter of the left main coronary artery is 9 mm. **c, d** Left ventricular angiography in diastole (*left*) and systole (*right*) shows left ventricular hypertrophy. Note: the patient was 23 years old and asymptomatic. The diagnosis was made after a routine medical examination that revealed a systolic murmur.

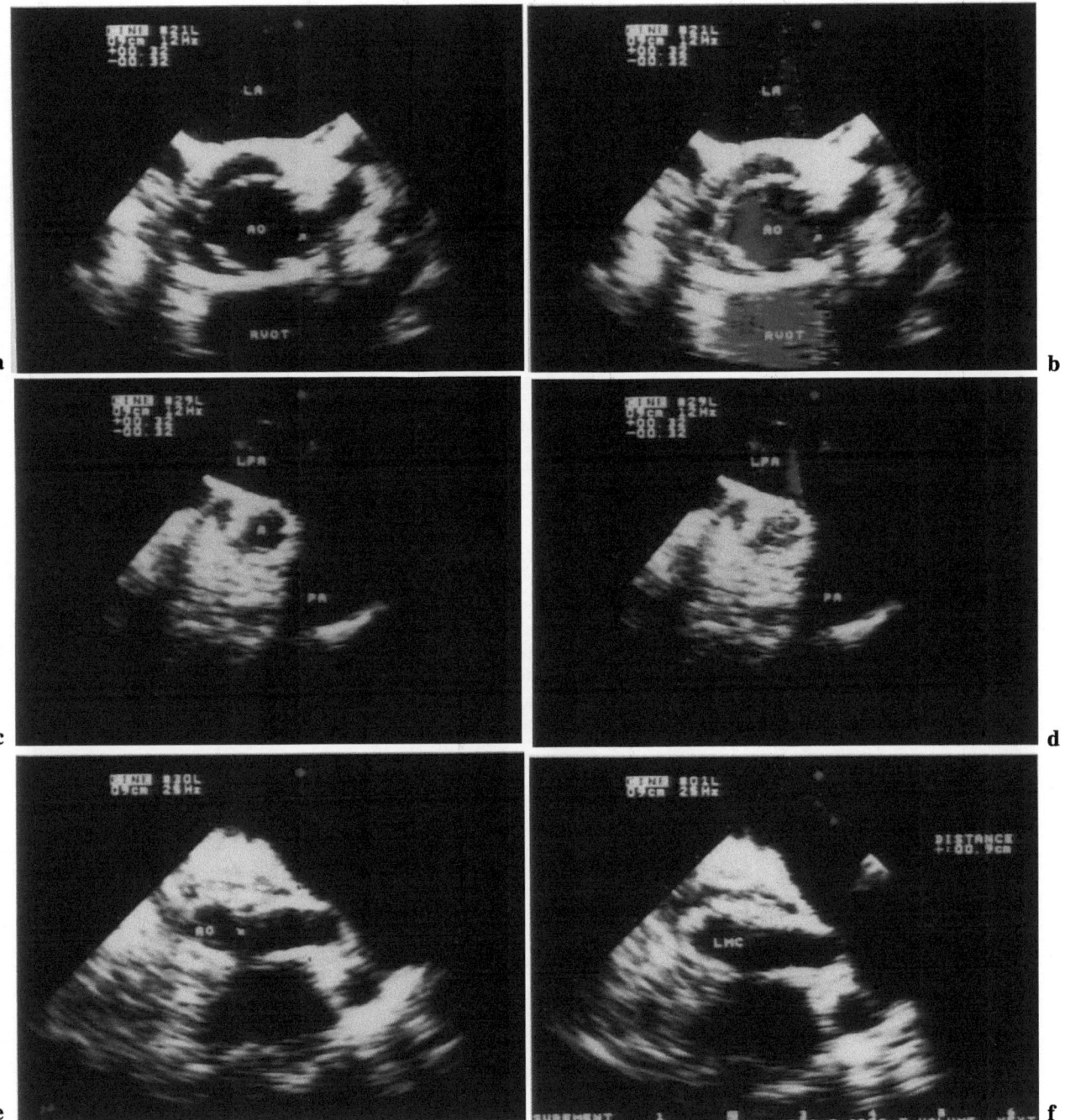

Fig. 3.57a–f. Supravalvular aortic stenosis. **a** Basal short-axis view shows a dilated aortic root with dysplastic aortic valve. A dilated left main coronary artery (*arrow*) arises from the aorta, proximal to the obstruction. **b** Color Doppler shows normal systolic ejection flow in the aortic root, proximal to the narrowing. **c, d** The narrowing of ascending aorta (*A*) and the turbulent flow (*mosaic*) in the stenotic tract can be visualized by withdrawing the transducer farther toward the basis. **e, f** Basal short-axis view proximal to the obstruction shows enormous dilatation of the left main coronary artery (*LMC*) up to a diameter of 9 mm.

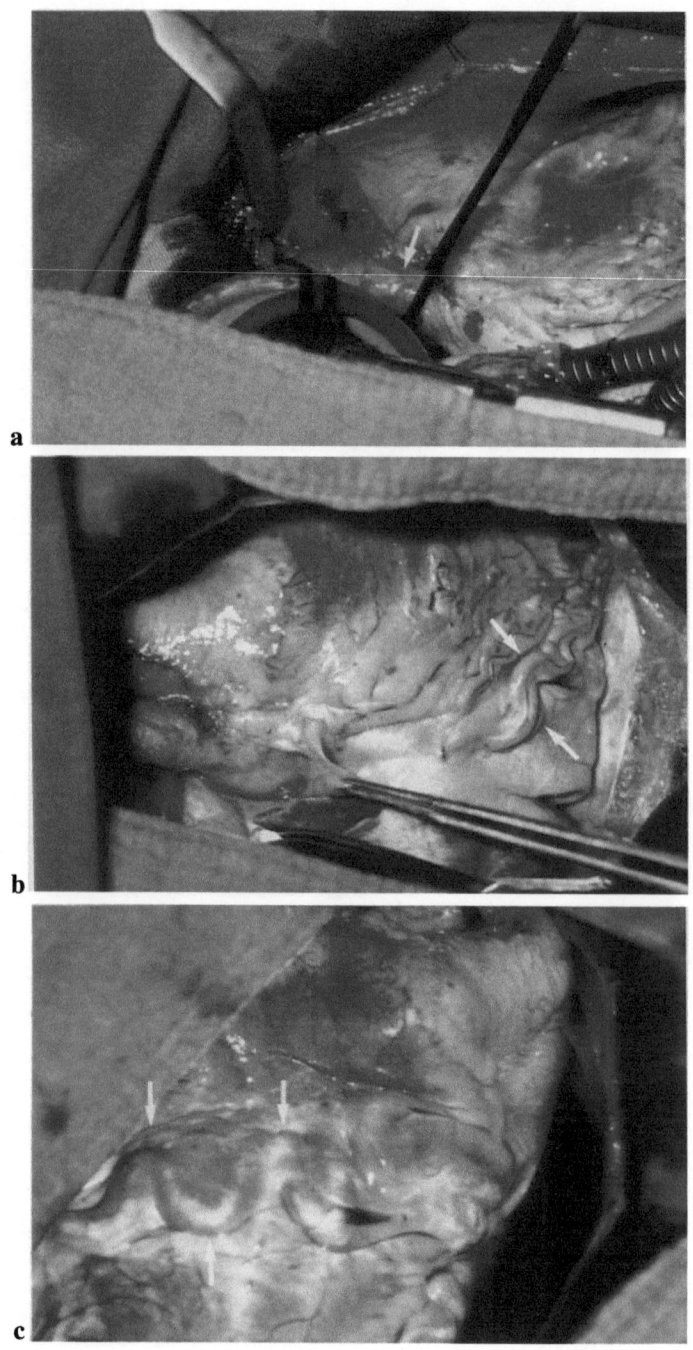

Fig. 3.58a–c. Supravalvular aortic stenosis, intraoperative view. **a** *Arrow*, tubular narrowing of the ascending aorta. **b, c** *Arrows*, highly dilated and tortuous left coronary artery.

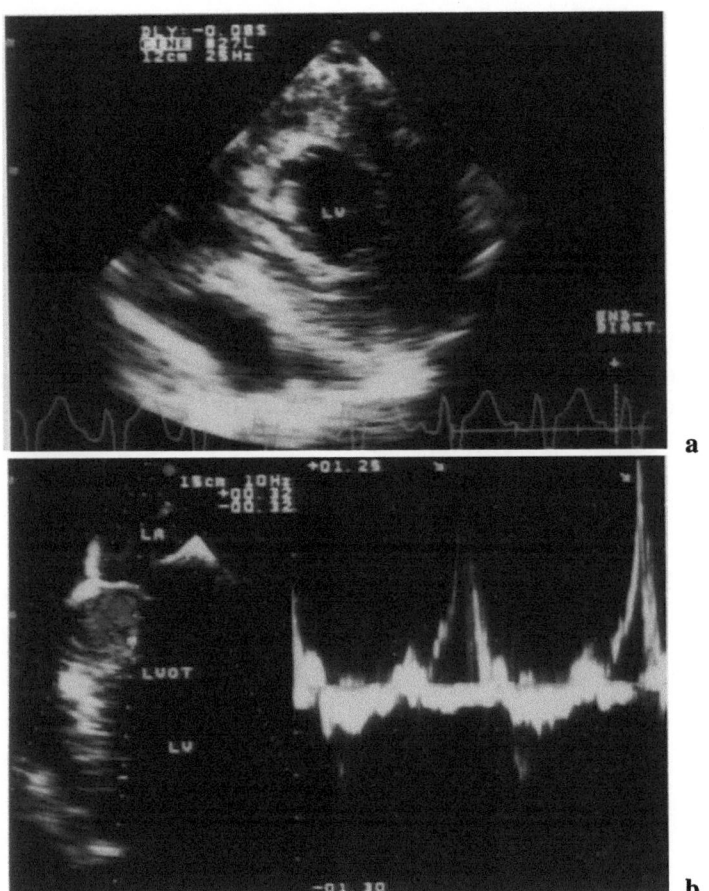

Fig. 3.59a, b. Supravalvular aortic stenosis. **a** Transgastric short-axis view shows hypertrophy of left ventricle. **b** Pulsed-wave Doppler. The sample volume is placed in the LVOT. The Doppler signal shows a delayed peak velocity of the left ventricular outflow occurring in late systole (*arrows*). This characteristic "daggerlike" waveform of the Doppler signal can be observed in the obstructions to LVOT, as well as hypertrophic obstructive cardiomyopathy.

Coarctation of the Aorta

Coarctation of the aorta is characterized by stenosis of the descending aorta, just distal to the left subclavian artery, close to the ductus arteriosus. TEE is useful for direct measurement of the descending aorta and assessment of the stenotic cross-sectional area.

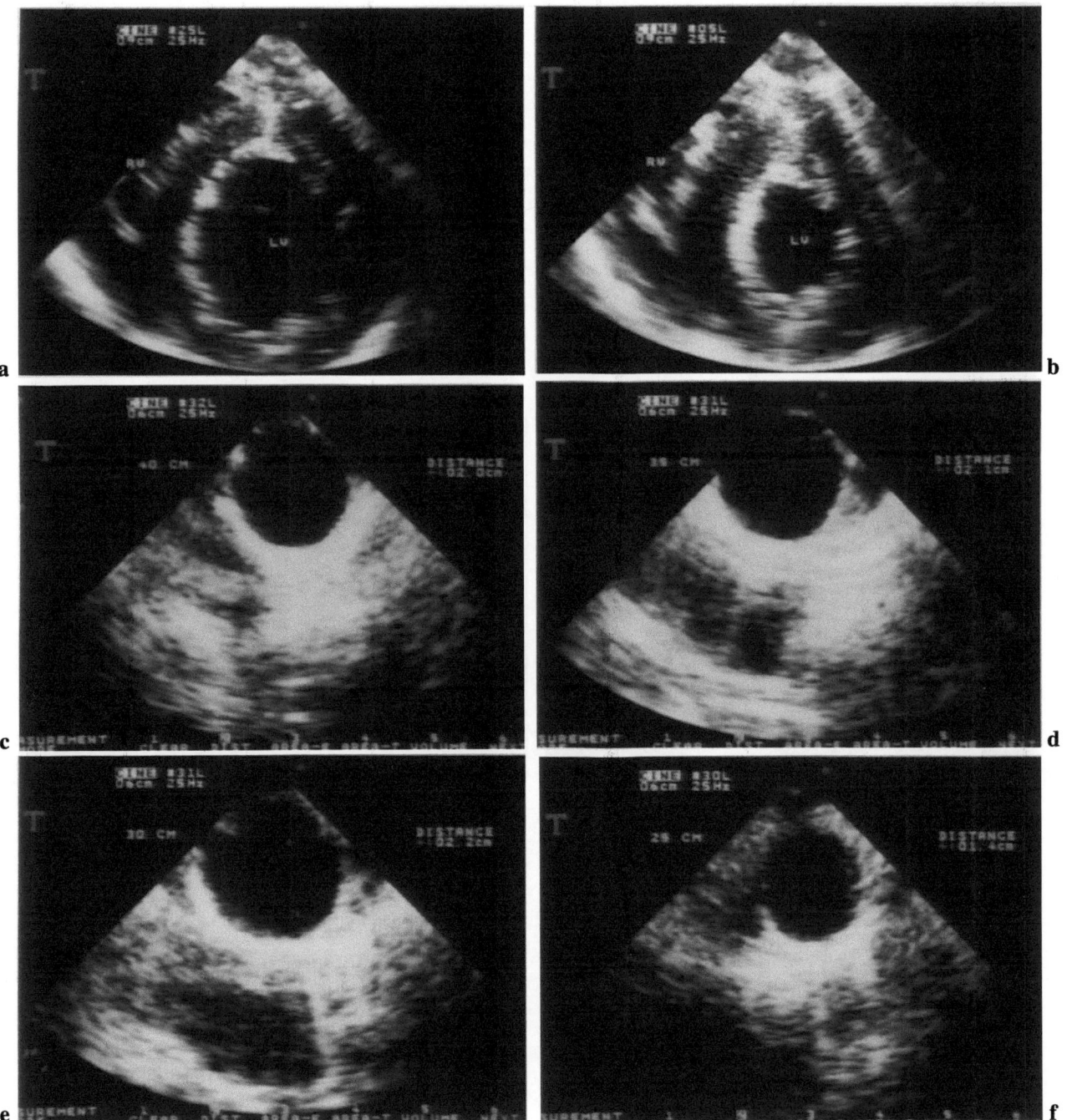

Fig. 3.60a–f. Coarctation of the aorta. **a, b** Transgastric short-axis view shows left ventricular hypertrophy, in diastole (*left*) and systole (*right*). **c–f** Transverse views of the descending aorta obtained by progressively withdrawing the esophagoscope from the stomach toward the basis. The distance of the transducer from the incisors is shown in each frame. At 40, 35, and 30 cm of depth the diameter of the descending aorta is 2, 2.1, and 2.2 cm, respectively. At 25 cm from the incisors the diameter of the aorta was reduced to 1.4 cm, indicating the aortic coarctation (**f**).

Ebstein's Anomaly

This heart malformation is characterized by downward displacement of the tricuspid valve into the right ventricle. The portion of right ventricle between the atrioventricular ring and the attachment of the tricuspid valve is "atrialized." The functional right ventricle is smaller than normal.

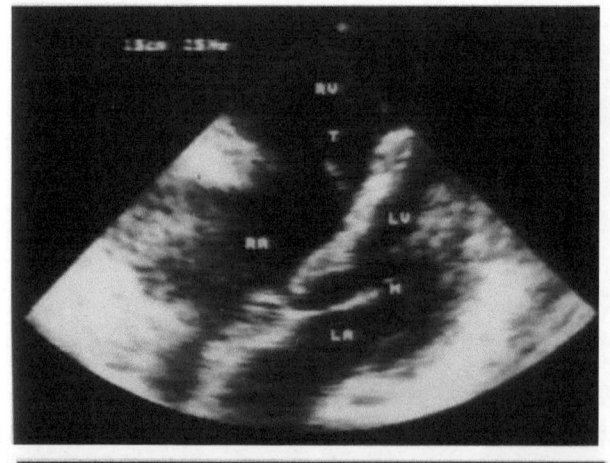

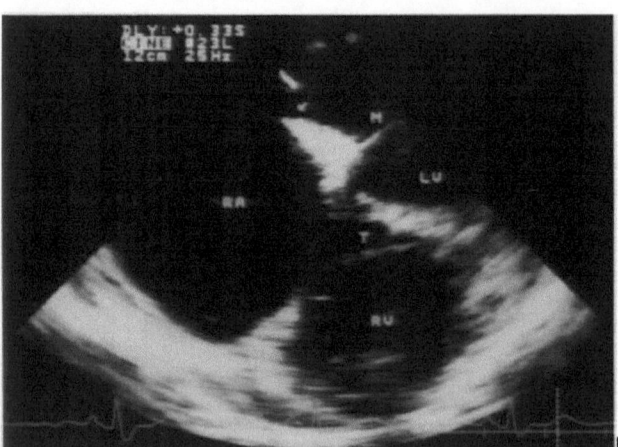

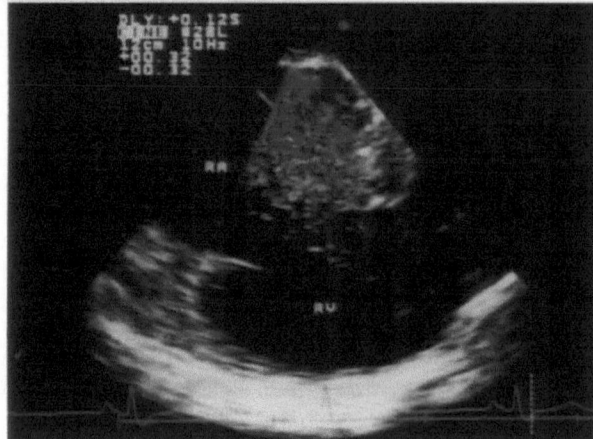

Fig. 3.61 a–c. Ebstein's anomaly. **a** Transthoracic echocardiography. Downward displacement of the septal leaflet of the tricuspid valve (*T*) and atrialization of the right ventricle are evident. **b, c** TEE. Displacement of the tricuspidal valve, dilatation of the right atrium, and the presence of an ASD (*arrow*) can be visualized. Color Doppler shows a large tricuspid regurgitant jet (*mosaic*) in the right atrium.

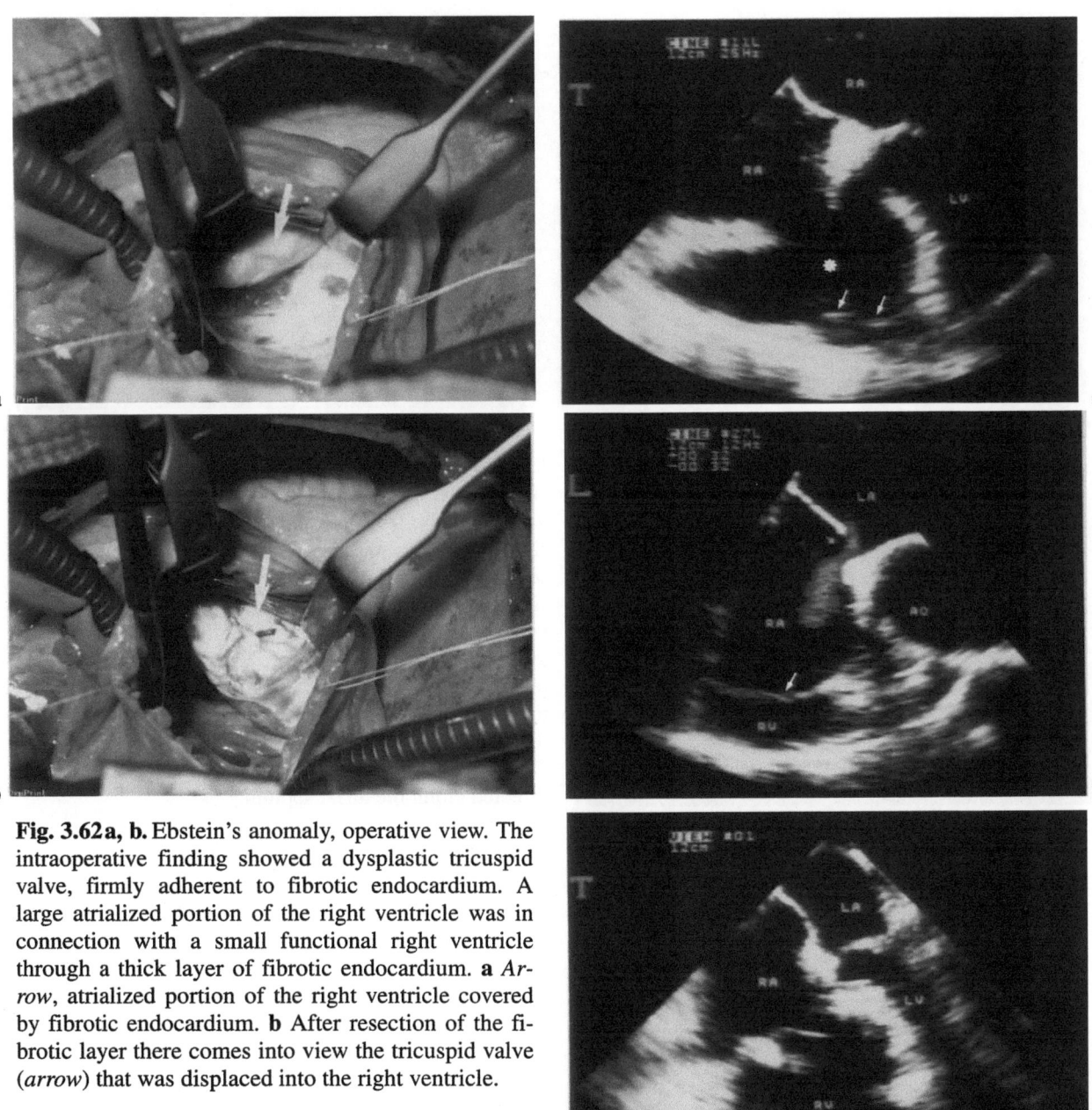

Fig. 3.62a, b. Ebstein's anomaly, operative view. The intraoperative finding showed a dysplastic tricuspid valve, firmly adherent to fibrotic endocardium. A large atrialized portion of the right ventricle was in connection with a small functional right ventricle through a thick layer of fibrotic endocardium. **a** *Arrow*, atrialized portion of the right ventricle covered by fibrotic endocardium. **b** After resection of the fibrotic layer there comes into view the tricuspid valve (*arrow*) that was displaced into the right ventricle.

Fig. 3.63a–c. Ebstein's anomaly; same patient as in Fig. 3.62. **a** Two-dimensional TEE, four-chamber view, shows the atrialized portion of the right ventricle (*). The tricuspid valve (*arrows*) was highly deformed, firmly adherent to fibrotic endocardium, and displaced downward in the right ventricle. **b** Longitudinal view shows ASD and left-to-right shunt (*blue*). *Arrow*, tricuspid valve. **c** After surgical repair. The fibrotic endocardium was resected and the atrialized portion plicated. A biological prosthetic valve (Hancock) was implanted. Note: in Ebstein´s anomaly the tricuspid annulus may be mistaken in echocardiography for normally positioned tricuspid leaflets.

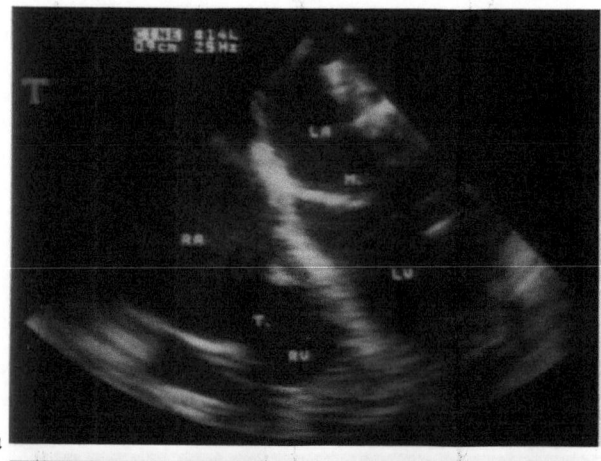

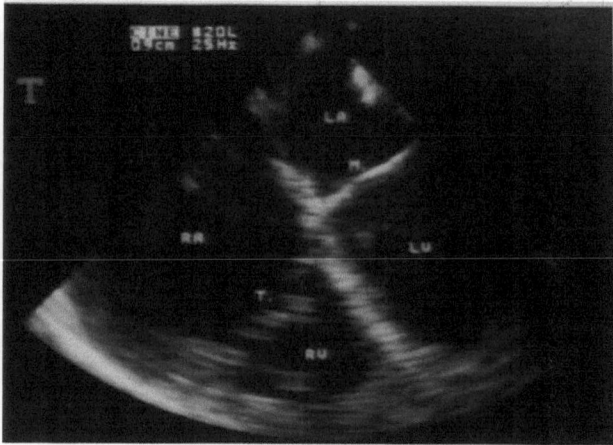

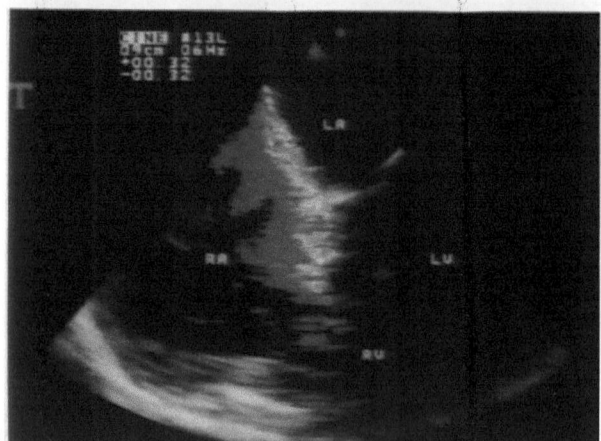

Fig. 3.64a–c. Ebstein's anomaly. The extent of tricuspid valve malformation in the Ebstein's anomaly varies widely, from minimal to severe. This patient shows a moderate form of Ebstein's anomaly with severe degree of tricuspid valve regurgitation. At surgical inspection the atrialized portion of the right ventricle could not be clearly identified. The septal leaflet was malformed. **a, b** Two-dimensional TEE, four-chamber view, shows that the attachment of the tricuspid valve leaflets is displaced at a level lower than the mitral valve. **a** Diastole. **b** Systole. **c** Color Doppler shows a regurgitant jet in the right atrium directed along the atrial septum.

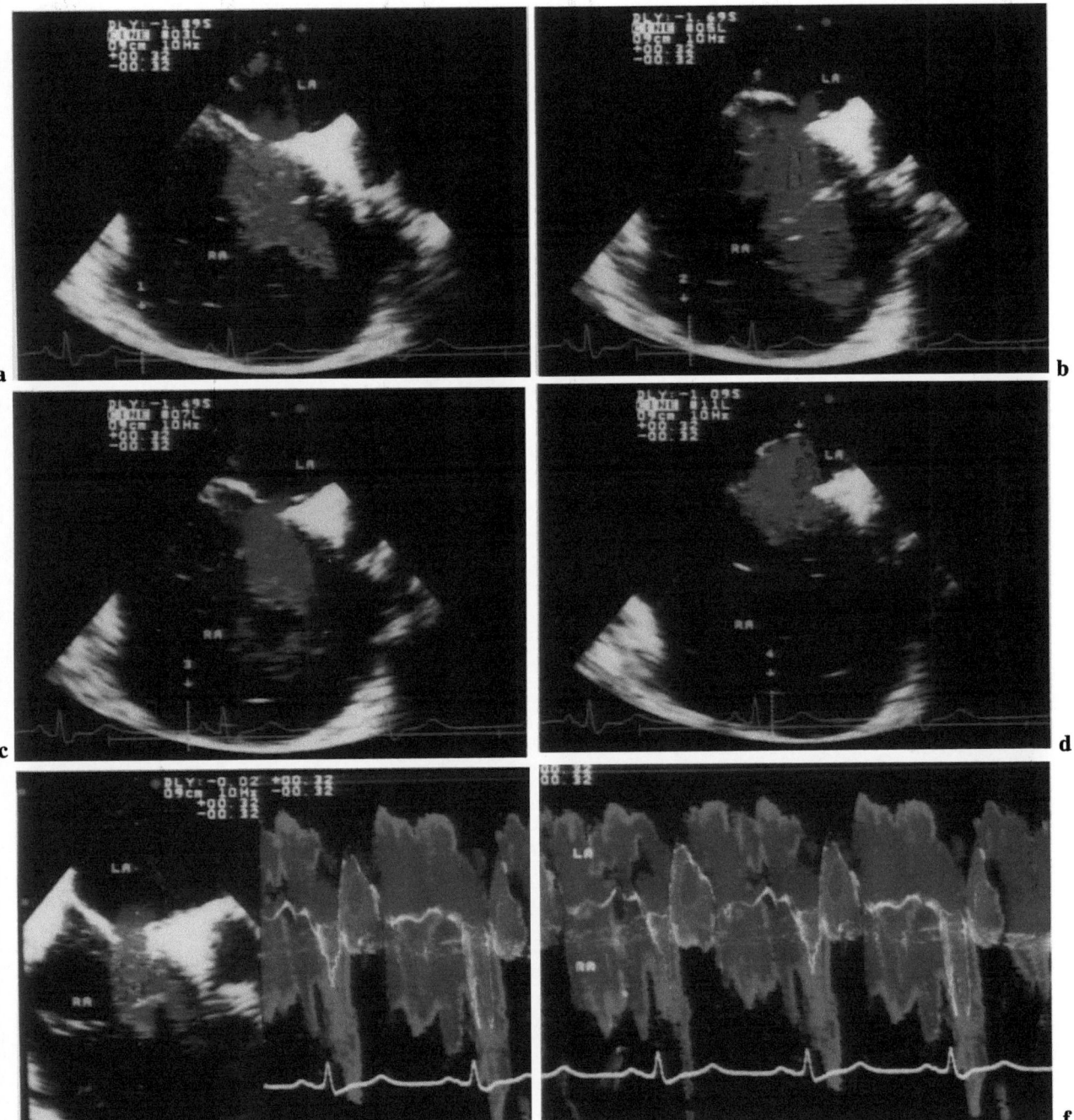

Fig. 3.65a–f. Ebstein's anomaly, bidirectional shunt at atrial level. **a–c** Color Doppler shows left-to-right shunt (*blue*) occurring during different phases of the diastole (*1, 2, 3* on ECG). **d** Right-to-left shunt (*red*) during the systole (*4* on ECG). *Arrow*, systolic bulging of the atrial septum. **e, f** Color M-mode shows the direction of the atrial shunt throughout the heart cycle. The right-to-left shunt (*red*) occurs only in systole. Note: the inversion of the shunt in systole is due to the tricuspid regurgitation.

Left Ventricular Function

TEE is widely used for intraoperative monitoring of global and regional left ventricular function during cardiac surgery. However, caution is necessary in assessing changes in left ventricular function before and after cardiopulmonary bypass because of the unequal loading conditions and the interference of catecholamine administration.

Transgastric View

The transgastric cross-sectional view of the left ventricle is particularly suitable for assessing global and regional left ventricular function. Diastolic and systolic changes in the cross-sectional area of the left ventricle and the percent shortening of the area provide an indirect index of ejection fraction.

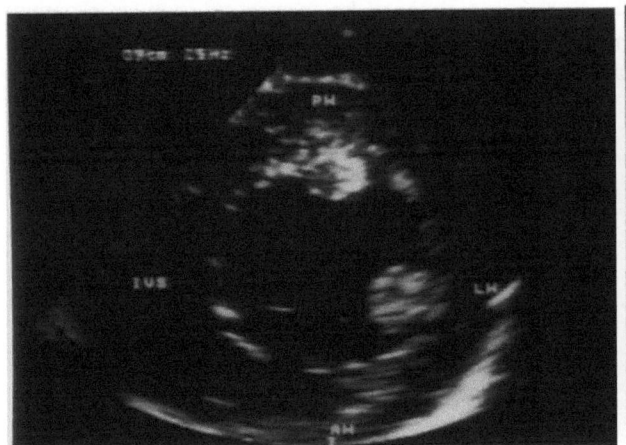 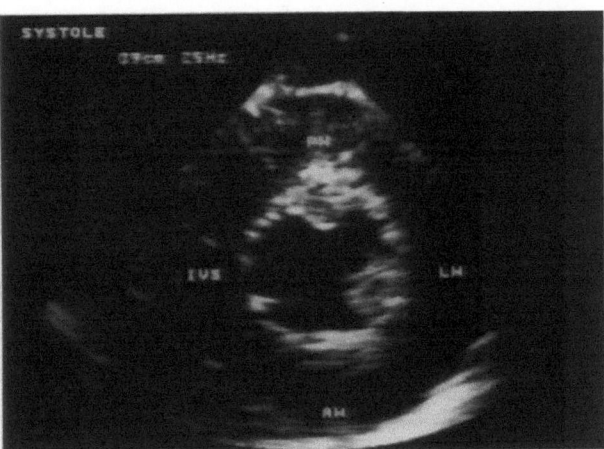

a   b

Fig. 4.1a, b. Transgastric short-axis view. This view is usually used for monitoring left ventricular function. These panels show the contraction of a normal heart. *Left*, cross-sectional view of left ventricle in diastole; *right*, in systole. Regional wall motion can also be assessed. *PW*, Posterior wall; *LW*, lateral wall; *AW*, anterior wall; *IVS*, interventricular septum.

4 Other Application of TEE

Since the introduction of echocardiography into the surgical theater is still fairly recent, many of its potential applications have not yet been investigated. This section describes new applications of TEE in heart surgery. The use of TEE in patients undergoing heart transplantation and in experimental heart surgery, such as in patients with dynamic cardiomyoplasty, has revealed new aspects of these diseases and contributed to their surgical treatment.

M-Mode Echocardiography

M-mode echocardiography allows highly accurate measurements of systolic and diastolic diameters of the left ventricle and of the changes in wall thickness during the cardiac cycle. Fractional shortening of the short diameter, measured at the level of the chordae tendineae, provides a simple and highly reproducible parameter for the assessment of left ventricular function.

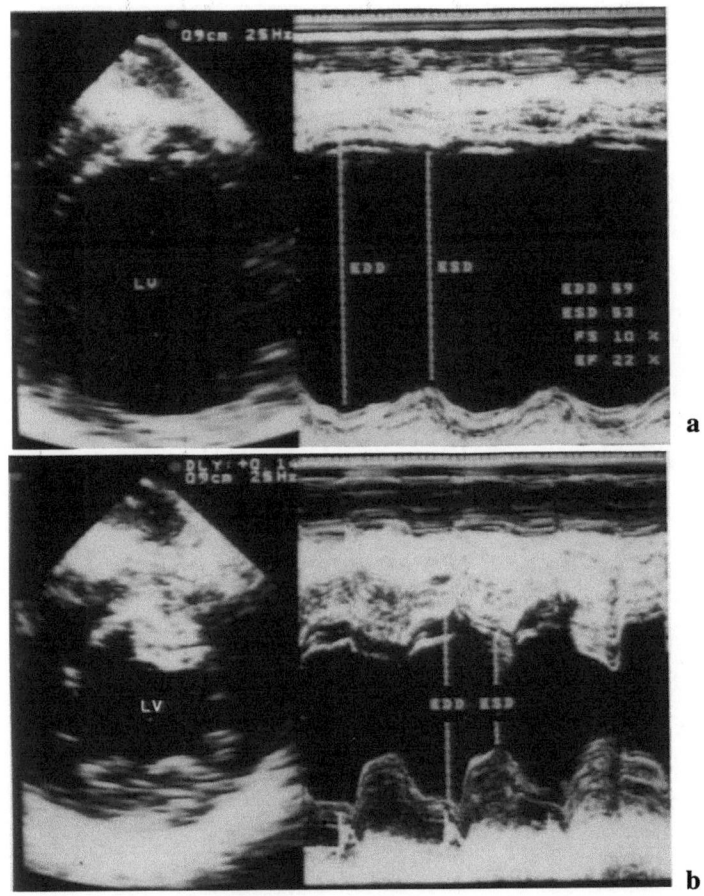

Fig. 4.2a, b. M-mode echocardiography, patient with dilated cardiomyopathy undergoing heart transplantation. **a** Impaired fractional shortening (*FS*) of left ventricle prior to heart transplantation. **b** Normal fractional shortening of the left ventricle of the transplanted heart immediately after weaning off cardiopulmonary bypass. *EDD*, End-diastolic diameter; *EDS*, end-systolic diameter; *EF*, ejection fraction.

Diastolic Function

Echocardiography provides only indirect parameters of diastolic function. Doppler curves of flow velocity of diastolic filling have been proposed for the study of diastolic function. Isovolumetric relaxation time can be calculated from the pulsed Doppler curve measured in a region between the inflow and the outflow of the left ventricle.

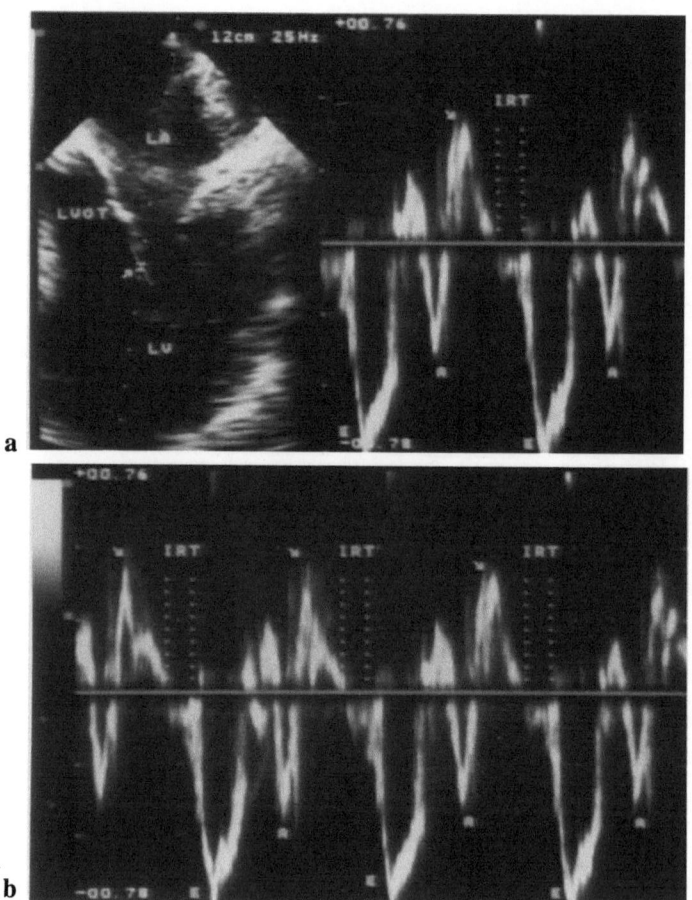

Fig. 4.3a, b. Assessment of diastolic ventricular function, pulsed Doppler at the level of the tip of anterior mitral leaflet. An estimate of isovolumetric relaxation time (*IRT*) can be measured from the end of left ventricular outflow (*arrow*) to the beginning of left ventricular inflow. *E*, Early diastolic filling; *A*, atrial diastolic filling of left ventricle.

Heart Transplantation

The peculiar anatomic characteristics of the transplanted heart and the function of the atrioventricular valves can be accurately visualized and investigated by TEE.

Atrial Anatomy

The anastomoses of donor and recipient portions of the atria create an "hourglass" configuration of the transplanted heart. The atria are enlarged, and the suture lines protrude into the atrial cavities. The distortion of the atrioventricular annulus may be due to the deformation of atrial geometry.

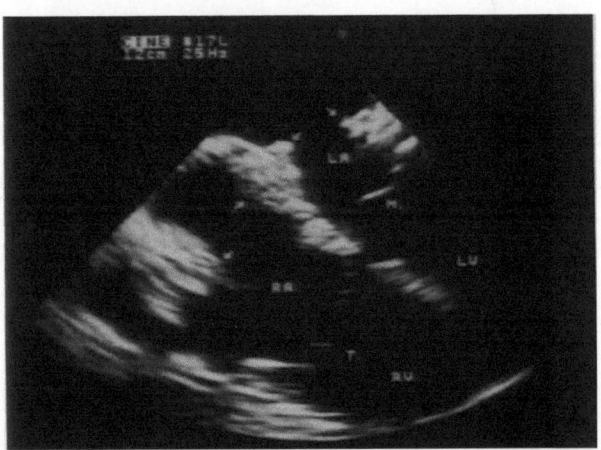

a

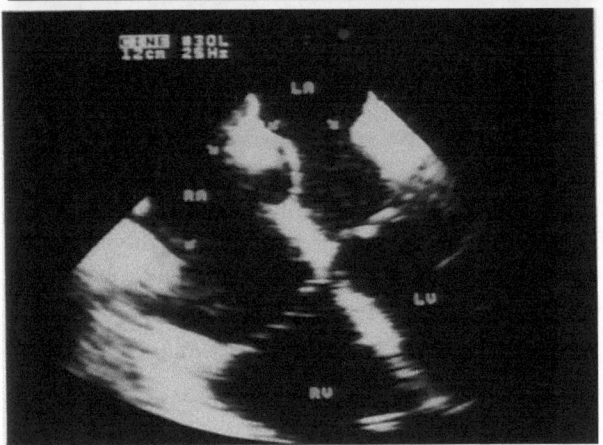

b

Fig. 4.4a, b. Orthotopic heart transplantation, atrial anatomy. Two-dimensional TEE, four-chamber view. *Arrows*, anastomoses between recipient and donor portions of the atria.

Pseudoaneurysm of the Atrial Septum

A cyclic bulging of the atrial septum has been
described in orthotopic heart transplantation. The
systolic bulging of the atrial septum toward the left
atrium may be due to tricuspid valve regurgitation,
which is a frequent occurrence in transplanted hearts.

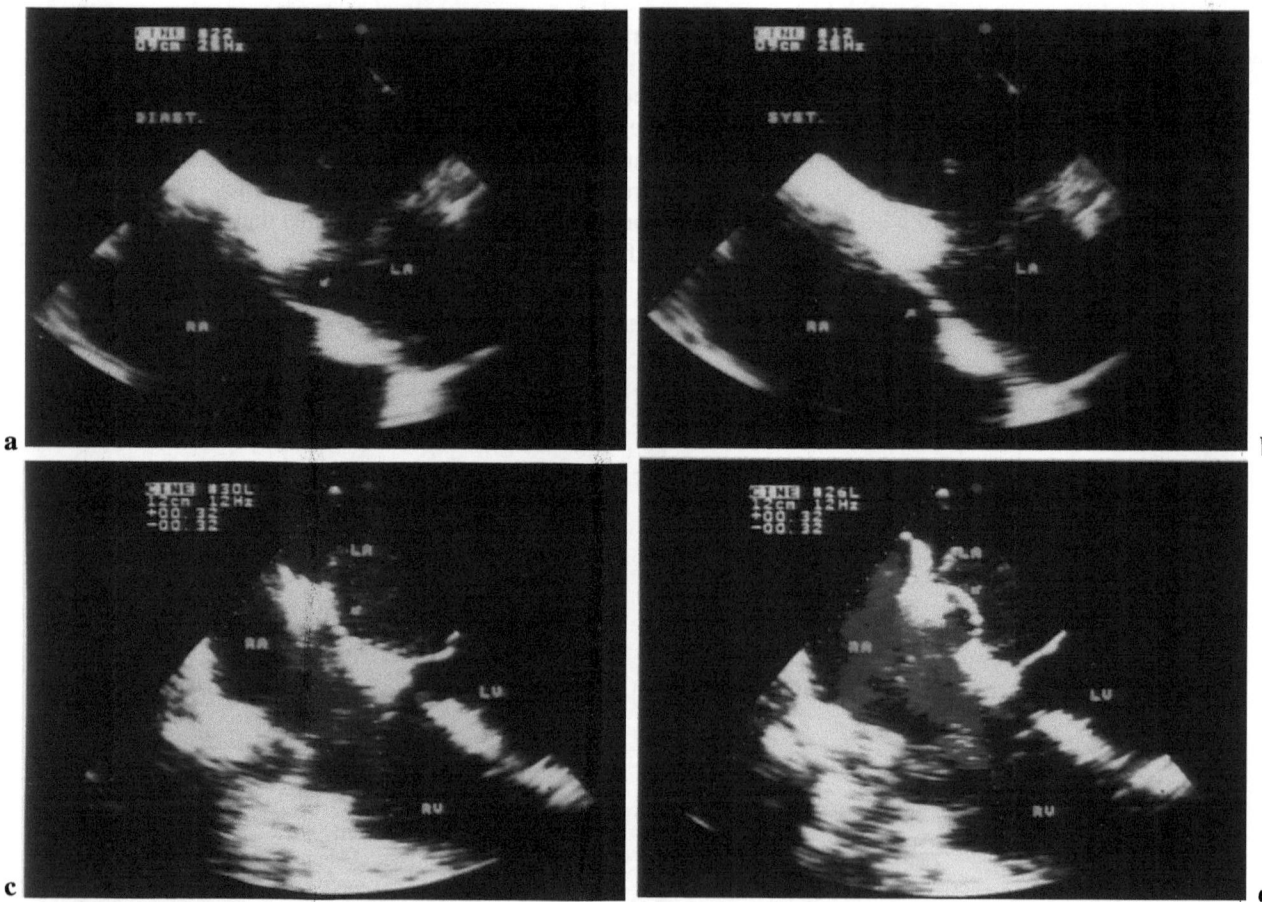

Fig. 4.5a–d. Orthotopic heart transplantation, pseudoaneurysm of the atrial septum. Two-dimensional
TEE, four-chamber view. Magnification of the atria.
The donor portion of the atrial septum shows phasic
excursions during the cardiac cycle. **a, b** *Arrows*,
bulging of the atrial septum toward the right atrium
in diastole (*left*), and left atrium in systole (*right*). **c,
d** Color Doppler in diastole (*left*) and in systole
(*right*).

Atrioventricular Valve Function

Mitral and tricuspid valve incompetence is common in patients after orthotopic heart transplantation. The etiology of this phenomenon is still not clear. The major factors involved include distortion of atrioventricular annulus and deformation of atrial geometry.

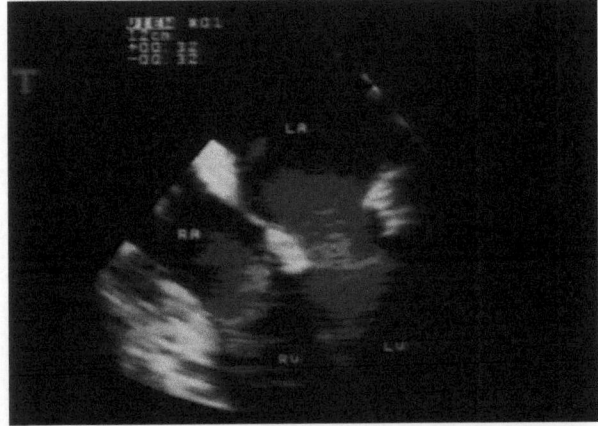

a

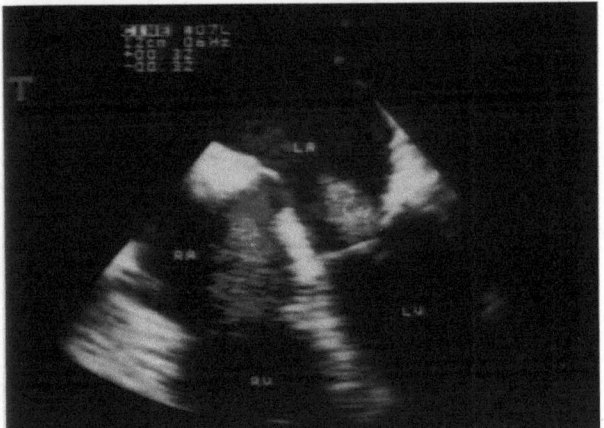

b

Fig. 4.6a, b. Orthotopic heart transplantation, atrioventricular valve function. Color Doppler TEE, four-chamber view. **a** Normal diastolic flow (*blue*) across the tricuspid and mitral valves. **b** Mitral and tricuspidal regurgitant jets in the left and the right atria (*mosaics*). The etiology of atrioventricular valve incompetence of the transplanted heart is still controversial. Note: the tricuspidal regurgitant jet is directed toward the atrial septum, which bulges into the left atrium in systole.

Tricuspid Valve Insufficiency

Tricuspid valve regurgitation occurs in about 90% of transplanted hearts. Its etiology is still controversial. We have found the geometry of the right atrium to be correlated with the incidence and severity of tricuspid insufficiency. The degree of tricuspid regurgitation shows a significant correlation with the ratio between the area of the recipient portion (R) and the area of the donor portion (D) of the right atrium. Patients with a higher R/D ratio show a greater degree of tricuspid regurgitation.

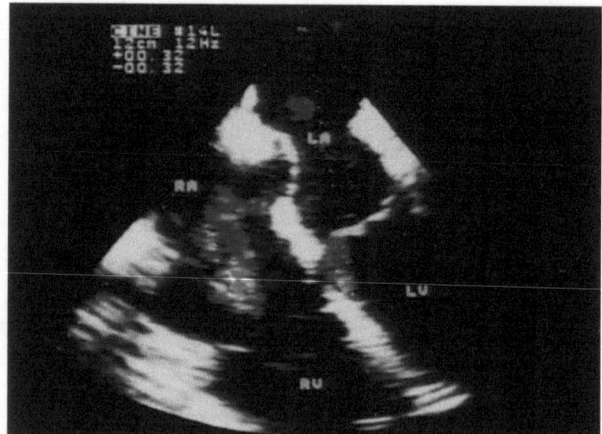

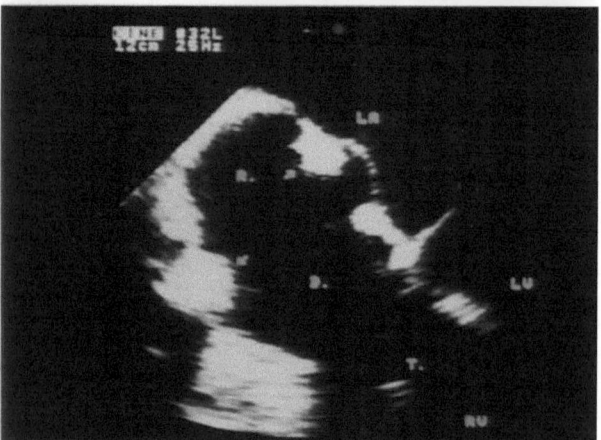

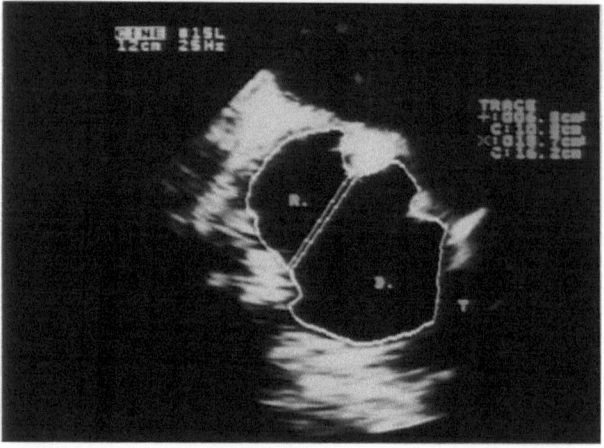

Fig. 4.7a–c. Orthotopic heart transplantation, tricuspid valve regurgitation and atrial geometry. **a** Tricuspid valve regurgitation occurring immediately after cardiopulmonary bypass. **b** *Arrows*, anastomoses between recipient and donor portions of the right atrium. **c** Cross-sectional area of the recipient (*R*) and of the donor (*D*) portion of the right atrium, measured at the sites of the atrial anastomoses.

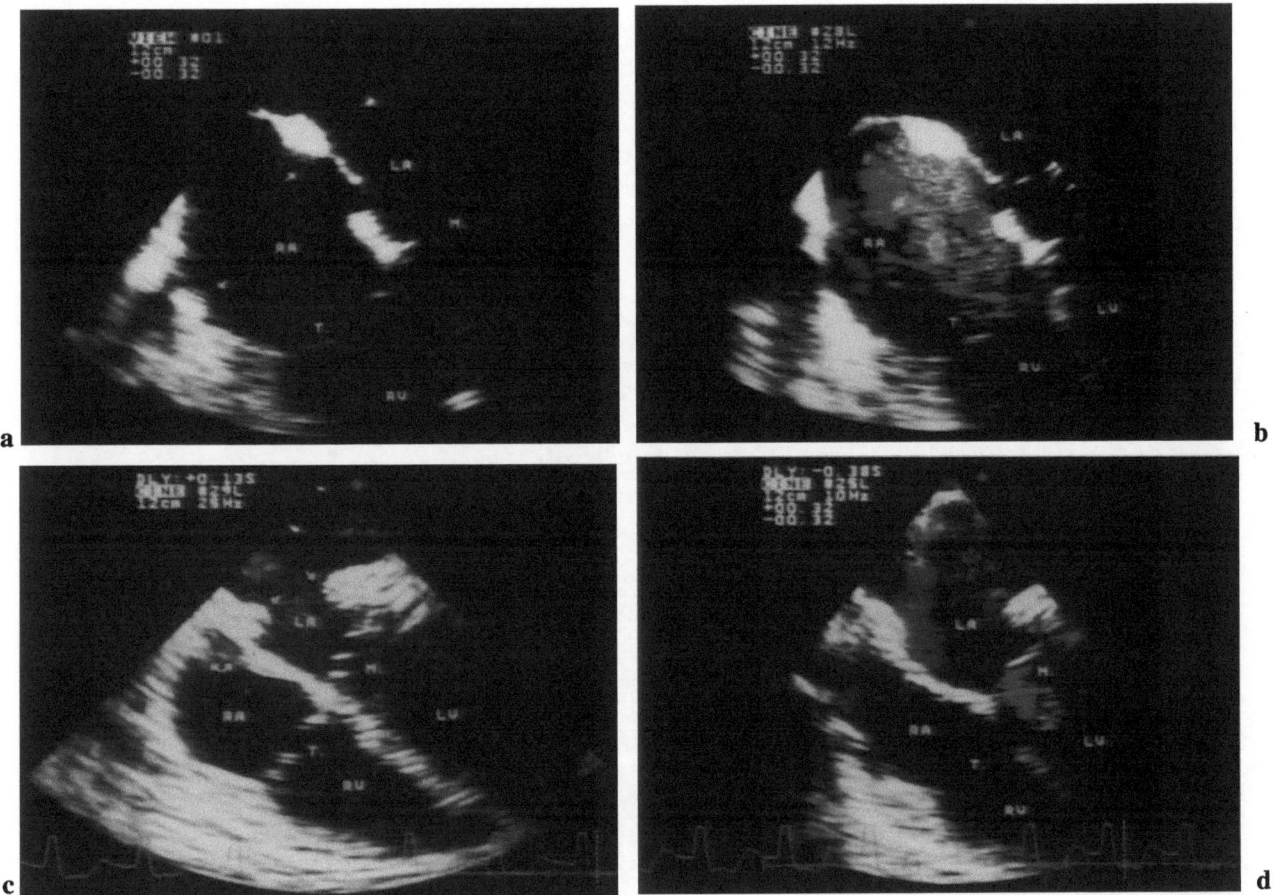

Fig. 4.8a–d. Orthotopic heart transplantation, tricuspid valve regurgitation and atrial geometry. Patients with larger recipient portion of the right atrium show a greater degree of tricupid valve regurgitation. **a, b** This patient shows a large recipient portion of right atrium (R/D ratio, 1.2). *Left*, *arrows*, sites of the atrial anastomoses. *Right*, important tricuspid valve regurgitation (jet area, 12.8 m²). **c, d** This patient shows an almost insignificant R/D ratio. No tricuspid regurgitation was found.

Mitral Valve Insufficiency

Mitral valve regurgitation occurs in about 50% of transplanted hearts. The degree of regurgitation is not correlated with the R/D ratio.

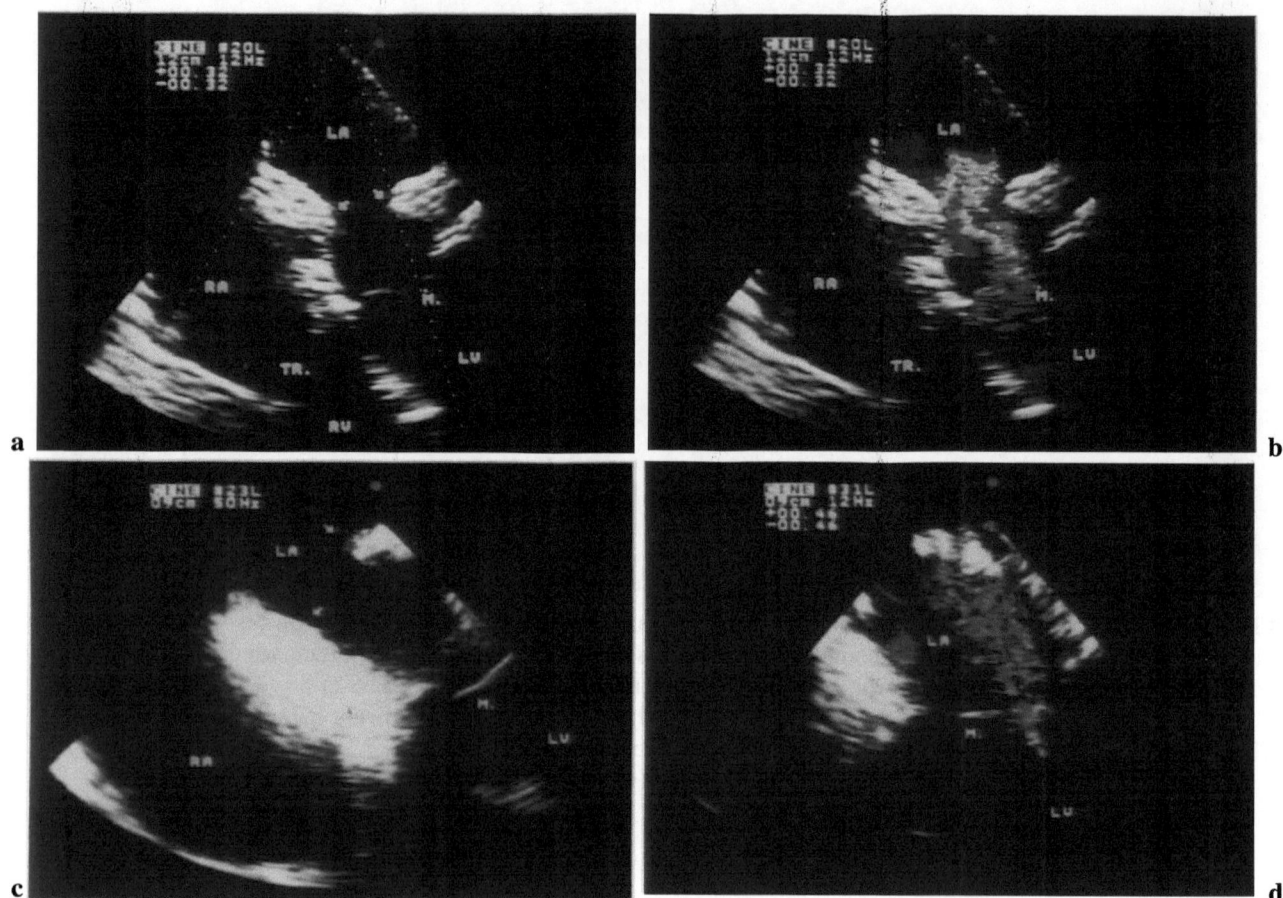

Fig. 4.9a–d. Orthotopic heart transplantation, mitral valve regurgitation and atrial geometry. Mitral valve regurgitation occurs in about 50% of transplanted hearts. The degree of mitral regurgitation is not cor- related with the geometry of left atrium. *Left, arrows*, sites of the anastomoses. *Right*, corresponding de- grees of mitral valve regurgitation.

Left Ventricular Inflow

Obstruction to left ventricular diastolic flow is a relatively common complication of heart transplantation.

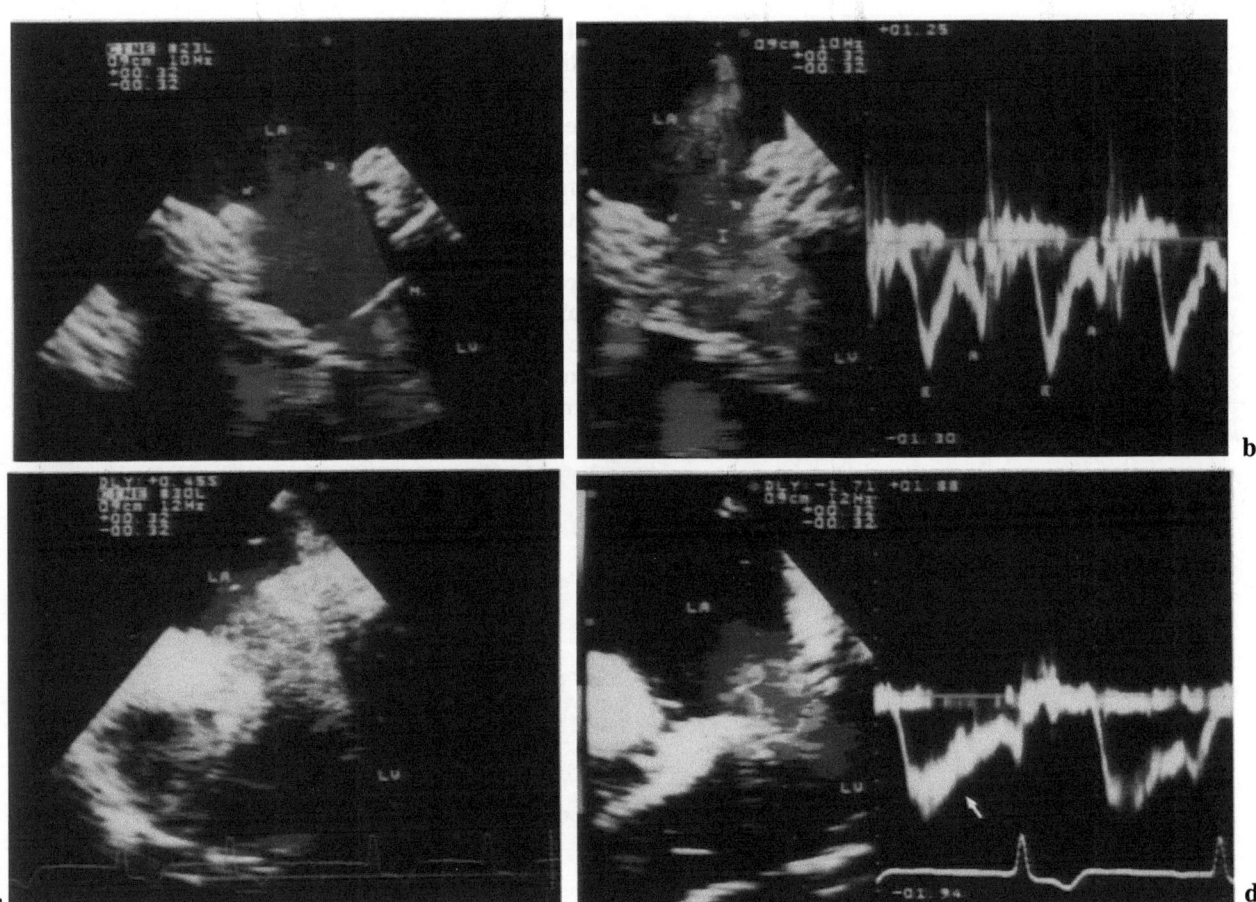

Fig. 4.10a–d. Orthotopic heart transplantation, left ventricular inflow. Protrusion of the atrial anastomosis into the left atrium may hinder the diastolic flow through the mitral valve. **a, b** *Left*, color Doppler shows normal diastolic flow across the suture sites (*arrows*) in the left atrium; *right*, pulsed-wave Doppler shows a normal diastolic flow pattern. *E*, Early diastolic filling; *A*, late diastolic filling. **c, d** *Left*, color Doppler shows turbulent diastolic flow across the mitral valve; *right*, pulsed-wave Doppler at the level of the mitral valve. The tracing shows delayed decay of the early diastolic flow velocity (*arrow*), a typical pattern of obstruction to ventricular diastolic filling.

Acute Rejection

Two-dimensional echocardiography has been proposed as a potential noninvasive diagnostic technique for recognizing acute cardiac rejection. The acute phase of heart transplant rejection is characterized by interstitial edema, which increases the refractility of myocardial walls. Heart transplant rejection can be recognized by the analysis of brightness of the echo signal from the myocardial walls.

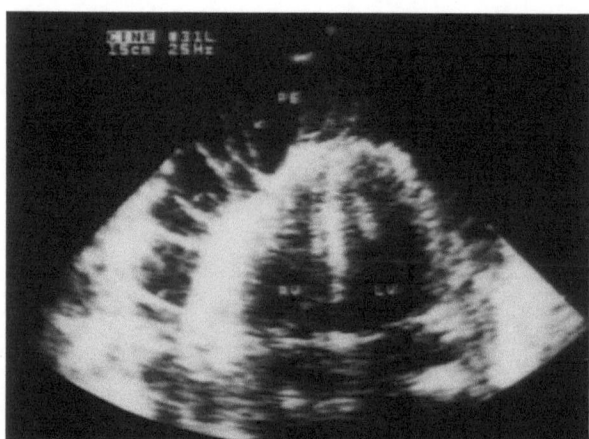

a

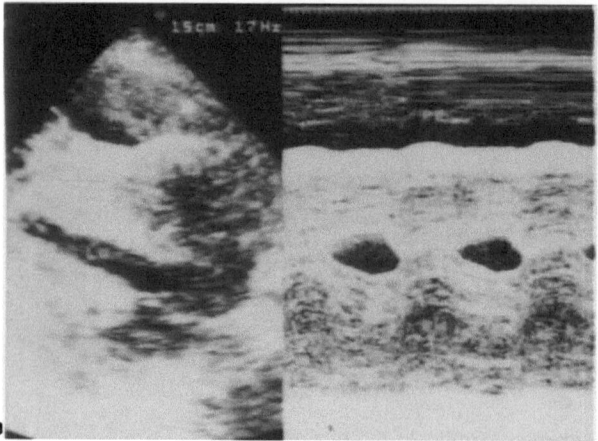

b

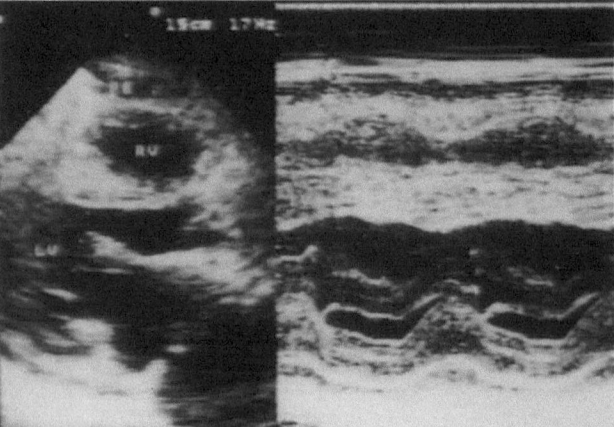

c

Fig. 4.11a–c. Orthotopic heart transplantation, acute rejection. Transthoracic echocardiography. **a** Apical view showing a large pericardial effusion (*PE*) and thickened, hyperrefractile myocardium during acute rejection. *Arrows*, fibrinous pericardial adhesions. The free wall of the right ventricle appears thicker than the lateral wall of the left ventricle. **b** M-mode echocardiography during acute rejection. Increased thickening of the myocardial walls. The myocardium appears hyperrefractile due to interstitial infiltration. **c** The same patient as in **b** after the remission of cardiac rejection. The thickness of the myocardial walls is markedly reduced.

Dynamic Cardiomyoplasty

Dynamic cardiomyoplasty is a surgical procedure in which the skeletal latissimus dorsi muscle is wrapped around the heart to assist myocardial contraction. The skeletal muscle is stimulated by a pacemaker synchronous with the ventricular systole. Dynamic cardiomyoplasty is performed at our institution in patients with severe heart failure. Echocardiography has proven useful in evaluating the efficacy of this new surgical procedure.

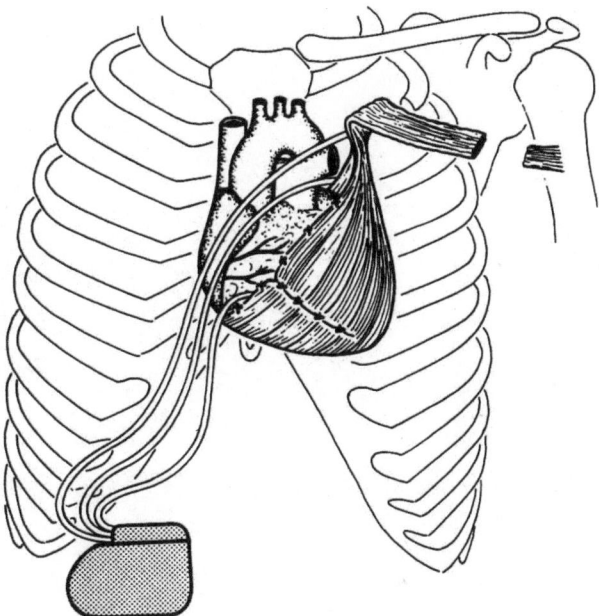

Fig. 4.12. Dynamic cardiomyoplasty. Schematic diagram showing the latissimus dorsi muscle wrapped around the heart and the position of the pacemaker.

Wall Motion

Two-dimensional and M-mode echocardiography provides a useful noninvasive diagnostic tool for assessing left ventricular function and wall motion after dynamic cardiomyoplasty.

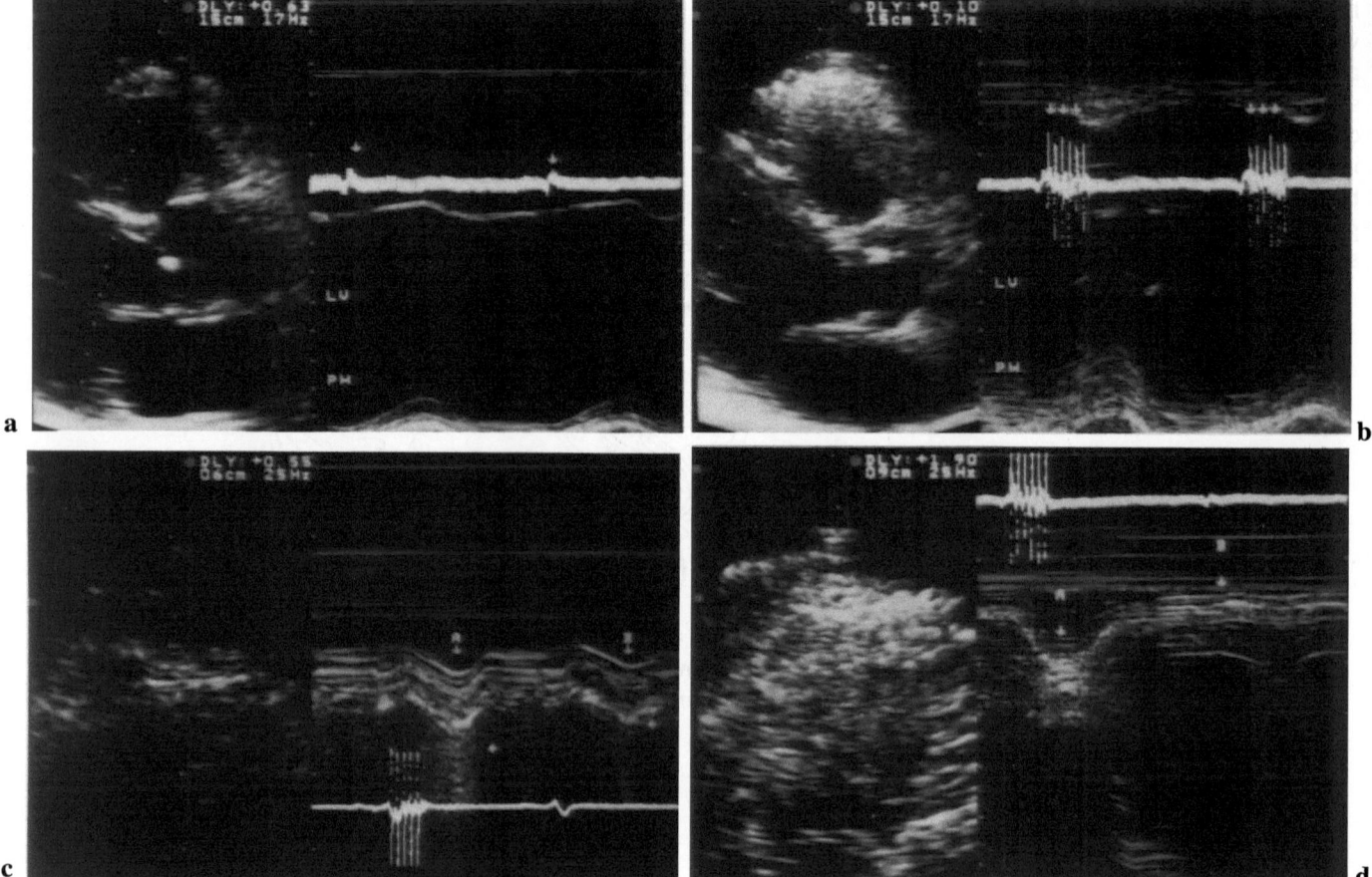

Fig. 4.13a–d. Dynamic cardiomyoplasty, wall motion. Transthoracic echocardiography, parasternal long-axis view. M-mode of left ventricle in a patient with cardiomyoplasty. **a** Nonstimulated contraction of left ventricle (*arrows* on the ECG). Note the impaired motion of the posterior wall (*PW*). **b** During the muscle stimulation (*arrows* on the ECG), a mar- ked increase in motion of the posterior wall (*PW*) can be observed. **c, d** Magnification of the M-mode tracing of the anterior wall of the right ventricle. Beat *A* (paced) shows greater wall motion than beat *B* (not paced). The spikes on the ECG indicate the paced beats.

Doppler Echocardiography

The effects of muscle contraction of paced beats can be evaluated by Doppler examination of intracardiac blood flow in patients who have undergone dynamic cardiomyoplasty.

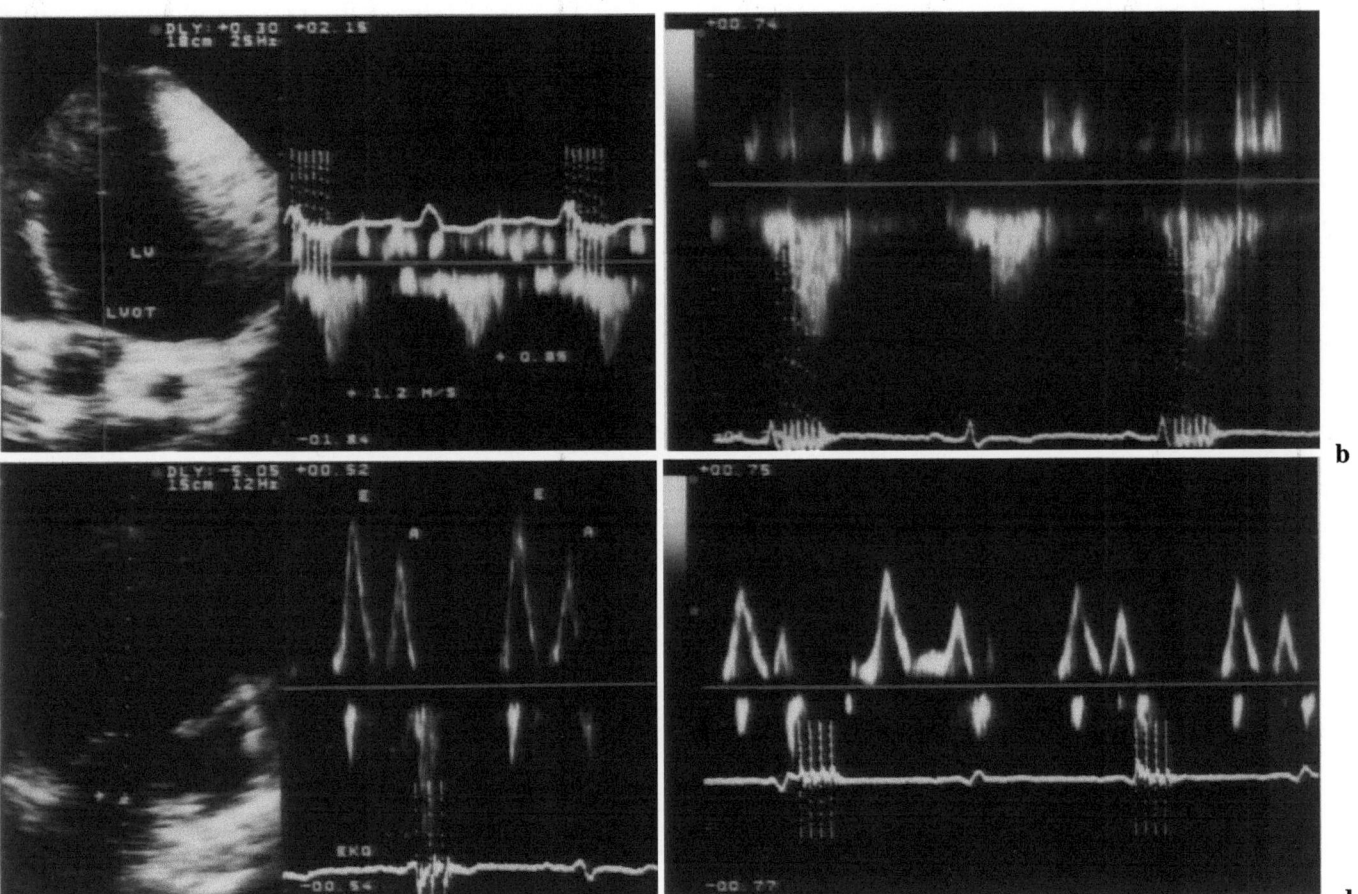

Fig. 4.14a–d. Dynamic cardiomyoplasty, Doppler-echocardiography. Transthoracic echocardiography, apical views. **a, b** Continuous-wave Doppler placed along the left ventricular ejection flow. On the Doppler tracings the paced beats show higher peak ejection flow velocity than the nonpaced beats. **c, d** Pulsed-wave Doppler at the level of the mitral valve. The delay of the muscle burst was adjusted on the basis of the diastolic flow tracings. The first burst occurred at the end of diastolic filling, just after completion of the left ventricular diastolic filling.

Bibliography

Two-Dimensional TEE

Abel MD, Nishimura RA, Callahan MJ, Rehder K, Ilstrup DM, Tajik AJ (1987) Evaluation of intraoperative transesophageal two dimensional echocardiography. Anesthesiology 66:64–68

Cohen GI, Chan KL (1991) Biplane transesophageal echocardiography: clinical applications of the long-axis plane. J Am Soc Echocardiogr 4:155–163

Cohen GI, Chan KL, Walley VM (1990) Anatomic correlations of the long-axis views in biplane transesophageal echocardiography. Am J Cardiol 66:1007–1012

Cucchiara RF, Nugent M, Seward JB, Messik JM (1984) Air embolism in upright neurosurgical patients: detection and localization by two dimensional transesophageal echocardiography. Anesthesiology 60:353–355

Currie P (1989) Transesophageal echocardiography: intraoperative applications. Echocardiography 6:403–414

De Simone R, Jeserich M, Ruffmann K, Kübler W (1988) Doppler-echocardiographic assessment of left ventricular filling parameters before and after coronary angioplasty. Eur Heart J 9:376

De Simone R, Lange R, Brachmann J, Vahl C, Saggau W, Hagl S (1990) Transesophageal Doppler echocardiographic evaluation of cardiac function during the implantation of an internal defibrillator (abstract) In: 4th meeting of the European Association for Cardio-Thoracic Surgery. Naples, 17–19 Sept 1990. Volume abstracts, p 212

Decoodt P, Kacenelenbegen R, Bar JP, Salmon K, Peperstraete B, Telerman M (1992) Clinical usefulness of biplane transesophageal echocardiography. Echocardiography 9: 257–275

Deutsch HJ, Curtius JL, Leischik R, Borowski A, Huttarsch H, de Vivie ER, Hilger HH (1991) Diagnostic value of transesophageal echocardiography in cardiac surgery. Thorac Cardiovasc Surg 39:199–204

Dubroff JM, Clark M, Wong CYH (1983) Left ventricular ejection fraction during cardiac surgery: a two dimensional echocardiographic study. Circulation 68:95–99

Frazin L, Talano JV, Stephanides L, Loeb HS, Kopel L, Gunnar RM (1976) Esophageal echocardiography. Circulation 54:102–108

Hisanaga K, Hisanaga A, Nagata K, Yoshida S (1977) A new transesophageal real time two-dimensional echocardiographic system using a flexible tube and its clinical application. Proc Jpn Soc Ultrason Med 32:43–44

Klein AL, Steward WC, Cosgrove DM, Salcedo EE (1990) Intraoperative epicardial echocardiography: technique and imaging planes. Echocardiography 7:241–251

Kuroda T, Kinter TM, Seward JB, Yanagi H, Greenleaf JF (1991) Accuracy of three-dimensional volume measurement using biplane transesophageal echocardiographic probe: in vitro experiment. J Am Soc Echocardiogr 4:475–484

Leung J, Schiller N, Mangano D (1989) Transesophageal echocardiographic assessment of left ventricular function. J Cardiac Imaging 5:63–70

Lindenbaum GA, Jacobs LE, Morris M, Bell-Thomson J, Kotler MN (1989) Perioperative surface and transesophageal color-flow Doppler evaluation of post-traumatic intracardiac shunt. Am Heart J 119:193–196

Matsumodo M, Oka Y, Strom J Frishman W, Kadish A, Becker RM, Frater RWM, Sonnenblick EH (1980) Application of transesophageal echocardiography to continuous intraoperative monitoring of left ventricular performance. Am J Cardiol 46:95–105

Meloni L, Abbruzzese PA, Cardu G, Aru GM, Loriga P, Ricchi A, Martelli V, Cherchi A (1990) Detection of microbubbles released by oxygenators during cardiopulmonary bypass by intraoperative transesophageal echocardiography. Am J Cardiol 66:511–514

Miyatake K, Okamoto M, Kinoshita N, Izumi S, Owa M, Takao S, Sakakibara H, Nimura Y (1984) Clinical applications of a new type of real-time two-dimensional Doppler flow imaging system. Am J Cardiol 54:857–868

Mohl W, Simon P, Neumann F (1990) Intraoperative echocardiography in the cardiac emergencies. Echocardiography 7:193–200

Omoto R (1990) New trend in transesophageal echocardiographic technology. Use of biplane transesophageal probe. Editorial comment. Circulation 82:1507–1509

Omoto R, Yokote Y, Takamoto S, Kyo S, Ueda K, Asano H, Namekawa K, Kasai C, Kondo Y, Koyano A (1984) The development of real-time two-dimensional Doppler Echocardiography and its clinical significance in acquired valvular disease:with specific reference to the evaluation of valvular regurgitation. Jpn Heart J 25:325–340

Omoto R, Kyo S, Matsmura M, Shah PM, Adachi H, Matsunaka T (1989) Biplane color Doppler transesophageal echocardiography:its impact on cardiovascular surgery and further technological progress in the probe, a matrix phased-array biplane probe. Echocardiography 6:423–429

Omoto R, Kyo S, Matsumura M, Maruyama M, Ykote Y (1991) Future technical prospects in biplane transesophageal echocardiography. Use of adult and pediatric biplane probes. Echocardiography 8:713–720

Omoto R, Kyo S, Matsumura M, Shah PM, Adachi H, Yokote Y, Kondo Y (1992) Evaluation of biplane color Doppler transesophageal echocardiography in 200 consecutive patients. Circulation 85:1237–1247

Pearlman AS, Gardin JM, Martin RP, Parisi AF, Popp RL, Quinones MA, Stevenson JG (1987) Guidelines for optimal training in echocardiography. Recommendations of the American Society of Echocardiography Committee for Physician Training in Echocardiography. Am J Cardiol 60:158–163

Richardson SG, Weintraub AR, Schwarz SL, Simonetti J, Caldeira ME, Pandian NG (1991) Biplane transesophageal echocardiography utilizing transverse and sagittal imaging planes. Echocardiography 8:293–309

Roelandt J, Thomson I, Vletter W, Brommersma P, Bom N, Linker D (1992) Multiplane transesophageal echocardiography: latest evolution in an imaging revolution. J Am Soc Echocardiogr 361–367

Roizen MF, Beaupre PN, Alpert RA, Kremer P, Cahalan MK, Shiller N, Sohn YJ, Cronnelly R, Lurz FW, Ehrenfeld WK, Stoney RJ (1984) Monitoring with two dimensional transesophageal echocardiography: comparison of myocardial function in patients undergoing supraceliac, suprarenal-infraceliac, or infrarenal aortic occlusion. J Vasc Surg 1: 300–303

Schlüter M, Langenstein BA, Polster J, Kremer P, Souquet J, Engel S, Hanrath P (1982) Transesophageal cross-sectional echocardiography with a phased array transducer system. Technique and initial clinical results. Br Heart J 48:67–72

Schlüter M, Hinrichs A, Thier W, Kremer P, Schräder S, Cahalan MK, Hanrath P (1984) Transesophageal two-dimensional echocardiography: comparison of ultrasonic and anatomic sections. Am J Cardiol 53:1173–1178

Seward JS, Khandheria BK, Oh JK, Abel MD, Hughes RW, Edwards WD, Nichols BA, Freeman WK, Tajik AJ (1988) Transesophageal echocardiography: technique, anatomic correlations, implementation, and clinical applications. Mayo Clin Proc 63:649–680

Seward JB, Khandheria BK, Edwards WD, Oh JK, Freeman WK, Tajik AJ (1990) Biplanar transesophageal echocardiography: anatomic correlations, image orientation, and clinical applications. Mayo Clin Proc 65:1193–1213

Shintani H, Nakano S, Matsuda H, Sakai K, Taniguchi K, Kawashima Y (1990) Efficacy of transesophageal echocardiography as a perioperative monitor in patients undergoing cardiovascular surgery. J Cardiovasc Surg 31:564–570

Souquet J, Hanrath P, Zitelli L, Kremer P, Langstein BA, Schlüter M (1982) Transesophageal phased array for imaging the heart. IEEE Trans Biomed Eng 29:707–712

Stümper O, Fraser AH, Ho SY, Anderson RH, Chow L, Davies MJ, Roelandt JRTC, Sutherland GR (1990) Transesophageal echocardiography in the longitudinal axis: correlation between anatomy and images and its clinical implications. Br Heart J . 64:282–288

Thier W, Schlüter M, Kremer P, Hausdorf G, Krebber HJ, Shräder S, Hanrath P (1983) Transesophageal 2-dimensional echocardiography: better demonstration of intra-atrial structures. Dtsch Med Wochenschr 108:1903–1907

Wang XF, Li ZA, Cheng TO, Deng YB, Wang JE, Yang Y (1992) Biplane transesophageal echocardiography: an anatomic-ultrasonic-clinical correlative study. Am Heart J 123:1027–1038

Zabalgoitia M, Gandhi DK, Evans J, Mehlman DJ, McPhearson DD, Talano JV (1991) Transesophageal echocardiography in the awake elderly patient: its role in the decision-making process. Am Heart J 120:1147–1153

Valvular Heart Disease

Castello R, Lenzen P, Aguirre F, Labovitz A (1992) Quantitation of mitral regurgitation by transesophageal echocardiography with Doppler color flow maping: Correlation with cardiac catheterization. J Am Coll Cardiol 19:1516–1521

Currie P, Stewart W (1990) Intraoperative echocardiography for surgical repair of the aortic valve and left ventricular outflow tract. Echocardiography 7:273–288

Czer LSC, Maurer G (1990) Intraoperative echocardiography for surgical repair of the aortic valve and left ventricular outflow tract. Echocardiography 7:305–322

Czer LS, Maurer G, Bolger AF, De Robertis M, Kleinman J, Gray RJ, Chaux A, Matloff JM (1989) Tricuspid valve repair. Operative and follow-up evaluation by Doppler color flow imaging. J Thorac Cardiovasc Surg 98:101–111

Dahm M, Iversen S, Schmid X, Drexler M, Erbel R, Oelert H (1987) Intraoperative evaluation of reconstruction of the atrioventricular valves by transesophageal echocardiography. Thorac Cardiovasc Surg 35:140–142

De Simone R, Lange R, Saggau W, Hagl S (1992a) Intraoperative echocardiography during De Vega's annuloplasty. A new application to reduce residual regurgitation. Eur Heart J 13(1):237

De Simone R, Lange R, Tanzeem A, Gams E, Saggau W, Hagl S (1992b) Intraoperative transesophageal echocardiography for the evaluation of mitral, aortic and tricuspid valve repair. A tool to optimize the surgical outcome. Eur J Cardiothorac Surg 6:665–673

De Simone R, Lange R, Tanzeem A, Gams E, Hagl S (1993) Adjustable tricuspid valve annuloplasty assisted by intraoperative transesophageal color Doppler echocardiography. Am J Cardiol 71:926–931

Drexler M, Erbel R, Dahm M, Mohr-Kahaly S, Oelert H, Meyer J (1986) Assessment of successful valve reconstruction by intraoperative transesophageal echocardiography (TEE). Int J Card Imaging 2:21–30

Goldman M, Guarino T, Mindich B (1990) Intraoperative evaluation of valvular regurgitation: comparison of echocardiographic techniques. Echocardiography 7:201–208

Helmcke F, Nanda NC, Hsiung MC, Soto B, Adey CK, Goyal RG, Getewood R (1987) Color Doppler assessment of mitral regurgitation with orthogonal planes. Circulation 75:175–183

Himelman RB, Kusumoto F, Oken K, Lee E, Calahan MK, Shah PM, Schiller NB (1991) The flail mitral valve: echocardiographic findings by precordial and transesophageal imaging and Doppler color flow maping. J Am Coll Cardiol 17:272–279

Hoffmann T, Kasper W, Meinertz T, Spillner G, Schlosser V, Just M (1987) Determination of aortic valve orifice area in aortic valve stenosis by two-dimensional transesophageal echocardiography. Am J Cardiol 59:330–335

Johnston SR, Freeman WK, Schaff HV, Tajik AJ (1990) Severe tricuspid regurgitation after mitral valve repair: diagnosis by transesophageal echocardiography. J Am Soc Echocardiography 3:416–419

King H, Csicsko J, Leshnower A (1980) Intraoperative assessment of the mitral valve following reconstructive procedures. Ann Thorac Surg 29:81–83

Kurlansky P, Rose EA, Malm JR (1987) Adjustable annuloplasty for tricuspid insufficiency. Ann Thorac Surg 44:404–406

Matsumura M, Kyo S, Shah PM, Adachi K, Yokote Y, Omoto R (1989) A new look at mitral valve pathology with biplane color Doppler transesophageal probe. J Am Soc Echocardiogr 2:215

Maurer G, Czer L (1991) Intraoperative color Doppler assessment in valve repair surgery. Echocardiography 8:263–271

Maurer G, Czer LS, Chaux A, Bolger AF, De Robertis M, Resser K, Kass RM, Lee ME, Matloff JM (1987) Intraoperative Doppler color flow mapping for assessment of valve repair for mitral regurgitation. Am J Cardiol 60:333–337

Miyatake K, Izumi S, Okanmoto M, Kinoshita N, Asonuma H, Nakagawa H, Yamamoto K, Takamiya M, Sakakibara H, Nimura Y (1986) Semiquantitative grading of severity of mitral regurgitation by real-time two-dimensional Doppler flow imaging technique. J Am Coll Cardiol 7:82–88

Nishimura R, Abel M, Housmans P, Warnes C, Tajik J (1989) Mitral flow velocity curves as a function of different loading conditions: evaluation by intraoperative transesophageal Doppler echocardiography. J Am Echocardiogr 2:79–87

Omoto R, Yokote Y, Takamoto S, Kyo S, Ueda K, Asano H, Namekawa K, Kasai C, Kondo Y, Koyano A (1984) The development of real-time two-dimensional Doppler Echocardiography and its cilnical significance in acquired valvular disease: with specific reference to the evaluation of valvular regurgitation. Jpn Heart J 25:325–340

Perry GJ, Helmcke F, Nanda NC, Byard C, Soto B (1987) Evaluation of aortic insufficiency by Doppler color flow mapping. J Am Coll Cardiol 9:952–959

Reichert SLA, Visser CA, Moulijn AC, Suttorp MJ, Brink RBA, Koolen JJ, Jaarsma W, Vermeulen F, Dunning AJ (1990) Intraoperative transesophageal color coded Doppler echocardiography for evaluation of residual regurgitation after mitral valve repair. J Thorac Cardiovasc Surg 100:756–761

Schlüter M, Kremer P, Hanrath P (1984) Transesophageal 2D echocardiographic features of flail mitral leaflet due to ruptured chordae tendineae. Am Heart J 108:609–610

Sheikh K, Bruijn N, Rankin S, Clements F, Stanley T, Wolfe W, Kisslo J (1990) The utility of transesophageal echocardiography and Doppler color flow imaging in patients undergoing cardiac valve surgery. J Am Coll Cardiol 15:363–372

Smith MD, Harrison MR, Pinton R, Kandil H, Kwan OL, De Maria AN (1991) Regurgitant jet size by transesophageal echocardiography compared with transthoracic Doppler color flow imaging. Circulation 83:79–86

Steward WJ, Currie PJ, Salcedo EE, Lytle BW, Gill CC, Schiavone DO, Debbie AA, Cosgrove DM (1990) Intraoperative Doppler color flow mapping for decision-making in valve repair for mitral regurgitation. Technique and results in 100 patients. Circulation 81:556–566

Takamoto S, Kyo S, Adachi H, Matsumura M, Yokote Y, Omoto R (1985) Intraoperative color flow mapping by real time two dimensional Doppler echocardiography for evaluation of valvular and congenital heart disease. J Thorac Cardiovasc Surg 90:802–812

Toma Y, Matsuda Y, Matsuzaki M, Anno Y, Uchida T, Hiroyama N, Tamitani M, Murata T, Yonezawa F, Moritani K, Katayama K, Ogawa H, Kusukawa R (1983) Determination of atrial size by esophageal echocardiography. Am J Cardiol 52:878–880

Zamorano J, Erbel R, Mackowsky T, Alfonso F, Meyer J (1992) Usefulness of transesophageal echocardiography for diagnosis of mitral valve prolapse. Am J Cardiol 69:419–422

Prosthetic Valves

Alam M, Rosman HS, Lakier JB, Kemp S, Khaja F, Hautamaki K, Magilligan DJ, Stein PD (1987) Doppler and echocardiographic features of normal and dysfunctioning bioprosthetic valves. J Am Coll Cardiol 10:851–858

Alam M, Serwin JB, Rosman HS, Sheth m, Sun I, Silverman NA, Goldstein S (1990) Transesophageal color flow Doppler and echocardiographic features of normal and regurgitant St. Jude Medical prostheses in the mitral valve position. Am J Cardiol 66:871–873

Cassidy M, Smith M, Gurley J, Booth D, Cater A, Salley R (1992) Detection of trombosis of St. Jude Medical prostheses by transesophageal echocardiography. Am Heart J 122:1466–1469

Chen YW, Kan MN, Chen JS, Lin WW, Chan MK, Hu WS, Hwang DS, Lee DY, Hwang SL, Chiang BN (1990) Detection of prosthetic mitral valve leak: a comparative study using transesophageal echocardiography, transthoracic echocardiography and auscultation. J Clin Ultrasound 18:557–561

Daniel L, Grigg L, Weisel R, Rakowski H (1990) Comparison of transthoracic and transesophageal assessment of prosthetic valve dysfunction. Echocardiography 7:83–95

De Simone R, Lange R, Saggau W, Tanzeem A, Hagl S (1992) Intraoperative evaluation of prosthetic valve function by transesophageal color Doppler echocardiography (abstract) in: 6th Annual Meeting of the European Association for Cardio-Thoracic Surgery, Geneva, 14–16 Sept 1992. Volume abstracts, p 204

Deutsch H, Bachmann R, Sechtem U, Curtius J, Jungfehülsing M, Schicha H, Hilger H (1992) Regurgitant flow in cardiac valve prostheses: diagnostic value of gradient echo nuclear magnetic resonance imaging in reference to transesophageal 2-D color Doppler echocardiography. J Am Coll Cardiol 19:1500–1507

Dzavik V, Cohen G, Chan KL (1991) Role of transesophageal echocardiography in the diagnosis and management of prosthetic valve thrombosis. J Am Coll Cardiol 18:1829–1833

Effron KM, Popp RL (1983) Two-dimensional echocardiographic assessment of bioprosthetic valve dysfunction and infective endocarditis. J Am Coll Cardiol 2:597–606

Gindea AJ, Schwinger M, Freedberg RS, Colvin ST, Kronzon I (1989) Dehiscence of a Carpentier mitral ring: diagnosis by transesophageal echocardiography. Am Heart J 841–843

Gorscan J, Kenny WM, Diana P, Berhard KA, Marone GC (1991) Transesophageal continuous-wave Doppler to evaluate mitral prosthetic stenosis. Am Heart J 121:911–914

Khanderia BK, Seward JB, Oh JK, Freeman WK, Nichols BA, Sinak LJ, Miller FAJr, Tajik AJ (1991) Value and limitations of transesophageal echocardiography in assessment of mitral valve prostheses. Circulation 83:1056–1068

Matsuda H, Sato H, Hosokawa Y, Yamamoto S, Nakamura K (1991) Closed stuck valve diagnosed by echocardiogram immediately after mitral valve replacement: a case report. Kyobu Geka 44:864–866

Meloni L, Aru GM, Abbruzzese PA, Cardu G, Martelli V, Cherchi A (1992) Localization of mitral periprosthetic leaks by transesophageal echocardiography. Am J Cardiol 69:274–276

Mohr-Kahaly S, Kupferwasser I, Erbel R, Oelert H, Meyer J (1990) Regurgitant jet in apparently normal valve prostheses: improved detection and semi-quantitative analysis by transesophageal 2-D color-coded Doppler echocardiography. J Am Soc Echocardiogr 3:187–195

Nellessen U, Schnittger I, Appleton CP, Masuyama T, Bolger A, Fischell TA, Tye T, Popp RL (1988) Transesophageal 2-dimensional echocardiography and color Doppler flow velocity mapping in the evaluation of cardiac valve prostheses. Circulation 78:848–855

Scott PJ, Ettles DF, Wharton GA, Williams GJ (1990) The value of transesophageal echocardiography in the investigation of acute prosthetic valve dysfunction. Clin Cardiol 13:541–544

Sprecher DL, Adamick A, Adams D, Kisslo J (1989) In vitro color flow, pulsed and continuous wave Doppler ultrasound masking of flow by prosthetic valves. Am J Cardiol 9:1306–1310

Tanaka M, Abe T, Takeuchi T, Watanabe T, Tamaki S (1991) Intraoperative echocardiography of a dislodged Bjärk-Shiley mitral valve disc. Ann Thorac Surg 51:315–316

Van den Brink RBA, Visser CA, Basart DCG, Duren DR, de Jong AP, Dunning AJ (1989) Comparison of transthoracic and transesophageal color Doppler flow imaging in patients with mechanical prostheses in the mitral valve position. Am J Cardiol 63:1471–1474

Williams GA, Labovitz AJ (1985) Doppler hemodynamic evaluation of prosthetic (Starr-Edwards and Bjärk-Shiley) and bioprosthetic (Hancock and Carpentier-Edwards) cardiac valves. Am J Cardiol 56:325–332

Endocarditis

Ballal RS, Mahan EF, Nanda NV, Sanyal R (1991) Aortic and mitral valve perforation: diagnosis by transesophageal echocardiography and Doppler color flow imaging. Am Heart J 121:214–217

Birmingham G, Rahko P, Ballantyne F (1992) Improved detection of infective endocarditis with transesophageal echocardiography. Am Heart J 3:777–780

Daniel WG, Schräder E, Mügge A, Lichtlen PR (1988) Transesophageal echocardiography in infective endocarditis. Am J Card Imaging 2:78–85

Daniel WG, Mügge A, Martin PR, Lindert O, Hausmann D, Nonnast-Daniel B, Laas J, Lichtlen PR (1991) Improvement in the diagnosis of abscesses associated with endocarditis by transesophageal echocardiography. N Engl J Med 324:795–800

Erbel R, Rohmann S, Drexler M, Mohr-Kahaly S, Gerzharz CD, Iversen S, Oelert H, Meyer J (1988) Improved diagnostic value of echocardiography in patients with infective endocarditis by transesophageal approach. Eur Heart J 9:43–53

Foster E, Kusumoto FM, Sobol SM, Schiller NB (1990) Streptococcal endocarditis temporally related to transesophageal echocardiography. J Am Soc Echocardiogr 3:424–427

Giannoccaro P, Ascah J, Sochowsky RA, Chan KL, Ruddy TD (1991) Spontaneous drainage of paravalvular abscess diagnosed by transesophageal echocardiography. J Am Soc Echocardiogr 4:379–400

Kan MN, Chen YT, Lee AYS (1991) Comparison of transesophageal to transthoracic color Doppler echocardiography in the identification of intracardiac mycotic aneurysms in infective endocarditis. Echocardiography 8:643–648

Karalis DG, Chandrasekaran K, Wahl JM, Ross J, Mintz GS (1990) Transesophageal echocardiographic recognition of mitral valve abnormalities associated with aortic valve endocarditis. Am Heart J 119:1209–1211

Klodas E, Edwards WD, Khanderia BK (1989) Use of transesophageal echocardiography for improving detection of valvular vegetations in subacute bacterial endocarditis. J Am Soc Echocardiogr 2:386–389

Polak PE, Gussenhoven W, Roelandt JR (1987) Transesophageal cross-sectional echocardiographic recognition of an aortic valve ring abcess and a subannular mycotic aneurysm. Eur Heart J 8:664–666

Porklab FL, Weinbaum DL, Lerberg DB, Phillips JC (1990) The source of recurrent bacteremia identified by transesophageal echocardiography. Ann Intern Med 112:628–629

Rohmann S, Erbel R, Darius H, Makowsky T, Mohr-Kahaly S, Nixdorff U, Drexler M, Meyer J (1991a) Prediction of rapid versus prolonged healing of infective endocarditis by monitoring vegetation size. J Am Soc Echocardiogr 4:465–474

Rohmann S, Seifert T, Erbel R, Jakob H, Mohr-Kahaly S, Makowsky T, Gärge G, Oelert H, Meyer J (1991b) Identification of abscess formation in native-valve infective endocarditis using transesophageal echocardiography: implications for surgical treatment. Thorac Cardiovasc Surg 39:273–280

Rohmann S, Erbel R, Darius H, Makowski T, Jensen P, Fischer T, Meyer J (1992a) Spontaneous echo contrast imaging in infective endocarditis: a predictor of complications? Int J Card Imaging 8:197–207

Rohmann S, Erbel R, Gärge G, Makowsky T, Mohr-Kahaly S, Nixdorff U, Drexler M, Meyer J (1992b) Clinical relevance of vegetation localization by transesophageal echocardiography in infective endocarditis. Eur Heart J 13:446–452

Roudaut R, Dupas JY, Gosse P, Dallocchio M (1991) Transesophageal echocardiographic visualization of leaflet destruction in two patients with suspected endocarditis. Echocardiography 8:357–361

Schwinger ME, Tunick PA, Freedberg RS, Kronzon I (1990) Vegetations on endocardial surfaces struck by regurgitant jets: diagnosis by transesophageal echocardiography. Am Heart J 119:1212–1215

Shively BK, Gurule FT, Roldan CA, Leggett JH, Schiller NB (1991) Diagnostic value of transesophageal compared with transthoracic echocardiography in infective endocarditis. J Am Coll Cardiol 18:391–397

Taams M, Gussenhoven E, Bos E, de Jaegere P, Roelandt JR, Sutherland GR, Bom N (1990) Enhanced morphological diagnosis in infective endocarditis by transesophageal echocardiography. Br Heart J 63:109–113

Teskey RJ, Chan KL, Beanlands DS (1989) Diverticulum of the mitral valve complicating bacterial endocarditis: diagnosis by transesophageal echocardiography. Am Heart J 118:1063–1065

Winslow T, Foster E, Adams J, Schiller N (1992) Pulmonary valve endocarditis: improved diagnosis with biplane transesophageal echocardiography. J Am Soc Echocardiogr 5:206–210

Coronary Artery Disease

Beaupre PN, Kremer PF, Cahalan MK, Lurz FW, Schiller NB, Hamilton WK (1984) Intraoperative detection of changes in left ventricular segmental wall motion by transesophageal two-dimensional echocardiography. Am Heart J 107: 1021–1023

Erbel R (1991) Transesophageal echocardiogaphy. A new window to coronary arteries and coronary blood flow. Circulation 83:339–341

Hong YO, Orihashi K, Oka Y (1990) Intraoperative monitoring of regional wall motion abnormalities for detecting myocardial ischemia by transesophageal echocardiography. Echocardiography 7:323–332

Iliceto S, Marangelli V, Memmola C, Rizzon P (1991) Transesophageal Doppler echocardiographiy evaluation of coronary blood flow velocity in baseline conditions and during dipyridamole-induced coronary vasodilation. Circulation 83:61–69

Matsuzaki M, Matsuda Y, Ikee Y, Takahashi Y, Sasaki T, Toma Y, Ishida K, Yorozu T, Kumada T, Kusukawa R (1981) Esophageal echocardiographic left ventricular antero-lateral wall motion in normal subjects and patients with coronary artery disease. Circulation 63:1085–1092

Pearce FB, Sheikh KH, deBrujin P, Kisslo J (1989) Imaging of coronary arteries by transesophageal echocadiography. J Am Soc Echocardiogr 2:276–283

Reichert SLA, Visser CA, Koolen JJ, Chapman JV, Angelsen BJ, Meyne MN, Dunning AR (1990) Transesophageal examination of the left coronary artery with a 7.5 MHz annular array 2-D color flow Doppler transducer. J Am Soc Echocardiogr 3:118–124

Simon P, Mohl MD (1990) Intraoperative echocardiographic assessment of global and regional myocardial function. Echocardiography 7:333–341

Taams MA, Gussenhoven J, Cornel JH, The SHK, Roelandt J, Lancee CT, van den Brand M (1988) Detection of left coronary artery stenosis by transesophageal echocardiography. Eur Heart J 9:1162–1166

Topol EJ, Weiss JL, Guzman PA, Dorsey-Lima S, Blanck TJJ, Humprey LS, Baumgartner WA, Flaherty JT, Reitz BA (1984) Immediate improvement of dysfunctional myocardial segments after coronary revascularization by intraoperative transesophageal two dimensional echocardiography. J Am Coll Cardiol 4:1123–1134

Yamaghishi M, Yasu T, Ohara K, Kuro M, Miyatake K (1991) Detection of coronary blood flow associated with left main coronary artery stenosis by transesophageal Doppler color flow echocardiography. J Am Coll Cardiol 17:87–93

Yamagishi M, Miyatake K, Beppu S, Kumon K, Suzuki S, Tanaka N, Nimura Y (1988) Assessment of coronary blood flow by transesophageal two-dimensional pulsed Doppler echocardiography. Am J Cardiol 15:641–645

Zwicky P, Daniel W, Mügge A, Lichtlen P (1988) Imaging of coronary arteries by color-coded transesophageal echocardiography. Am J Cardiol 15:639–644

Aortic Dissection

Börner C, Erbel R, Henkel B, Meyer J (1984) Evaluation of the thoracic aorta by transesophageal echocardiography. Circulation 70:II–293

DeMaria AN, Bommer W, Neumann A, Weinert L, Bogren H, Mason DT (1979) Identification and localization of aneurysms of the descending aorta by cross-sectional echocardiography. Circulation 59:755–761

De Simone R, Haberbosch W, Iarussi D, Iacono A (1990) Transesophageal echocardiography for the diagnosis of thoracic aorta aneurysms and dissections. Cardiologia 35: 387–390

Engberding R, Bender F, Grosse W, Eckardt M, Müller U, Bramann H, Schneider D (1987) Identification of dissection or aneurysm of the descending thoracic aorta by conventional and transesophageal two-dimensional echocardiography. Am J Cardiol 59:717–719

Erbel R, Mohr-Kahaly S, Rennollet H, Brunier J, Drexler M, Wittlich N, Iversen S, Oelert H, Thelen M, Meyer J (1987) Diagnosis of aortic dissection: the value of transesophageal echocardiography. Thorac Cardiovasc Surg: 35:126–133

Erbel R, Daniel W, Visser C, Engberding R, Roelandt J, Rennolet J (1989) Echocardiography in the diagnosis of aortic dissection. Lancet I:457–461

Erbel R, Bednarczyk I, Pop T, Todt M, Henrichs KJ, Brunier A, Thelen M, Meyer J (1990) Detection of dissection of the aortic intima and media after angioplasty of coarctation of the aorta. An angio-

graphic, computer tomographic and echocardiographic comparative study. Circulation 81:805–814

Erbel R et al for the European Cooperative Study Group on Echocardiography (1993) Effect of medical and surgical therapy on aortic dissection evaluated by transesophageal echocardiography. Implications for prognosis and therapy. Circulation 87:1604–1615

Granato JE, Dee P, Gibson RS (1985) Utility of two-dimensional echocardiography in suspected ascending aortic dissection. Am J Cardiol 56:123–129

Kyo S, Takamoto S, Adachi H, Matsumura M, Kimura S, Yokotre Y, Omoto R (1989) Intraoperative evaluation of repair of aortic dissection: surgical decision making. Int J Card Imaging 4:49–50

Mohr-Kahaly S, Erbel R, Steller D, Bärner N, Drexler M, Meyer J (1987) Aortic dissection detected by transesophageal echocardiography. Int J Card Imaging 2:31–35

Mohr-Kahaly S, Erbel R, Rennolet J, Wittlich N, Drexler M, Oelert H, Meyer J (1989) Ambulatory follow-up of aortic dissection by transesophageal 2-D and color-coded Doppler echocardiography. Circulation 80:24–33

Troianos CA, Savino JS, Weiss RL (1991) Transesophageal echocardiographic diagnosis of the aortic dissection during cardiac surgery. Anesthesiology 75:149–153

Cardiac Tumors

Alam M, Sun I (1991) Transesophageal echocardiographic evaluation of left atrial mass lesions. J Am Soc Echocardiogr 4:323–330

Awad M, Dunn B, Halees Z, Mercer E, Akahtar M, Hainau B, Duran C (1992) Intracardiac rhabdomyosarcoma: transesophageal echocardiography finding and diagnosis. J Am Soc Echocardiogr 5:199–202

Ezekowitz MD, Smith ED, Rankin R et al (1983) Left atrial mass: diagnostic value of transesophageal 2-dimensional echocardiography and indium-111 platelet scintigraphy. Am J Cardiol 51:1563–1564

Lestuzzi C, Nicolosi G, Mimo R, Pavan D, Zanuttini D (1992) Usefulness of transesophageal echocardiography in evaluation of paracardiac neoplastic masses. Am J Cardiol 70: 247–251

Mügge A, Daniel WG, Haverich A, Lichtlen PR (1991) Diagnosis of noninfective cardiac mass lesions by two-dimensional echocardiography. Circulation 83:70–78

Obeid A, Marvasti M, Parker F, Rosenberg J (1989) Comparison of transthoracic and transesophageal echocardiography in the diagnosis of left atrial myxoma. Am J Cardiol 63: 1006–1008

Reeves WC, Chitwood WR Jr (1989) Assessment of left atrial myxoma using transesophageal two-dimensional echocardiography and color flow Doppler. Echocardiography 6: 547–549

Rey M, Tunon J, Compres H, Rabago R, Fraile J, Rabago P (1991) Prolapsing right atrial myxoma evaluated by transesophageal echocardiography. Am Heart J 122:875–877

Turlapati RV, Jacobs LE, Kotler MN (1990) Right atrial myxoma causing total distruction of the tricuspid valve leaflets. Am Heart J 120:1227–1231

Vargas-Barron J, Romero-Cardenas A, Villegas M, Keirns C, Gomez-Jaume A, Delong R, Malo Camacho R (1991) Transthoracic and transesophageal echocardiographic diagnosis of myxomas in the four cardiac cavities. Am Heart J 121:931–933

Cardiomyopathies

De Simone R, Gualtieri S, Coppolino P, Cittadini A, Iarussi D, Iacono A (1989) Echocardiographic features of cardiac amyloidosis. Cardiovascular Imaging 1(4):61–64

Ius P, Salandin V, Zussa C, Valfre C (1991) Surgical treatment of left-ventricular outflow-tract obstruction guided by intraoperative transesophageal echocardiography. Thorac Cardiovasc Surg 39:205–207

Mügge A, Daniel W, Wolpers H, Kläpper J, Lichtlen P (1989) Improved visualization of discrete subvalvular aortic stenosis by transesophageal color-coded Doppler echocardiography. Am Heart J 117:474–475

Pearson AC, Gudipati CV, Labovitz AJ (1988) Systolic and diastolic flow abnormalities in elderly patients with hypertensive hypertrophic cardiomyopathy. J Am Coll Cardiol 12(4):989–995

Schwinger M, Kronzon I (1988) Improved evaluation of left ventricular outflow tract obstruction by transesophageal echocardiography. J Am Soc Echocardiogr 2:191–194

Pericardial Effusion

Hogue CW, Plati M, Barzilai B, Kaiser LR (1991) Intraoperative use of transesophageal echocardiography with pulsed-wave Doppler: evaluation of ventricular filling dynamics during pericardiotomy. Anestesiology 75:701–704

Kochar GS, Jacobs LE, Kotler MN (1990) Right atrial compression in postoperative cardiac patients: detection by transesophageal echocardiography. J Am Coll Cardiol 16: 511–516

Simpson IA, Munsch C, Smith EEJ, Parker DJ (1991) Pericardial haemorrhage causing right atrial compression after cardiac surgery: role of transesophageal echocardiography. Br Heart J 65:355–356

Torelli J, Marwick TH, Salcedo EE (1991) Left atrial tamponade: diagnosis by transesophageal echocardiography. J Am Soc Echocardiogr 4:413–414

Vilacosta I, San Roman Calvar JA, Prieto EI, Recio MG, Elbal LM (1991) Transesophageal echocardiography features of atrial septum in constrictive pericarditis. Am J Cardiol 68: 271–273

Congenital Heart Disease

Cyran SE, Kimball TR, Meyer RA, Bailey WW, Lowe E, Balisteri WF, Kaplan S (1989) Efficacy of intraoperative transesophageal echocardiography in children with congenital heart disease. Am J Cardiol 63:594–598

De Simone R, Iarussi D, Haberbosch W, Scialdone A, Irace L, Iacono A (1989) Clinical utility of Doppler-echocardiographic method for estimating intracardiac shunts. Combined Doppler and hemodynamic evaluation. Cardiologia 34:689–694

Fram DB, Missri J, Therrien ML, Chawla S (1991) Assessment of Ebstein anomaly and its surgical repair using transesophageal two-dimensional echocardiography and Doppler color flow maping. Echocardiography 8:367–371

Fyfe DA, Kline CH, Sade RM, Greene CA, Gillette PC (1991) The utility of transesophageal echocardiography during and after Fontan operations in small children. Am Heart J 122:1403–1415

Gnanapragasam JP, Houston AB, Northridge DB, Jamieson MPG, Pollock JCS (1991) Transesophageal echocardiographic assessment of primum, secundum and sinus venosus atrial septal defects. Int J Cardiol 31:167–174

Hanrath P, Schlüter M, Langestein BA, Polter J, Engel S, Kremer P, Krebber HJ (1983) Detection of ostium secundum atrial septal defects by transesophageal cross-sectional echocardiography. Br Heart J 49:350–358

Kaulitz R, Stümper O, Gueskens R, Narayanswami S, Elzenka NJ, Chan CK, Burns JE, Godman MJ, Hess J, Sutherland GR (1990) Comparative values of the precordial and transesophageal approaches in echocardiographic evaluation of atrial baffle function after an atrial correction procedure. J Am Coll Cardiol 16:686–694

Lam J, Neirotti RA, Nijveld A, Schuller JL, Blom-Muilvijk CM, Visser CA (1991) Transesophageal echocardiography in pediatric patients: preliminary results. J Am Soc Echocardiogr 4:43–50

Langholz D, Louie EK, Konstadt SN, Rao TLK, Scanlon PJ (1991) Transesophageal echocardiographic demonstration of distinct mechanisms of right and left shunting across a patent foramen ovale in the absence of pulmonary hypertension. J Am Coll Cardiol 18:1112–1117

Lin SL, Tin CT, Hsu TL, Chen CH, Chang MS, Chen CY, Chiang BN (1992) Transesophageal echocardiographic detection of atrial septal defect in adults. Am J Cardiol 69: 280–282

Ludomirsky A, Erickson C, Vick GW, Cooley DA (1990) Transesophageal color flow Doppler evaluation of cor triatriatum in an adult. Am Heart J 120:451–454

Mehta RH, Helmcke F, Nanda NC, Hsiung M, Pacifico AD, Hsu TL (1990) Transesophageal Doppler color flow mapping assessment of atrial septal defect. J Am Coll Cardiol 16:1010–1016

Mehta RH, Helmcke F, Nanda NC, Pinheiro L, Samdarshi T, Shah V (1991) Uses and limitations of transthoracic echocardiography in the assessment of atrial septal defect in the adult. Am J Cardiol 67:288–294

Morimoto K, Matsuzaki M, Tohma Y, Ono S, Tanaka N, Michishige H, Murata K, Anno Y, Kusukawa R (1990) Diagnosis and quantitative evaluation of secundum-type atrial septal defect by transesophageal Doppler echocardiography. Am J Cardiol 66:85–91

Mügge A, Daniel G, Kläpper J, Lichtlen PR (1988) Visualization of foramen ovale by transesophageal color-coded Doppler echocardiography. Am J Cardiol 62:837–838

Muhuideen IA, Robertson DA, Silvermann NH, Haas G, Turley K, Calahan MK (1990) Intraoperative echocardiography in infants and children with congenital cardiac shunt lesions: transesophageal versus epicardial echocardiography. J Am Coll Cardiol 16:1687–1695

Muhiudeen IA, Roberson DA, Silverman NH, Haas G, Turley K, Cahaklan MK (1992) Intraoperative echocardiography for evaluation of congenital heart defects in infants and children. Anesthesiology 76:165–172

Nemec JJ, Davidson MB, Marwick TH, Chimowitz MI, Stoller JK, Klein AL, Salcedo EE (1991a) Detection and evaluation of intrapulmonary vascular shunt with contrast Doppler transesophageal echocardiography. J Am Soc Echocardiogr 4:79–83

Nemec JJ, Marwick TH, Lorig RJ, Davidson MC, Chimowitz MI, Litowitz H, Salcedo EE (1991b) Comparison of transcranial Doppler ultrasound and transesophageal contrast echocardiography in the detection of intraatrial right-to-left shunts. Am J Cardiol 68:1498–1502

Oh JK, Seward JB, Khanderia BK, Danielson, Tajik AJ (1988) Visualization of sinus venosus atrial septal defect by transesophageal echocardiography. J Am Soc Echocardiogr 1: 275–277

Patt MV, Obeid AI (1991) Cor triatriatum with isolated pulmonary venous stenosis in an adult: diagnosis with transesophageal two-dimensional echocardiography. J Am Soc Echocardiogr 4:185–188

Ritter SB (1990) Transesophageal echocardiography in children: new peephole to the heart. J Am Coll Cardiol 16: 447–450

Ritter SB (1991) Transesophageal real-time echocardiography in infants and children with congenital heart disease. J Am Coll Cardiol 18:569–580

Robertson D, Muhiudeen IA, Calahan M, Silvermann N, Haas GS, Turley K (1991a) Intraoperative transesophageal echocardiography of ventricular septal defect. Echocardiography 8:687–697

Robertson DA, Muhiudeen IA, Silverman NH, Turrley K, Haas GS, Cahalan MK (1991b) Intraoperative transesophageal echocardiography of atrioventricular septal defect. J Am Coll Cardiol 18:537–545

Schlüter M, Langestein BA, Thier W, et al (1983) Transesophageal echocardiography in the diagnosis of cor triatriatum in the adult. J Am Coll Cardiol 2:1011–1015

Seward JB, Tajik AJ, Edwards WD, Hagler DJ (eds) (1987) Two-dimensional echocardiographic atlas, vol 1. Congenital heart disease. Springer, New York

Sheeram N, Sutherland GR, Geuskens R, Stümper OFW, Taams M, Gussenhoven EJ, Hess J, Roelandt JRTC (1991) The role of transesophageal echocardiography in adolescents and adults with congenital heart defects. Eur Heart J 12:231–240

Siostrzonek P, Lang W, Zageneh M, Gässinger H, Stümpflen A, Rosenmayr G, Heinz G, Schwarz M, Zeiler K, Mässlacher H (1992) Significance of left-sided heart disease for the detection of patent foramen ovale by transesophageal contrast echocardiography. J Am Coll Cardiol 19:1192–1196

Stern H, Erbel R, Schreiner G, Henkel B, Meyer J (1987) Coarctaction of the aorta: quantitative analysis by transesophageal echocardiography. Echocardiography 4:387–395

Stümper OFW, Elzenka NJ, Hess J, Sutherland GR (1990) Transesophageal echocardiography in children with congenital heart disease: an initial experience. J Am Coll Cardiol 16:433–441

Stümper OFW, Narayanswami S, Elzenka NJ, Sutherland GR (1990) Diagnosis of atrial situs by transesophageal echocardiography. J Am Coll Cardiol 16:442–446

Stümper OFW, Sutherland GR, Gueskens R, Roelandt J, Bos E, Hess J (1991) Transesophageal echocardiography in evaluation and management after a Fontan procedure. J Am Coll Cardiol 17:1152–1160

Takamoto S, Kyo S, Adachi H, Matsumura M, Yokote Y, Omoto R (1985) Intraoperative color flow mapping by real time two dimensional Doppler echocardiography for evaluation of valvular and congenital heart disease. J Thorac Cardiovasc Surg 90:802–812

Ungerleider RM (1990) The use of intraoperative echocardiography with Doppler color flow imaging in the repair of congenital heart disease. Echocardiography 7:289–304

Ungerleider RM, Kisslo JA, Greeley WJ, Van Trigt P, Sabiston DC (1989) Intraoperative prebypass and postbypass epicardial color flow imaging in the repair of atrioventricular septal defects. J Thorac Cardiovasc Surg 98:90–100

Ungerleider RM, Greeley WJ, Sheikh KH, Philips J, Pearce FB, Kern FHK, Kisslo JA (1990) Routine use of intraoperative epicardial echocardiography and Doppler color flow imaging to guide and evaluate repair of congenital heart lesions. A prospective study. J Thorac Cardiovasc Surg 100:297–309

Wienecke, Fyfe DA, Kline CH, Greene CA, Crawford FA, Sade RM, Gillette PC (1991) Comparison of transesophageal echocardiography to epicardial imaging in children undergoing ventricular septal defect repair. J Am Soc Echocardiogr 4:607–614

Heart Transplantation

Angermann CE, Spes CH, Tammen A, Stempfle HU, Schztz A, Kemkes BM, Theisen K (1990) Anatomic characteristics and valvular function of the transplanted heart: transthoracic versus transesophageal findings. J Heart Transplant 9: 331–338

Bhatia SJ, Kirshenbaum JM, Shemin RJ, Cohn LH, Collins JJ, Disesa VJ, Yaing PJ, Mudge GH, Sutton MH (1987) Time course of reduction of pulmonary hypertension and right ventricular remodeling after orthotopic cardiac transplantation. Circulation 76:819–826

Haverich A, Albes JM, Fahrenkamp G, Schäfers HJ, Wahlers T, Heublein B (1991) Intraoperative echocardiography to detect and prevent tricuspid valve regurgitation after heart transplantation. Eur J Cardio-thorac Surg 5:41–45

Herrmann G, Simon R, Haverich A, Cremer J, Dammenhayn L, Schäfers H-J, Wahlers T, Borst HG (1989) Left ventricular function, tricuspid incompetence and incidence of coronary artery disease late after orthotopic cardiac transplantation. Eur J Cardiothorac Surg 3:111–117

Lambertz H, Sigmund M, Hoffmann R, Flachskamp FA, Messmer BH, Hanrath P (1991) Transesophageal Doppler analysis of pulmonary venous flow in cardiac transplant recipients. Am Heart J 121:623–626

Lange R, Sack FU, Saggau W, De Simone R, Hagl S (1991) Performance of dynamic cardiomyoplasty related to the functional state of the heart. J Card Surg 6:225–235

Ulstad V, Braunlin E, Bass J, Shumway S, Molina E, Homans D (1992) Hemodynamically significant suture line obstruction immediately after heart transplantation. J Heart Lung Transplant 11:834–836

Appendix

About "Atlas of TEE Demo"

This Atlas is also available as an electronic book: *"Interactive Atlas of Transesophageal Color Doppler Echocardiography and Intraoperative Imaging"* published on CD-ROM by Springer-Verlag. The enclosed disk *"Atlas of TEE Demo"* contains a reduced version of the CD-ROM. In this short version you may access only some pages. The items in italics in the indexes are not available. The chapter *"Two-dimensional TEE"* contains two special pages (22, 30) which demonstrate the transversal and the longitudinal views respectively. These pages show a diagram of the heart and the great arteries with different positions of the transducer in the esophagus on the left side, and the corresponding imaging planes on the right side of the screen. Click on the view plane or on the transducers to display the corresponding echocardiographic view on the right side of the screen. This program will help you to locate and recognize the standard transversal and longitudinal imaging views and their spatial orientation. In addition, you may access the first page of each section and some examples containing movies, such as the first page of *"Valvular Heart Disease"* and *"Cor Triatriatum"*.

How to install "Atlas of TEE Demo"

- Insert the disk into the disk drive.
- Double click on *"Atlas of TEE Demo.sea"*.
- The installer will copy the files to the hard disk in a new folder named *"Atlas of TEE Demo"*.
- Open this new folder and double click on the file *"Atlas of TEE Demo"* to start the program.

If QuickTime™ is not installed in the extension folder, the movies will not run. If you want to display the movies, copy QuickTime™ to the extension folder and reinstall the program *"Atlas of TEE Demo"*.

This demo version runs exactly like the full version. The instructions in the following pages are related to the CD-ROM version of the Atlas. Please refer to them, but remember that some features are not available due to the limited space on the floppy disk.

About "Interactive Atlas of TEE" (CD-ROM)

This *Atlas* was written to communicate to other cardiologists, cardiac surgeons, and students the experience achieved in the use of color Doppler transesophageal echocardiography at the Department of Cardiac Surgery, University of Heidelberg, Germany. The *Atlas* includes a comprehensive collection in cardiac pathology selected from routine perioperative examinations.

This type of data is usually shown as color photographs in journals and in books, and this work was also initially intended to be organized in this way. It is in fact available as a book from the same publisher. However this format is far from ideal since echocardiographic examinations are typically dynamic data, i.e., video sequences. Although in many cases it is possible to select frames which particularly well represent specific sequences, much information is necessarily lost in the process, and in general the observation cannot be effectively reproduced. The alternative option, i.e. the use of videotapes to record the sequences, has obvious limitations: it does not allow random access, and it prevents easy association of pictures, text, and movies. In this CD-ROM based *Atlas* we try to take advantage of the large storage capacity of the CD-ROM and of the graphics capabilities of the Macintosh to create an "animated book", which, while retaining the usual structure of a book as much as possible, allows the additional feature of displaying movies. They can be carefully examined in slow motion or frame by frame, as is normally done on the echocardiograph. The use of this type of media also allows the addition of useful features, such as the ability to click on the indexes to find the related data, or remembering the recently observed pages, to go back quickly. This CD-ROM includes 277 pages, more than 500 echocardiographic figures, and 136 movies of digitally recorded video sequences, showing real TEE examinations.

The creation of this Atlas on CD-ROM was not without complications: the screen is smaller and has much lower resolution than the page of a book, and the speed requirements of echocardiographic movies (25 frames per second, large screen sizes) are presently at the limit of the capabilities of many personal computers. Compression techniques had to be chosen carefully to preserve the quality of the graphics while allowing performance, and special care had to be devoted to avoiding unnecessary delays in accessing the slow CD-ROM medium. In particular, we tried to reduce to a minimum the time in which the computer is busy and the user is not in control, as was too often the case observed on many early CD-ROMs. In its present form the *Atlas* runs on every Macintosh which allows the use of color. Movies run at full speed even on slower machines, such as Mac IIcx or PowerBooks. Starting and quitting the program takes only a few seconds. The *Atlas* does not take over the computer; system menus may be activated at any time and the *Atlas* may be run at the same time as other programs, within the limits of the available RAM. The time for going from page to page varies according to the number of figures, but it is usually kept within 1-2 seconds. If the Atlas is transferred to a hard disk on a faster 68040 Macintosh, this time is typically reduced to less than 1 second.

How the *Atlas* is organized

The *Atlas* is organized as a tree. It is composed of six main sections: Introduction, Techniques, Acquired Heart Disease, Congenital Heart Disease, Other Applications of TEE, and References. Each of these is further divided into smaller subsections, termed as follows:

Section	*Example:* Acquired Heart Disease
Chapter	*Example:* Valvular Heart Disease
Topic	*Example:* Mitral Valve
Subtopic	*Example:* Mitral Valve Prolapse

How to use the *Atlas*

I. Browse the *Atlas*

The *Atlas* may be read as if it were a conventional printed book. You can go from page to page by using the arrows, choose topics in index or subindex pages, or go directly to the beginning of the various sections, by clicking on their names. You can even go at random to any page in the *Atlas* by moving the triangular cursor at the bottom of the page. You can use the "Up" arrow to go to the beginning of the higher order subdivision, for example, the chapter which includes the present topic. You can return to the previously visited page with the "Back" arrow. The observed pages are retained in memory, and you can trace back all the pages in the order in which you have seen them by repeatedly pressing the "Back" arrow button.

Pages are composed of text, figures, and, unlike a printed book, movies. Movies are identified by a small movie icon in the top right corner. You can activate the movies by clicking on them once, and stop them by clicking again. Only one movie at a time may be active; therefore if you click on a movie while another is running, the former is activated while the latter stops.

II. Examine movies

The pages of the *Atlas* have been edited so that only the central part of the movie is displayed. Double-click on the movie to go to the page where the full size movie is displayed, together with the technical details of the original recording. Data such as type of recording, projection, type of probe, and depth setting of the echocardiographic examinations are reported. Click on them to see additional information.

The movie may run at variable speed, corresponding to heart rates between 30 and 120 beats per min by using the cursor in the bottom right of the page. Click once on the movie to stop it and look at the single frames. Length measurements may be done by dragging the mouse over the stopped movie frames.

III. Self-teaching assessment

By pressing the button "Self Test" a movie is picked at random and displayed in a page similar to the movie page described above. All functions are available, but the title of the movie indicating the diagnosis is not displayed, and the triangular cursor at the bottom is also hidden.

You are expected to study the movie, compare the corresponding projections by clicking on "View", and make guesses. You can press the button "Show Hint" to display the cursor indicating the section of the *Atlas* in which the movie is contained. This gives a generic indication of the type of pathology. This last action also reveals a new button, "Show Diagnosis". Press it to display the title of the movie. Press the "Up" arrow button to go to the page where the movie is described.

For further information please contact:

Springer-Verlag
Electronic Media
Tiergartenstraße 17
69121 Heidelberg, FRG
Phone: 0049-6221-487665
FAX: 0049-6221-487366
internet: em-helpdesk@springer.de

In the US and Canada:

Springer-Verlag
Electronic Media
175 Fifth Avenue
New York, NY 10010, USA
Phone : 001-212-4601682
FAX: 001-212-4736272
internet: lange@spint.compuserve.com

Subject Index

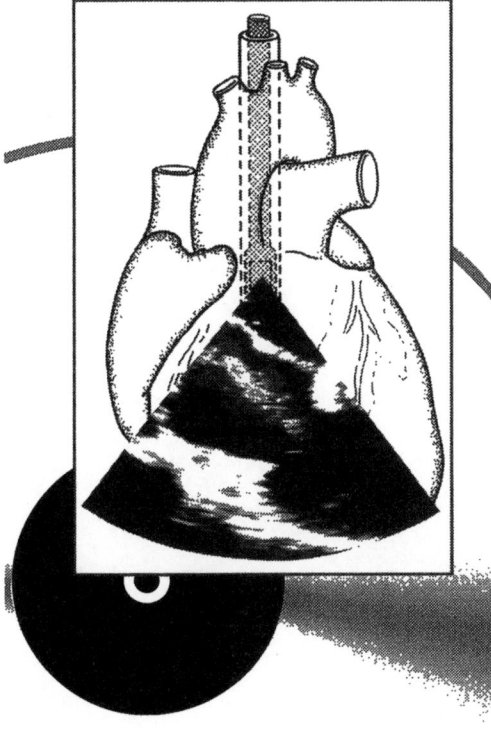

R. De Simone

Interactive Atlas of Transesophageal Color Doppler Echocardiography and Intraoperative Imaging
CD-ROM for Macintosh

With the assistance of **G. Paolella**

With contributions by **R. Lange**, **S. Hagl**

1994. CD-ROM for Macintosh, booklet with approx. 10 pp. ISBN 3-540-14179-0

The **Interactive Atlas of Transesophageal Doppler Echocardiography and Intraoperative Imaging** is the new multimedia application that provides an interactive educational tool in transesophageal echocardiography (TEE). This electronic manual of TEE will introduce the user to the diagnostic possibilities of this new technique and will enable him to recognize and diagnose a wide range of acquired and congenital heart diseases. The CD-ROM includes 505 high-quality echocardiographic figures and 136 movies, i.e. digitally recorded video sequences, showing real echocardiographic examinations. This program represents a complete interactive course of TEE for cardiologists, cardiac surgeons, anesthetists and internists. A randomized self-test program gives extra value to the interactive atlas.

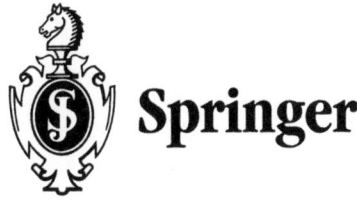

Springer

Springer-Verlag
and the Environment

We at Springer-Verlag firmly believe that an international science publisher has a special obligation to the environment, and our corporate policies consistently reflect this conviction.

We also expect our business partners – paper mills, printers, packaging manufacturers, etc. – to commit themselves to using environmentally friendly materials and production processes.

The paper in this book is made from low- or no-chlorine pulp and is acid free, in conformance with international standards for paper permanency.

MIX
Papier aus verantwortungsvollen Quellen
Paper from responsible sources
FSC® C105338

Printed by Libri Plureos GmbH
in Hamburg, Germany